the OVER 40 WOMEN'S FITNESS BOOK

Leisure Press
P.O. Box 3
West Point, NY 10996

the *OVER 40* WOMEN'S FITNESS Book

Carol Spilman

A publication of Leisure Press.
P.O. Box 3, West Point, N.Y. 10996
Copyright © 1982 Carol Spilman
All rights reserved. Printed in the U.S.A.

ISBN: 0-88011-009-0
Library of Congress Number: 81-85633

Photography by Lawrence Ruggeri
Cover Layout: Diana J. Goodin

CONTENTS

INTRODUCTION

What is so special about the age of forty? Why do many suffer "rites of passage," others breeze by in total oblivion, while **some** choose to fall apart completely? Choose they do, whether consciously or not, because what the mind proposes, the body tends to obey.

What is inevitable, and what can we do either as a preventative or a therapy? Your mother may have been "matronly" at the age of 41, had arthritis, constipation, insomnia and "nerves." Her mother did before her; so you feel your destiny is set.

Certainly, genetics play a role in aging and disease as it does in other aspects of physiology; however, many deleterious effects can be ameliorated by simple changes in the life style, especially diet, activity, and stress. Many of life's constant stresses we can directly influence, such as excessive intake of alcohol, caffein, tobacco, sugar, salt, fat and FOOD. We can select forms of relaxation that are healthful rather than detrimental, benefiting not only ourselves, but others with whom we have contact.

We are not puppets! We have the power of choice, regardless of Aunt Minnie's flab and mother's bowels!

The need and desire to reward ourselves for coping with the myriad complex problems facing women today is real, but our rewards may, in truth, be another form of punishment. Eventually we pay for overindulgence, by losing our looks, our youth, and our friends. It is possible to have pastimes and habits that bring pleasure and relaxation and are beneficial at the same time.

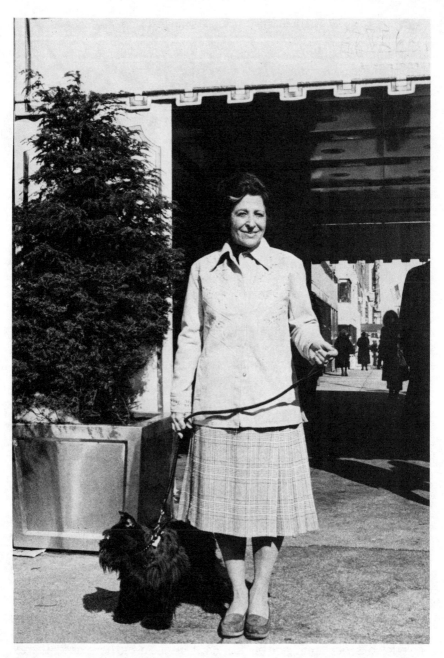

It is possible to have pastimes and habits that bring both pleasure and relaxation and are beneficial at the same time.

My special treat is a quiet walk in a local park. I watch the seasons evolve from the earliest cherry blossom to the last astor in the fall. Here one experiences space and serenity in beautifully landscaped ponds, formal and informal gardens. The senses are stimulated by a myriad of textures, colors, sounds and scents. When our sensory organs are keen, we are aware of the world both within and around us, and we are "alive" no matter what our age.

"Staying Alive," as the BeeGees sing, is the name of the game. The older people in my classes love that song; for them it has a special meaning, as it can for us at any age.

I know of no way to eliminate aging. Whoever comes up with that secret will be the most sought after person in the world! In my classes I have seen old people in their twenties and young ones in their eighties. One woman aged 80-plus could bend foreward from the hips and with straight knees touch her palms to the floor. She was also currently learning how to read and write the Greek language. A young mind with a young body — they go together.

Changes due to aging are inevitable, the degree, variable. Some may have already happened to you, some may never. Many changes occur in the 40's or earlier, such as changes in hair and skin color and texture, demineralization of the bones, aches and pains in the neck and other joints, loss of flexibility and muscle tone, a general downward shifting of the features and figure, a thickening of the waist, abdomen and hips, a need for reading glasses and more sleep, depression, menopause or pre-menopausal menorrhagia.

You may have tried one of the more common (or not so common) youth potions, or creams. One is Dr. Frank's "No Aging Diet" which consists of foods high in ribonucleic acids and other factors, or perhaps you've gone to Europe for live cell therapy or Gerivitol. (The FDA will not allow these techniques here, although Gerivitol (G.H.3) has been proven "safe and effective" for more than 25 years.) Many have attested to their efficacy, but we have to do with what we've got, so some of us experiment cautiously with the antioxidants, Vitamins E and C, and the mineral selenium. You can try ginseng, and staying out of the sun. Some rejuvenation tricks work for some of us some of the time, but as each of us is different, it is difficult to prescribe. One popular notion for retaining youth and vitality over forty is taking on a young lover. Again, that may or may not be for you!

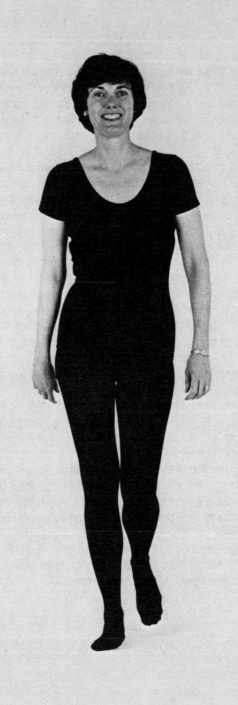

1
THE TIME IS NOW!

Ask active people if they get enough exercise, and most likely they will say no (because it rained last Thursday), while the sedentary person will swear she gets more than enough exercise (walking to the car). The truth is, those who are naturally active tend to have less body fat while sedentary people are often fatter and do everything at a slower pace. Do they move less because they are fat, or are they fat because they are less active? The answers are not all in yet, but both may be true. A woman doctor from Hungary speaking at a conference on aging at the National Institutes of Health (NIH) said that exercise should begin prenatally. Be that as it may, there is nothing we can do about that today, so we must begin where we are now.

Maintaining proper weight has not always been easy for me, as I am not one of those naturally tall, thin ectomorphs, nor am I a "born athlete". However, I have always been active, and prefer to participate rather than observe. I was fortunate that there was no one to drive us anywhere as children and that we walked for family recreation. I still love to walk, no matter how much other exercise I may get. Anywhere is fine, but hills, mountains and the seashore are special treats.

Don't wait until your summer vacation. The time to begin is now, the time to stop is never. If you are motivated, exercise will become a lifelong habit, and a pleasurable form of recreation.

Before we talk more about the simplest and most natural form of exercise, walking, let me say that whatever form of exercise you choose should be enjoyable, or you won't continue. One can also increase activity by modifications of behavior and habits. This means going up and down the stairs more often, walking those short distances instead of driving, getting things for yourself instead of sending the children. I'm sure you can think of many more ways to lift your body out of that chair!

Now that you're up, start moving. If you spend less than an hour a day on your feet, you are a certain candidate for obesity and related health problems. One should strive for a minimum of 2 hours; which need not be consecutive. How does one explain an overweight waitress, who may be on her feet for 8 hours?

For one thing, she may simply be overeating, or constantly snacking, and if you take in more than you burn up, the excess is stored as fat. The intensity of the activity plays a major role. For instance, walking at a slow stroll on a level road will only burn up 120 to 150 calories per hour. If you walk 3.5 miles per hour, you will use between 300-360 calories. Your calories burned over a week's period can be accumulated just as you accumulate the calories you take in. For example, if your increased activity equalled a 3,500 calorie expenditure in one week, you would lose one pound in that period of time. The easiest way to do it is to decrease your intake at the same time you increase your activity.

Chart 2-1 provides you with an idea of how many calories you are burning in one day. It is a good idea to keep a record for 3 days, at the same time recording the number of calories you are taking in. If you don't have a good calorie book, the Department of Agriculture will send you a copy of **"Nutritive Value of Foods"** or **Handbook Number 8**. There is a great deal of nutritional information in these books. If you are interested in the sodium content of food, handbook #8 is the one to get.

Once our body has adapted to a given amount of activity, we will not get "exercise value" unless we increase it. Eventually we reach our optimal level, and maintaining weight is easier. For instance, running allows me to eat more of my favorite foods.

Brisk walking tones the entire body, increases oxygen consumption, (distributing additional oxygen to all parts of the body, including the brain), relieves depression and firms the thighs and buttocks. Hill climbing is an excellent aerobic exercise (as can be walking). This, and climbing stairs, has an even better firming action on the buttocks-especially the gluteus maximus, the muscles you're sitting on right now. If you are out of condition, train by rapid walking on level ground before attempting Everest.

Some people have a naturally good walking stride; others may need to learn again. To increase the length of your stride, thus making walking more pleasurable and beneficial, move out from your hips. Let your arms swing freely with each step. Leave your purse at home and wear shoes that are comfortable, and not rubbing. Shoes are your only item of equipment, so they should be good ones. Other than for short distances, tennis shoes won't do. Enjoy your walk by observing the people and surroundings. Enjoy, but don't stop, as that will decrease the exercise benefits and increase your fatigue.

APPROXIMATE CALORIC COST FACTORS OF DAILY ACTIVITIES

Activity	Cal./min./lb.	Activity	Cal./min./lb.
Sleeping	.0078	Dressing	.0250
Resting in Bed	.0079	Showering	.0230
Sitting normally	.0080	Basketball	.0470
Sitting, reading	.0080	Volleyball	.0230
Sitting, lecture	.0110	Playing Ping-Pong	.0260
Sitting, eating	.0110	Calesthenics	.0330
Telephoning	.0110	Golf	.0360
Playing Cards	.0100	Tennis	.0460
Conversing	.0120	Squash	.0690
Writing	.0120	Running Long Distance	.1000
Washing Dishes	.0120	Bowling	.0440
Cooking	.0130	Making Bed	.0270
Listening to radio, TV	.0130	Ironing	.0280
Personal, toilet	.0130	Football	.0670
Singing	.0170	Dancing, Moderately	.0270
Playing Piano	.0180	Dancing, Fairly Vigorously	.0460
Standing, light activity	.0190	Playing with children	.0250
Driving car	.0190	Running 7 min. mile	.1030
Washing Clothes	.0190	Running 8.5 min. mile	.0930
Bicycling, downhill	.0180	Playing Pool	.0200
Bicycling on level	.0330	Swimming, sprinting	.1560
Bicycling up hill	.0410	Swimming, Breast stroke 20 yd./min.	.0320
Walking, level (indoors)	.0230	Swimming, Breast stroke 40 yd./min.	.0640
Walking, level (outdoors)	.0410		
Walking upstairs	.1330	Swimming, Backstroke 25 yd./min.	.0260
Walking downstairs	.0510	Swimming, Backstroke 40 yd./mn.	.0560
Walking uphill	.0560		
Archery	.0340	Swimming, Crawl 45 yd.	.0580

After walking, the next stages are hill climbing or roving. Roving is a combination of walking and jogging. Jog until you feel the need to walk, then walk until you feel like jogging again. One can cover many miles this way. There are three parameters to consider when exercising for aerobic conditioning: intensity, duration and frequency. One may be interchanged with the other; your personal goals will determine your specific training. Carbohydrates and fat are the chief sources of fuel for energy expenditure. When working near maximal capacity as competitive runners are, you are burning glycogen, or the sugar that is stored in the muscles and liver. Runners deplete glycogen when they "hit the wall" and replace it through a high carbohydrate diet. Interestingly, many elite runners do not hit the wall. When working at less than maximal effort, you burn sugar and fat, which is what we are interested in for weight reduction. Therefore it is preferable to walk or run for longer periods of time at a less than maximal effort. At this point, you may be burning 50-50, and 50% fat will be coming from fatty depots. A word about coffee: In large amounts, it can cause heart irritability and palpitations, and cause you to burn sugar when exercising, instead of fat. However, if you drink a cup or one and a half cups before exercising, you may have added energy and be more likely to burn fat. I am not recommending coffee if you do not already drink it; I am saying to limit the amount before exercising.

What is aerobic exercise, how do we get it, what good is it, and how much do we need? Before beginning any type of exercise or diet program, it is wise to consult with your physician. If you are lucky, he or she may know something about conditioning; if he does not, find someone who does. If you are over forty, an exercise stress test is advisable, to show the reaction of your heart and blood pressure to stress and to measure your vital capacity. If your doctor is not equipped to give one, check with a local college.

People have said to me that after running for two minutes, they become exhausted and quit. They feel the same when hiking. What they don't realize is that if they would hold out for four minutes or so, they would get a second wind, or steady state, and get into the aerobic cycle of energy.

Under four (4) minutes you are utilizing a combination of anaerobic energy (eight seconds or less) which depends on high energy stored phosphates; at ten to ninety seconds, phosphates and lactic acid; two to four minutes, lactic acid and aerobic; and finally, aerobic. Under certain conditions, you would use anaerobic (without oxygen) energy in your sport. The tennis serve, high jump, golf swing and volleyball spike are examples. If you don't utilize this type of energy, it is a waste of time training for it, and not useful for weight control and cardiovascular benefits.

During the first few minutes of exercise, you struggle because you are running at an oxygen deficit, that is, you are taking in less oxygen than you are using. When you get into the aerobic cycle of energy, the additional oxygen you bring in will break down carbohydrates into pyruvic acid, and utilizing fat and protein substances, break them down to carbon dioxide, water and energy. At this point, fatigue is minimal, and, with conditioning, exercise can continue for quite a while. Your aerobic capacity increases along with the functional capacity of the support systems for oxygen transport — the heart, lungs, and vascular system.

As you train aerobicly, the time you spend comfortably in this steady state will lengthen. At the end of your exercise period, you breathe heavily in the stage called "oxygen debt." You are replacing the oxygen you borrowed in the beginning. Conditioning not only increases your capacity, but shortens the length of recovery time. During recovery, your pulse will be dropping, but you need to cool down gradually by walking at a slower pace until your breathing is normal. This is just as important as warming up before you begin. Warm-ups and cool-downs should also include stretching of all of the muscles involved in the activity. This will not only help prevent injury, but also aid in the development of long, strong muscle fibers rather than short, bulky ones.

General rules for aerobic conditioning include starting within our own abilities, improving gradually, and maintaining consistency. Many forms of exercise can be aerobic, including disco dancing. In fact, dancing can be more strenuous than running! Generally, one needs to exercise three to five times a week for twenty to forty minutes. It is better to alternate hard days with easy ones. On your easy day, you could walk instead of run, or run for a shorter length of time.

I have found that women our age are usually not as competitive as men,

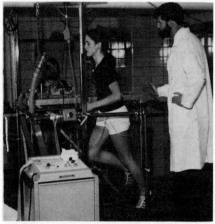

If you're over 40, an exercise stress test is advisable to show the reaction of your heart and blood pressure to stress and to measure your vital capacity.

therefore less likely to push past the pain and into injury. This may be due to our upbringing, but I think it is an advantage. Women are more tuned to their bodies and will admit pain or fatigue and heed warning signals. We also tend to be more flexible and willing to do stretching exercises.

There are some medical contraindications to exercise. Some are: acute infection, uncontrolled blood sugar, extreme anemia, some heart conditions, extremely high blood pressure, a resting heart rate over 100. Check with your doctor because some of these conditions can be corrected with exercise used judiciously. Adult onset diabetes, for instance, has in many cases been brought under control with weight loss and exercise alone. Exercise should not be thought of as a means to weight and figure control only. You can have a smashing figure and still be in lousy shape!

A few words about all aspects of physical conditioning before I tell you how to determine your own aerobic program: Along with cardiovascular endurance, we need to work on muscular strength and endurance, joint and muscular flexibility and balance. This is especially crucial for people who hold sedentary jobs, as all of these aspects deteriorate as we grow older; we cannot take any for granted. If our occupations don't demand it, we don't need the strength to carry hundred pound bags of feed. We do need to be able to carry our groceries, our children, and do other tasks requiring physical strength. We can't and shouldn't depend on others to do that which we should do ourselves.

Weight control is another reason for building muscular strength. Yes, you can add strength and tone without bulk! Our basal metabolic rate (B.M.R.) is the rate at which our body burns calories while sustaining life's processes. If someone has a low B.M.R. he or she tends to gain weight; the opposite is **usually** true if it is high. Every part of our body has a different B.M.R., the brain having the highest. Muscle is higher than fat, which is one reason why men burn more calories. A muscular person can burn more calories just sitting than an obese person walking. Our activites affect our B.M.R. As to be expected, it is the lowest when we are sleeping. There is a big difference between sitting and standing, which is why activity is so important in weight control.

Balance and flexibility are also important. These affect the way we move and all of the things we do, including sexual activity. If our balance and flexibility are poor, we are more likely to fall or injure ourselves, and we are putting limits and restraints on all of our activities. It never ceases to amaze when I see the improvement people experience in all aspects of fitness in just 5 days at my spa — this, plus weight loss. In addition to the many exercise options they are offered, they are encouraged to walk as much as possible, breathe in deeply the fresh air, drink freely of the mineral water between meals, and seek their own level of activity.

One of the most common benefits of exercise is relief from the symptoms of stress, which can be immediate and/or long term. You may be feeling worried, anxious, nervous or depressed, go for a walk or run, and come back feeling like a million. Most likely you will have more energy and a clearer mind with which to face your problems, and solutions may come during your run or walk. Often runners write poetry and other compositions, finding they are more creative.

Jane came to my spa with chronic stress-induced headaches, resulting in a trigger point in one of the cranial muscles. She had begged her doctor for tranquilizers, but he refused, suggesting exercise instead. The five days she spent with us were the longest she had gone symptom-free in years; she left looking and feeling like a new (and younger) person, a zealous convert to exercise.

Dr. Hans Kraus, world-renowned orthopedist and physical medicine doctor, has treated muscular and bone disorders for over half a century. His many books, such as **Backache, Stress, and Tension,** are the best on the subject. He states that at least 80% of backaches are caused by under-exercised muscles and tension. With Dr. Sonia Weber he developed the Kraus-Weber fitness tests which are given throughout the world to people of all ages to test for minimal fitness. Two of the tests, the sit-up and toe touch are given by one large corporation before they hire anyone for any job. If you have weak abdominal muscles and and an inflexible spine, you are likely to develop back problems; fail the tests and you don't get hired. Add tension to weak, shortened muscles and you have a prescription for pain and disability. We may not be aware of chronic muscular tension, or that we are clenching our jaws or fists, until we develop pain, trigger points or changes in the musculature or joints. Often the stooped, painful, limited movements of old age are the results of disuse begun in youth.

When we are under stress, our bodies prepare for "fight or flight." Adrenalin starts pouring, and there is no socially acceptable way to relieve this tension except through exercise. Exercise even releases the adrenalin stored in the heart muscle itself. Dr. Kraus believes in beginning and ending all of his exercise sessions with special tension reducing movements. Many have great difficulty in releasing tensions, as they have not consciously identified them, nor do they know ehre they are manifested in the body.

MORE ABOUT RUNNING

Running is addictive, both psychologically and physiologically. (It is theorized that one becomes addicted to the chemical Beta-Endorphin, whose production increases during aerobic exercise.) Deprive a runner of her sport for a day or so and she becomes nervous, irritable, has trouble sleeping, and experiences other symptoms of withdrawal. Running has been called a positive addiction because of its numerous benefits, but it can become negative when it is done to the detriment of health and life. Runners are seen competing with rush hour traffic; in fact, twenty were killed in the State of New Jersey last year.

Psychiatrists look at the situation from their perspective. Traditionally, physical work was used in psychiatric wards to treat depression, with poor results because the activity was meaningless to the patient. Running is a versatile exercise. It may be used differently each time. Sometimes we may be venting anger, another time releasing joy. Running is a pleasure to anticipate and an activity we can control. One may have trouble learning the necessary skills involved in tennis, but running comes naturally. The rhythmic movement is soothing, our minds become free and our thinking more creative; there is a sense of accomplishment when we have finished, which is helpful to our self-esteem.

All of these things don't necessarily occur the first time you go trotting down the road. It takes a while to adapt, and in the beginning, you may find no pleasure in running at all. Some people never do. It is not for them. For me, running is a natural extension of the walking and hiking I have done all my life and is relaxing and enjoyable.

There is evidence that aerobic exercise has biochemical effects on the body, influencing the central nervous system on a cellular level. Some researchers have looked into the balancing of the neurotransmitters serotonin and norepinephrine, and others not yet identified. In any case, running seems to be the aerobic exercise most often identified with addiction.

You may have read conflicting statements about running. Dr. Peter Steinchron has been quoted as saying he "never saw a happy runner." He never saw me! Some runners look unhappy because at that particular moment running may be uncomfortable. They may be running too hard, pushing past a pain, or having a bad day. If you are not overly competitive, these problems can be easily overcome, barring physical injury. This same doctor wrote twenty years ago that running was bad for the heart. Today, most cardiologists would take issue with that! Dr. Steinchron's name was brought up at a workshop that a cardiologist and I gave for senior adults. The doctor noted that Dr. Steinchron had not practiced medicine for twenty years, and therefore he questioned his judgment.

Perhaps you heard that running caused menstrual-like cramps in women because of a possible increase in prostaglandins. You may have also read that runniing relieves menstrual cramps, which happens to be true in my case. I repeat: we are unique, and the most important thing you can do for yourself is to know yourself!

Running, like other exercise, involves stressing the body, recovery from the stress, and the body adapting to greater stress. When you finish your run, you should have more energy, be more relaxed, and feel better about yourself than when you began. If you are fatigued for more than 15 minutes afterwards, you may have run too fast or too long at that particular time, or there may have been other stressing factors such as heat or cold. I suggest wearing a hat in the summer and running in the coolest part of the day, and in winter running in the warmest part of the day.

As the training effect takes place and our maximum oxygen output increases, we find that all of the everyday chores we used to find tiring are now easier. We have energy to spare for things we enjoy, like disco dancing, or playing with our children.

I believe that beginners should train at 60% of their maximum heart rate, eventually working up to 80%. It is dangerous to go higher unless you are a competing athlete, because the risks outweigh the benefits. To determine your own maximum heart rate, take the figure 220 and subtract your age. 60% of that is where you begin. For instance, a woman of forty would start out by training at a pulse rate of 108 beats per minute. AT 80% her pulse would be 144. Seniors need to increase their heart rate by no more than 20; thus they could begin their training at 100 and work up to no more than 120. It is easy to find the pulse in the carotid artery after exercising, just don't press too hard and never on both sides at once! Take your pulse for 10 seconds, and multiply by 6 to get the rate for one minute. As the pulse drops rapidly after exercising, take it immediately after your run, while you are still walking in your cool-down. Wait until your body has cooled, and your pulse and breathing are normal before taking a hot shower, as heat draws blood away from the heart and could cause you to pass out.

If you are seriously contemplating running, get a good book on the subject, and remember, your most important investment is your shoes. Two excellent books for women are **Women's Running** by Dr. Joan Ullyot, and **Aerobics for Women**, by Dr. Cooper.

One of my personal benefits of running is that I can eat more of the foods I enjoy, such as fruits and nuts and cheese. I admit I am hooked, but don't give up on exercise if you find that running is not for you. Perhaps walking, bicycling or dancing is just your thing. Swimming is excellent if you have joint problems, or are very obese.

The many benefits we derive from exercise are not restricted to runners, but the workout must be sufficiently strenuous to be of value. More benefits from exercise are: protection against stress—a delaying of the aging process, increase in density of the bones, less degenerative diseases, possible prevention of, or more rapid recovery from heart attack, and reduced convalescence time after surgery.

If you think running is for you, read on. If it is not, skip the next chapter.

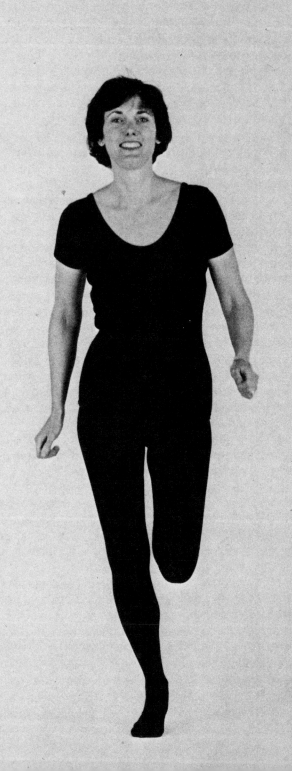

2
YOU WANT TO RUN!

To run or not is the question, and you have decided to give it a try. Your over forty body and mind are not quite sure what you are getting into. For me, there is no question at all. Running, not eating, is my psychiatrist. My mind relaxes with the first step, and I feel free of the hassles, tensions, and pressures of the day. Sure, it's in my mind, but so are many of our stresses, and when my mind relaxes, so does my body. The tension in my upper back disappears, and I start feeling GOOD.

Running is not for everyone. Even obesity may be a contraindication, because of the stress on the weight-bearing joints. Keep in mind the contraindications I mentioned, and check with your doctor. If you are really anxious to start running, go to a doctor who runs, or at least one who is trained in sports medicine. If the answer is no, stick with walking, bicycling, swimming or some other aerobic activity, and skip this chapter.

The walk and walk-run part of your program will take about thirty minutes per session and last about eight weeks. I emphasize ABOUT because of the differences in human physiology. This part of your training may take three months or more, but don't give up and think of yourself as a flabby failure. It took forty plus years for you to get in the shape you are in today; you are not going to change that overnight. Consistency is the key word. Do something every day, even just a little; if you are not overdoing, you will feel better, not worse. You are not competing with anyone, not even yourself, at this point. The time will come when you will be elatedly running fifteen minutes without stopping.

Let's backtrack and discuss what is helpful to a beginner, and what you will need. It is best, time-wise, if you can run from where you live or work. If time is not a problem, then by all means drive to a variety of safe and attractive running places. Allow time to do stretches before and after you run (five to ten minutes each), and leave time for a shower. An hour is usually more than enough.

Special clothing is not necessary, unless you want it. It makes sense to wear clothing that does not bind or rub, allows for circulation of air, and absorbs perspiration. Try to run in the coolest part of the day in the summer, and wear as little as possible. If you run in the sun, a loose-fitting hat will protect your head. A tennis skirt and elasticized halter are my hot weather favorites. In cold weather, removable layers are best, making sure your head, feet, and hands are covered warmly.

Remember, your body temperature will rise and you will perspire, even though it is cold. Clothing that is too restrictive or warm will cause further perspiration, causing over-cooling. Cotton socks, or tennis peds, are best for summer. Add some wool for winter, and make sure your socks don't bunch or slip, or you will get blisters.

There are two items of clothing that are important to a woman. One is a proper bra and the other, shoes. If you are small enough to go braless comfortably, and you prefer to, then don't be afraid to do so. For most women, myself included, a bra that is lightweight, elastic, and supports without riding or binding, is sufficient. Other women need additional comfortable support, and for this purpose several exercise or jogging bras have been developed. You can find these in sporting goods and department stores. Try them on and decide for yourself; keep in mind that padding can be hot, cotton absorbs perspiration, and bonding and hard closures can dig into tender flesh (some of this can be alleviated by a band-aid or tape).

Shoes, like bras, vary according to the individual. It is better to buy a lower-rated shoe that fits properly than one rated 5-Star (by Runner's World) that rubs.

Try on several pairs before you buy, and plan to spend around thirty dollars. Cheap imitations can destroy your incentive, feet, back and knees. Look for comfort first, making sure the shoes (try on both) firmly cradle the sides and back of the foot. Allow toe room for your socks and to accommodate any swelling caused by running. If you can, run around the store in them, or even down the street. Flexibility is important, and so is cushioning, which is necessary to protect the feet, knees and back from the impact of running on hard surfaces. I prefer nylon uppers because they are soft, lightweight and washable. Of course, you will check for flaws, such as missing eyelets or loose stitching.

Times have certainly changed. When I started running, all I could get were boy's track shoes. When running became popular, I switched to men's Adidas because they were narrow. Now there is a good selection of women's shoes, and women runners are taken seriously.

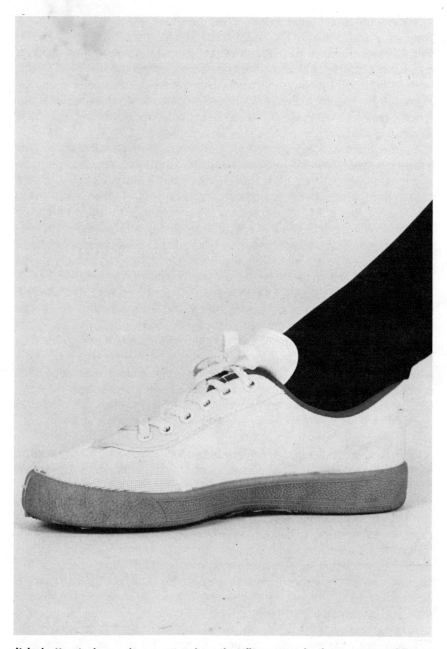

It is better to buy a lower-rate shoe that fits properly than one rated 5-star that rubs.

Some women continue to run when pregnant, if they have a normal pregnancy and feel well. The same holds true for menstruation; some feel better because of their run, others worse. Women who have had children may have a special problem if they have a prolapsed uterus or tend to be incontinent when running or jumping. Sometimes these problems can be alleviated by special exercises, surgery or other means. Again, this is a specific condition—don't feel that just because you have children you can't try running at all.

As you get into running, you will get to know your body, and if wise, you will heed its signals. Most likely you will need more, not less sleep, and perhaps an occasional nap. If you are fatigued after your run, you will know you have run too hard, and skip a day. However, beginners should plan to run every day, even if just a little. It is too easy for one "skipped" day to extend to forever. You will get to know which pains to ignore, and which require rest and treatment. You will know your heart rate without taking your pulse, and if you can't talk to your partner you are running too hard. You will have good days and bad, and some when you will feel you can run forever.

Because we are running for conditioning, weight loss, and pleasure, we look to increase our distance, rather than speed. Yes, pleasure! Once you get to the point where you can run easily for fifteen minutes, you will experience less strain and more enjoyment. Most runners don't enjoy the first mile or two, but that is not true for me, unless I'm having a bad day. I run in a variety of scenic areas and vary my speed and distances. If I feel especially good when running a "hard" day, I run farther. I always feel fantastic after my run. Some say you need to run long distances to effect the chemical changes that produce a true runner's high. But, running itself is an "upper", and all you really need to do is run.

When you are running at a comfortable pace, at least 50% of your energy is being supplied by fat. That is exactly what you are looking for in weight control. However, running is harder for the overweight. Maximal oxygen consumption (when work load grows more difficult, but oxygen consumption fails to increase) is directly related to weight as well as training. It is expressed in milliliters of oxygen per kilogram of body weight per minute, or ml/kg.min. A beginning lean runner may have higher levels of oxygen uptake than a fatter, more experienced runner. Stick with it, because the heavier you are, the more calories you are expending. For example, a woman weighing 120 pounds will burn up 76 calories running a ten-minute mile, and one weighing 160 will expend 100 calories. You may be working hard at running, but remember, one of the benefits of aerobic conditioning is that your sub-maximal work becomes easier. This means you will have more energy for everything else you do.

Always check with your doctor before running. A stress test is advisable;

however, the findings may not be accurate. Stress testing does not show the condition of your vascular system. For this reason, additional testing may be prudent. Your doctor may want to look at your blood lipids (triglycerides, total cholesterol, and high and low-density lipoproteins). The evidence shows exercise will decrease (in the long term) the triglycerides and low-density lipoproteins (the kind that forms plaques in the arteries) and increase the level of high-density lipoproteins (considered beneficial). This is one of the ways exercise decreases the risk of heart attack and stroke.

Another potential problem for the beginner is the knees. Assuming you are not extremely overweight or arthritic, look to simple measures for prevention. Naturally, you are going to start with good shoes that will absorb some of the stress at impact. You may want to run on a grass or dirt surface for a while, although with the new shoes this is not as important as it once was. Be aware of the camber of the road. Run in both directions, so as to stress the knees equally. Are your thighs (quads) weak? Running will strengthen them somewhat, but additional exercises will be helpful, especially if you are doing downhill running. True runner's knee is an inflammation on the underside of the kneecap. Possible causes are an old injury or pronation of the foot, which causes a rotation of the shin bone. The best advice is to see a sports podiatrist, who may fit you with an orthotic. If the pain is on the outside of the knee, it may be caused by the rubbing of tendons. On the inside, it could be bursitis or a stress fracture. If a mild pain becomes worse, and persists before, during and after your run, seek medical help, either from an orthopedist or podiatrist. As a rule, it takes as long for an injury to heal as it took for you to get in the injured state. In other words, if the pain was gradually getting worse over a period of 4 months, expect healing to take that long. You may not have to be totally inactive during that time, but you will certainly have to slow down.

Beginners don't need to worry about overtraining as long as they run within their current abilities and don't injure weak or improperly warmed up muscles. Stretching is most important for someone with inflexible muscles and joints, and warming up also means walking or slow jogging, especially in cold weather.

If you reach a point of chronic fatigue that is not helped by additional sleep and rest, check the possibility of allergic reactions (food, pollen), or chronic infection, such as sinusitis. Consider iron: it is possible to be out of iron stores without tests showing anemia, especially if you are still menstruating. Approximately 25% of menstruating women suffer from iron deficiency, if not anemia. Studies concerning "sports anemia" have been inconclusive. There are various theories about its causes, and a recent study showed that female athletes did not have a greater percentage of iron deficiency than other women. Iron is involved in the transport of oxygen to the muscles, which makes it important in an exercise program. Some consider the current standard of 18 mg. per day as being too little. Iron is found in green leafy vegetables and beans, as well as meat and liver; however, it is not readily absorbed from vegetable sources. Taking vitamin C with a meal, or eating foods high in C (citrus, green pepper, cabbage) enhances the availability and absorption of the iron in that meal. If necessary, take an iron supplement, preferably with vitamin C, and not with TEA, whole grains, milk or eggs. (See chapter on nutrition.)

What other foods or supplements are ergonic aids, that is, improve athletic performance? Many authorities say there are none, other than carbohydrates and adequate water. Most will say that all of the vitamins and minerals we need come from our food. This may be true if you are not lactose intolerant, have no food allergies, have no impaired absorption due to aging or other causes, eat a wide variety of fruits and vegetables fresh from the garden and in season, know that the soil your grains and produce are grown in is not mineral deficient, eat little or no coffee or sugar, are in perfect health, not under stress, don't smoke, breathe unpolluted air (inside and out), feel and look terrific, and are not dieting to the point of eliminating necessary nutrients.

Runners need adequate fluid, sodium, chloride, potassium and magnesium. Unless running in extreme conditions to which we are not acclimated, we get enough sodium chloride (salt) from our foods, without adding additional or eating obviously salty foods. The best sources of potassium are fruits and vegetables, especially oranges and bananas. Magnesium is the green color of chlorophyl, or green vegetables. It is also plentiful in seeds, nuts, whole grains, peanut butter, wheat germ and dolomite. Some sports physiologists also suggest 500 mgs. of vitamin C daily, and the B vitamins B1, B2, B6, B12, & Niacin. An overdose of niacin will keep you out of the fat cycle of energy, something you don't want! Vitamin E and selenium are helpful in smoggy weather (too much selenium can be toxic; more than 100 mcg. "micrograms" daily are not recommended).

Some coaches swear by erogenic aids. The Russians consider vitamin C to be one, along with the controversial calcium pangamate, or "vitamin" B-15. In this country, the research on B-15 shows conflicting results. (So, what's new?) Dr. Victor Herbert, chief of the Hematology and Nutrition Laboratory of the Bronx Veterans Administration Medical Center in New York City, along with Dr. Neville Coleman who also works in the laboratory, showed the ingredients in B-15 to be mutagenic, which means that it has a 90% chance of causing cancer. (Reported in the Journal of American Medicine.) Furthermore, the composition of various B-15 supplements varies from one manufacturer to another.

Pangamic Acid was discovered in apricot pits by E.T. Krebs, the man who also discovered Laetril. It occurs naturally where other B-complex vitamins are found, such as wheat germ, brewers yeast and liver, and was erroneously called vitamin B-15. The active ingredient of the original vitamin B-15 is N,N-Dimethylglycine (DMG) which acts as a metabolic enhancer by increasing the utilization of oxygen by the cellular tissue. Dr. Larry Lytle, a holistic-minded dentist in North Dakota, showed with his experiments on twelve high school athletes that the half that took B-15 had 30% lower lactic acid levels than those on placebos. Most members of the professional football teams take it as well.

My own experience and that of my friends who take it has been that if you have a respiratory illness, B-15 is remarkable. Until I took B-15, I could not get rid of a cough and low-grade fever that lingered for months after the flu; and within two days I was running again. I have tried several varieties of B-15, and found that the one that really seems to make a difference is the original formula put out by Food Science Labs, called AANGAMIK 15, a combination of calcium gluconate and DMG. The FDA has yet to approve the controversial B-15, so you must use your own judgment regarding it.

Other ergonic aids are brewers yeast, bee pollen and **raw** wheat germ oil. Dr. Thomas Cureton, one of the most respected exercise physiologists and trainers in the business, is still running at age eighty. He taught Roger Bannister to run the four-minute mile, encouraged doctors to exercise their heart patients, and has special insight into the fitness abilities of older people. He says you lose speed as you age, but with training you will not lose endurance and its related benefits to health.

Dr. Cureton has much interest in nutrition and diet as an aid in athletic performance, and, along with his colleagues at the University of Illinois, he has conducted 42 studies on wheat germ oil. The conclusion was that it did increase endurance, probably through stimulating the energy production of the muscle cells. It is not vitamin E that does it, however. The active ingredient is octocosanol, which is destroyed by heat. For this reason you should use raw, cold pressed wheat germ oil. He feels it is best taken with skim milk after a workout, when the body needs nutrition.

I have taken wheat germ oil off and on for over twenty years. I notice that when I first start taking it there is an immediate increase in energy, especially if I have been "dragging" for some time. Gradually the increased jolt of energy wears off, and there is a leveling effect. This appears to be true with most substances you put in your body: you become used to them, and the effect is reduced. The usual dosage is a teaspoon in a glass of skim milk; but if you can't stand the taste, you can get it in capsule form. The flavor should be nutty, not bitter (which means it is too old). Remember, it is an oil, therefore, high in calories.

Our needs and tolerances are individual, and large doses of vitamins may be toxic. The safest are the water-soluable, C and B vitamins, with the excess being secreted in the urine. One aid you WILL need is water. Drink before and after you run, and during it if you perspire profusely in hot weather. Drink small amounts at a time so you don't feel water-logged or nauseated. Water also helps prevent fatigue, and increases the absorption of minerals.

You are unlikely to get injured if you are reasonably careful. The most important things to consider are shoes, careful warm-ups, keeping within your present capabilities, and avoiding hazardous and uneven surfaces. If you run on grass, know in advance where the holes are: look about thirty feet ahead of you, instead of at your feet. Eventually, you will develop a sixth sense about dangers such as stones, holes, and grass; but until then, be careful. One runner I know blackened her eye during a running fall.

Shinsplints are a runner's injury that can and should be avoided. That pain in the front of the shin that some runners can run through some of the time, can also knock you out of running for a long time.

What are shinsplints? Doctors disagree. Some call it an inflammation of the periosteum, (the lining of the shin bone), or it may be an inflammation of the tendons or the muscle itself. Others feel it is pain preceding a stress fracture, or a loosening of minute muscle fibers from the tibia (large bone) and fibula (outside bone).

What causes them? Overuse is one cause, or structural imbalance. Overuse can be running thirty miles a week for one person, or ninety for another. Running on a hard surface with the wrong shoes may contribute, as well as running in a circle on a banked track or on a road where one leg is always short, and other pronated. Other factors are insufficient calf stretching, excessive hill running, leaning too far forward, and wearing shoes that are too large.

Common sense will help you prevent shinsplints, and women usually have more of this when it comes to sports than men do. You're not going to run beyond your present capabilities. If you laid off for a while, you are going to start again at a lower level, and not increase your distance too rapidly. Stretch your calf muscles for at least ninety seconds before your run, and hold the stretch (3 thirty-second stretches, for example). Strengthen the muscles on the front of your legs by lifting the toes and holding for a few seconds, or standing on a slant board with your toes pointed down and rolling up on the balls of your feet several times.

It is possible to run through shinsplints, but not through stress fractures unless you are willing to risk injury. How can you tell when to keep going and when to stop? This is highly individual, but certainly pain is telling you that something is wrong. If the pain doesn't go away after a few minutes, slow down, or stop. A stress fracture will be more painful than a shinsplint, and on a smaller area, but remember that shinsplints often precede them.

If you DO get a shinsplint, the first thing to do is to firmly run your hand

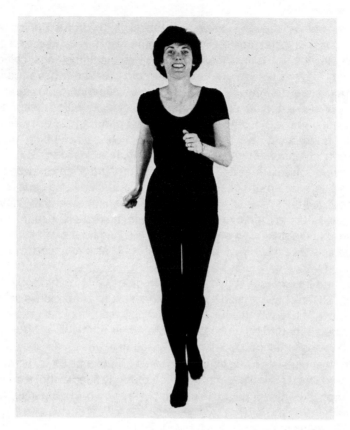

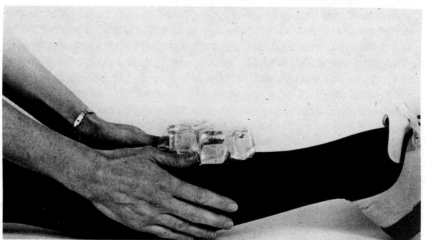

Common sense can help you prevent shinsplints.

along the area, as though pressing the muscle to the bone. Put ice on it for ten minutes and take some aspirin, or Ecotrin, which is coated, and passes through the stomach before dissolving. Stretch the hamstrings, calves and quadriceps several times a day, and make sure your shoes have cushioning and a good heel counter. If the pain persists, stop running for a couple of weeks, and see a doctor. You don't need to become a jellied mess because you are not running. You can exercise all other parts of your body, and keep up your endurance by bicycling, swimming, hill or stair climbing. If nothing else is available, don't forget that old stand-by, brisk walking.

Recurrent ankle sprains are another common injury. They may be caused by inadequate treatment of earlier injuries or structural imbalances. Here, too, good well-fitting shoes are important. Personally, because I have narrow heels, I like the Etonic running shoes with the extra lace that snugs the shoe around the ankle. An elastic support will also help a weak ankle, and with exercise (see the end of this chapter) it may be all you need to allow you to run pain-free.

Structural imbalances may be found in other parts of the body. For instance, you may have limited rotation in the hips, or a variation in the length of your legs. The result may be an alteration in the angle of gait, causing your body to be supported by muscular action, rather than efficient positioning. The imbalances may cause shinsplints or other injuries.

Treatment consists of flexibility exercises and exercises to increase the range of motion of the hip joints. Again, a properly fitted orthotic may make the difference between being able to run miles and not being able to run at all.

Ankle sprains may occur despite your efforts at prevention. It is primarily the ligaments that are injured in a sprain, and they may be partially or completely ruptured. The most common kind of ankle sprain is when the foot turns inward excessively, usually because you stepped on an uneven surface or into a hole. An eversion sprain, which occurs on the inside of the ankle, can be caused by a fall.

The immediate first aid is ice, to reduce swelling and relieve pain. Compression, such as an ace bandage, also helps. If you can stand and walk around comfortably within a few minutes, the chances are the sprain is slight. Exercise with caution until the ankle has returned to full strength. If you cannot put pressure on it, see a sports physician or podiatrist for proper treatment. This is important in order to prevent recurrent instability. Do not put off the examination in hopes the ankle will heal itself, as you will be doing further damage.

Some trainers use contrast baths as part of the treatment for ankle sprains. Ices are used for the first 48 to 72 hours, then baths alternating warm with cold, always finishing with cold. In addition, an elastic stocking (not an ace bandage) is used with sequential pneumatic pressure.

The contrast baths are given in any receptacle large enough to hold the injured extremity. The warm water is 98°-F. During the treatment, range of motion exercises are performed. You invert, evert, dorsiflex and plantarflex the ankle, and write your name with your big toe. The sequence of contrast baths is:

warm	5 minutes
cold	1 minute
warm	2 minutes
cold	1 minute
warm	2 minutes
cold	1 minute
warm	2 minutes
cold	1 minute

This is part of one form of treatment currently used for ankle sprains. It is important, however, for you to consult your own physician.

One does not usually give beginners body positioning for running, as it is best to do what feels natural and comfortable. However, there are a few rules of thumb that can apply to almost everyone.

Hold your arms comfortably around waist level or slightly below, as you will be wasting energy holding them in front of your chest. Arms should not swing across your body, as this may cause the hips to rotate inward, leading to improper positioning of the legs and feet. Keep your shoulders relaxed. If you feel tension there, periodically shrug, and shake your arms and shoulders loosely. Don't run on your toes, or you will get sore calves. Save that for the sprinters. Jogging is an extension of walking, so your gait will be similar, although not exactly the same as in walking. Don't try to lengthen your stride unnaturally, as this can lead to knee injury. Watch your posture. Leading with your belly will cause swayback and pain. Keeping your back flat utilizes your abdominal and gluteal (buttocks) muscles. Pushing off with your big toe helps, but you might want to save that for when you are more experienced. Some runners feel that an extra hard exhalation after six or so breaths is helpful. Listen to your body — if you feel the need to exhale hard, then do so.

If you are going to take your running seriously, you may want to factor in your own condition when taking your pulse, or you may use the formula I gave earlier. In either case, you take your pulse while walking, and within ten seconds of your run. The pulse is easy to find in the carotid, but press gently, on one side only; count to ten seconds, and multiply by six. The following is a formula using your own resting pulse to aid in determining your exercise heart rate. To find your resting pulse, take it first thing in the morning for one minute. Do this for three days, and use the average. For a similar method, see chapter on exercise.

MAXIMUM HEART RATES			
Age 31-40	Age 41-50	Age 51-60	Age Over 60, keep exercise heart rate no
187	185	178	higher than 120.

Maximum Heart Rate minus your resting H.R. times 70% plus Resting H.R. = **Exercise Level,** that is **your exercise pulse.** If you train at less, you are not getting full benefits; training more may place you in danger.

Of what sort of dangers are we speaking when we train beyond our target heart rate? First, let me say that the resting heart rate is not a constant, although training does tend to lower it. Many factors, other than illness, affect the pulse. Chronic and acute stress certainly can, even the stress caused by being happily excited. You will not find an accurate resting heart rate when you are excited by being near someone who turns you on, nor would it be "normal" when driving in rush hour or struggling to meet a deadline. Coffee, cigarettes, food allergies, an overactive thyroid, a heavy meal, can all elevate the heart rate. Running adds additional stress to what may already be a stressful situation and should be taken in moderate doses at these times. That does not mean that one should abstain altogether, because running relieves many of the psychological and physiological effects of stress. Speaking of a reduced heart rate, I don't believe the published reports that President Carter's rate was reduced from 60 to 40 — that of a top athlete — after one year of jogging.

Based on epidemiological studies, the American Heart Association has identified lack of exercise as one of the most significant risk factors in coronary artery disease. However, because of the difficulty in isolating the influence of other factors, there is some controversy among medical professionals. There is no evidence that exercise will prevent a heart attack in the case of pre-existing disease. It is felt, however, that it will reduce the severity, and increase the likelihood of survival.

Increasing the intensity of your training gradually — as I have suggested — is extremely important, especially if you are beginning in the middle years. There may be additional fat which will reduce your maximum performance, and the effects of training will be achieved more slowly. If, for instance, an untrained person undertakes a sudden bout of vigorous exercise, the result would be extreme shortness of breath and fatigue. The heart rate would be greatly elevated and take a long time (half an hour to an hour) to return to resting, and the systolic blood pressure would be elevated.

Many factors cause this, including a rise in body temperature which increases the heart rate, and an increase in hormones. An untrained person can collapse after sudden and extreme exercise. This occurs because of virtual cessation of venous return to the heart. Remaining in an upright position, the leg veins in an untrained person do not contract as well as those in a trained person, allowing the blood to pool, rather than sending it back to the heart, and this causes a sudden drop in blood pressure. An untrained person's heart will also have greater difficulty in expelling an adequate stroke volume. For these and other reasons it is important to increase your training gradually, finish your runs with a walk so that the leg muscles can assist in the return of blood to the heart, and postpone your hot shower until your body is returned to normal respiration and heart rate.

Although it may take some time to see cardiovascular training effects, the nervous system responds quickly, as norepinephrine levels are lower with the second bout of exercise.

In conclusion, let's review some of the most important effects of training on women:

- Training effects: an increase in the efficiency of the heart; an increase in cardiac output; a drop in resting blood pressure; a slowing of the resting heart rate; a stabilization of cardiac rhythm; perhaps a reduction in the risk and severity of heart attack; the tone of the veins is increased, and with training, less blood is needed by the skin and more can be used by the working muscles.

- It takes longer for an older person to see a training effect. The greatest effect occurs early, after perhaps as little as two or three weeks, with the biggest improvement seen in those the least fit. Training can continue over several years, if the work load is increased progressively.

- Women respond to training in the same way as men. Their extra fat (up to a point) may be helpful as a source of energy in long distances. A certain minimal amount of muscular strength is necessary.

- Running reduces body fat, thereby reducing total cholesterol and uric acid levels.

- Running improves self image and relieves depression.

- The beneficial effects of running are quickly reversed. You don't store fitness, only fat.

Beginning to run may mean crossing a large hurdle both physically and psychologically for the woman over forty. This is especially true if she has been sedentary and subjugated. If your doctor approves, and your mind is willing, your body will be able. Just remember to start with brisk walking and proceed to walking-running before you become a runner.

Here are some psychic aids in making your run easier and more fun:

Color affects both our minds and bodies. Wear a bright, warm color that is both pleasing and energizing to you, and mentally suffuse your whole body with it. Run with your thumb and forefingers together and take a deep breath. This helps to recircuit our body energies. Have a lively song going through your head, and run in step with it. Write a poem or enjoy the scenery and the people you are passing. Hold an interesting conversation with a running friend or a stranger.

Finally, run in places that are reasonably safe. Streets and highways are for cars. If you run along the edge, stay well out of the way of traffic, and wear fluorescent lighting at night. The very presence of runners seems to antagonize some drivers; so be alert. If you run alone, know your neighborhood. You may want to carry a police whistle on a chain, or run with your dog. Dogs can also pose a threat: if you know where the mean ones are, avoid them! Last, but most important, RUN FOR FUN!

EXERCISES FOR RUNNERS

The tighter and more inflexible your muscles and joints are, the more you need to stretch before your run. In cold weather, warm up with a very slow jog before you stretch. Stretching afterwards is important, too, because then the warm muscles can actually be lengthened by a stretch you hold for twenty seconds or more. Injury is most likely to occur when muscles and joints are tight and cold, and cosmetically, most women prefer the look of long, strong muscles as opposed to short, bulky ones.

The muscles is the back of the body may become tight and shortened with running if stretching is not included in your routine. The following exercises should be done once or twice before and after your run. Do the stretches **SLOWLY**, hold the stretch, and **DON'T BOUNCE.**

ACHILLES TENDON AND CALF STRETCHERS

Stand facing a wall, about 3 feet away. Palms on the wall at shoulder level. KEEP YOUR BACK STRAIGHT as you slowly bend your elbows, bringing your head toward the wall. **Keep the heels on the floor.** If it is painful, bend your knees slightly. Anytime you flex your foot, that is, pull your toes toward your face, you are stretching your calf and Achilles. You can do this in a variety of ways. One, walk barefooted in carpeting, on your heels, with your feet flexed. Sit on a chair with your legs straight out in front of you. Flex your feet, bend forward SLOWLY, and hold the stretch.

TOE TOUCH

The toe touch stretches everything from head to the heels. If you are very tight, or have any kind of back problem, it should always be done with the

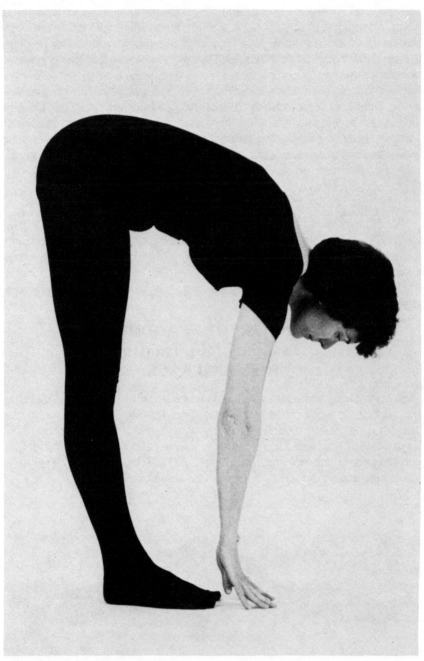

Stretching exercises should be performed slowly, without bouncing.

knees BENT. Take a deep breath, and as you exhale, bend your head towards the floor, then your neck, and then the rest of your spine until you are hanging loosely from your hips with the top of your head pointing towards the floor. DON'T BOUNCE, just hang there breathing deeply. Visualize your hands getting closer to the floor each time you exhale. You will find that as your body relaxes it will stretch, especially if the muscles are warm. **Never force your body; just allow it to happen.** If you can already touch your fingertips to the floor, work towards getting your palms down. If you get dizzy when bending forward, eliminate this exercise. Bend your knees and roll back up to a standing position, one vertebra at a time, keeping knees bent until you are all the way upright.

HAMSTRING STRETCH

Standing straight, clasp your hands behind your back. KEEP YOUR BACK STRAIGHT and bend forward from the hips. The head should stay in line with the rest of the spine. Hold your stretch! You should feel the stretch down the back of your legs. If you feel discomfort in your back, discontinue the exercise, as you are probably doing it incorrectly. Return **slowly** to a standing position.

STRETCH FOR THIGH ADDUCTORS
(Insides of the Thighs)
HIPS AND BACK

Sit on the floor and spread your legs as far apart as you comfortably can. For the most effective stretch, the legs should be straight; however, if your back and hamstring muscles are very tight, let your knees bend slightly. Take a deep breath, and as you exhale, slowly lean forward from the hips as you slide your hands forward. HOLD THE STRETCH, breathing deeply and visualizing your head touching the floor as you stretch.

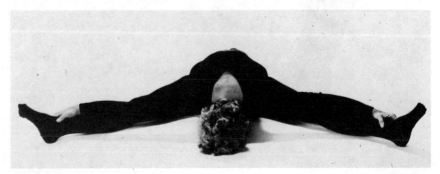

Thigh adductors feet flexed.

Return to the starting position, and keeping the knee pointing towards the ceiling, SLOWLY stretch over the right leg. HOLD THE STRETCH; then repeat it with the foot flexed. Try to touch your knee with your head. Repeat with the other leg.

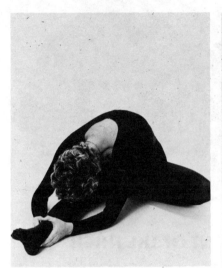

Back and legs forward stretch.

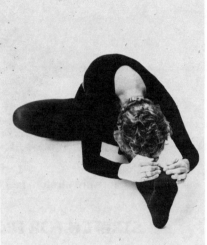

Back and legs foot flexed.

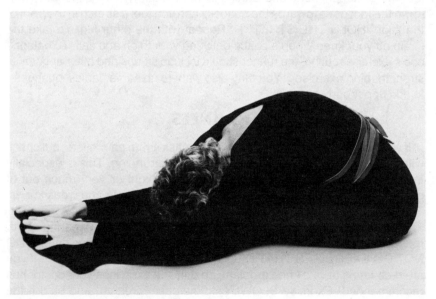

Back and legs; forward stretch.

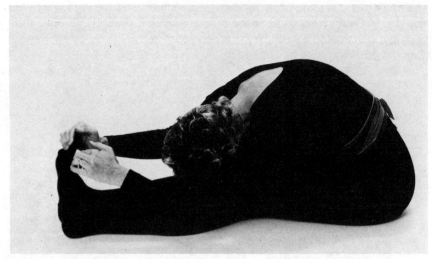

Back and legs; forward stretch; feet flexed.

STRETCH FOR FRONT OF THE THIGH

Holding onto a support with your left hand, if necessary, grasp your right foot with your right hand and leaning forward slightly, pull the foot back and up so the foot goes towards the buttocks and you feel a stretch in the front of the thigh. HOLD THE STRETCH. Repeat with the other leg. To take the strain off your knee, keep a space between your thigh and calf. To balance one's exercise routine, the runner should include sit-ups and other abdominal strengthening exercises. You may also want to do some "ladies' pushups," to add upper body strength.

THE KNEES

If you have persistent knee pains, don't mask it with pain killers, but check with your sports physician before you continue running. This is especially true if you have had knee surgery, are overweight or very much out of condition. Weak thighs and hamstrings lead to unstable and weak knees. The following exercises are helpful to strengthen the knees.

Precautions: If you are suffering from Chondromalacia, (a wearing down, roughening or cracking of the articular cartilage) or a dislocated patella, DO NOT DO EXERCISES THAT REQUIRE BENDING OF THE KNEE. If you are recovering from a knee problem, do only the exercises your doctor has recommended. Exercise SLOWLY, to increase strength, and stop if the exercise causes pain.

ISOMETRICS FOR
FRONT AND BACK OF THE THIGHS

Lie with your right knee bent, and your left leg straight. Tighten the **front** of the thigh muscles by trying to push the back of the left knee towards the floor. Place your hand on your thigh and be aware of it contracting. HOLD THE CONTRACTION FOR 5 SECONDS ONLY. Rest for 5 seconds, and repeat. To strengthen the hamstrings (back of the thigh), push down with the heel instead of the back of the knee. Hold 5 seconds. Never hold an isometric contraction for more than 5 seconds, and exhale as you contract. Counting the seconds out loud is a good way to accomplish this.

FRONT AND INNER THIGH

Sit in a chair, with your legs in front of you, heels resting on the floor. Push your legs together as hard as you can, and **hold for 5 seconds.** Do it 3 times, twice a day, working up to 5 times daily. Work this one in any time you are seated. These exercises will give you firm, attractive thighs, as well as help support and stabilize your knees. You also will find that all of your walking and stair climbing, etc., will be easier.

SINGLE LEG LIFTS

Lie flat on your back with your left knee bent. Tense the thigh muscle in the right leg, then SLOWLY lift the right leg about 24 inches off the floor, keeping the leg STRAIGHT. Lower SLIGHTLY, rest, and repeat. To strengthen the muscles on the inner thigh as well, do the same exercise with the leg slightly rotated so the foot is pointing outwards as you slowly lift and lower your leg. It is important also to stretch these muscles. Repeat exercises on the other leg.

LEG STRAIGHTENING

Sit in a chair with the knees bent. Place a towel under the working knee. SLOWLY lift your foot until your knee is completely straight. Hold for 3 seconds; lower slowly. After a few weeks the exercise will become easy. Make it harder by gradually adding weights. You may start your resistance exercises by wearing boots, then by lifting your pocketbook with the strap, eventually making it heavier. You may also use the opposite leg as resistance. Cross at the ankles, and RESIST with the top leg. Bicycle riding strengthens the thighs. Move the seat up or down to vary the bend in the knee. These exercises are suggested as general strengthening for the thighs. Check with your doctor first if you have pain or orthopedic problems.

THE FEET AND ANKLES

As with the previous exercise, if you have pain or other problems, check with your doctor before exercising. An orthotic or special shoes may be part of your therapy.

ANKLES

Rotate your ankles OUTWARD several times. Repeat, circling them INWARD. Alternate pointing your toes with flexing your feet, (they are pulled back in a fish-hook position). Roll your feet inward so the soles are touching, then roll them out in the opposite direction. Repeat.

FEET, ANKLES, and CALVES

Stand with the balls of your feet on a step or board and your heels on the edge. Hold onto the wall for balance, if necessary. SLOWLY roll up on the balls of your feet, then slowly lower back down so your heels are below the surface and you feel a stretch in your Achilles and calf. Repeat 5 times, working up to 10. Optional activities include:
- Roll up a piece of cloth with your toes several times.
- Pick up marbles with your toes, and walk across the floor with them.
- Alternating warm and cool foot soaks helps stimulate the circulation and restore lagging energy.

MEDICAL INSTRUCTIONS FOR RUNNERS

TEMPERATURE AND HUMIDITY

Temperature and humidity can substantially affect the performance and safety of runners. When the temperature exceeds 70°F (21°C) and/or humidity is greater than 50%, the incidence of heat-related injury markedly increases. The race medical team will monitor these conditions and post colored flags at the starting line to alert runners to the weather situation.

FLAG COLOR CONDITION

Red Temperature is over 75°F or humidity is over 50%. Runners who are sensitive to heat or humidity should carefully consider participation.

Yellow Temperature is over 70°F or humidity is over 45%. Since both are likely to rise during the race, runners should be able to recognize significant changes in physical status. (See below).

Green Temperature is below 70°F and humidity is below 45%.

PREVENTION OF PHYSICAL PROBLEMS

- Runners attempting to participate in a race of this distance should have trained adequately. This should include at least two long-distance runs within the previous month that are at least two-thirds the length of this race.
- Elevate your legs when they are tired, and talk someone into giving you a foot massage with warm oil. GREAT!
- Avoid running to exhaustion within the week preceding the race.
- Remember, you will be running on yesterday's meals. We suggest a light meal no less than two hours before the race. Avoid fatty foods on race day. Emphasize carbohydrate intake the day before the race.
- Maintenance of adequate hydration is the most important preventive measure. If you become thirsty, you are behind in fluids. Drink two 8-oz glasses of fluid (preferably water) within 10 to 15 minutes of race time. Drink continuously throughout the run. Unless you are totally committed to time, stop to drink; finishing is the goal. There will be water stations at the start as well as along the course.
- Pre-run warm-up must include stretching exercises of the calf, hamstring, quadriceps, groin, and trunk muscles. If you begin to feel muscle tightness or cramps, stop and stretch.
- Blisters can be prevented by wearing wellfitted, broken-in shoes and soft lightweight socks. Powder in shoes and socks will reduce friction. Remove pebbles immediately. Nails should be trimmed. If you feel a hot spot developing, stop at an aid station for care. They will be positioned every 2.5 miles.
- Chafing occurs where clothing rubs against the skin. It can be prevented by wearing loose-fitting clothing and applying petroleum jelly or protective bandaging in susceptible areas such as nipples, armpits, neckline, and groin.
- You will be one of many runners, so run defensively. Stay to the right. Watch out for other runners and yield if necessary.
- Pace yourself. Don't burn yourself out by starting too quickly. Common sense is the key.

RECOGNITION OF PHYSICAL PROBLEMS

While every runner will experience varying degrees of discomfort, significant changes in physical status should be recognized. If in doubt, stop to ask for advice. Medical personnel, identifiable by red caps, will be positioned at all aid stations.

- Symptoms of overexertion: nausea, vomiting, extreme breathlessness, dizziness, unusual fatigue, headache.
- Symptoms of heat injury: piloerection (hair on end or gooseflesh) on the chest or upper arms, chilling, headache or throbbing pressure, unsteadiness, vomiting or nausea, labored breathing, faintness, muscle cramps. Continuing the race with these symptoms may result in collapse or unconsciousness. Stop. Get help.
- Not only can blisters be painful, but infection can result and be literally life-threatening. Have them treated at an aid station.
- If stretching does not relieve cramps, stop at an aid station.
- Abrasions (skin scrapes, "strawberries") may become infected. Have them treated.

Report significant injuries or downed runners to medical personnel. A field hospital will be established at the finish line. Injured runners will be transported there.

3
BEHAVIOR
MODIFICATION

Up until the last ten years or so most dieters were unsuccessful, because as soon as the weight was lost they resumed old habits, regaining the lost pounds and usually some additional. In 1967 a behavioral psychologist instituted a breakthrough with what is known as behavior modification. Through counseling sessions, the obese patients learned the whys, wheres and whens of their eating habits and instead of experiencing the usual up and down yo-yo syndrome, their weight stayed off.

The principles of behavior modification are:

- Description of behavior to be modified.
- Replacement with more desirable behavior.
- Development of techniques to control behavior.
- Positive reinforcement, or rewards.

These principles apply both to caloric intake and expenditure. The calories you expend, or your amount of activity, is as important as your diet. In fact, many obese people do not eat more than their non-obese counterparts; they are simply more sedentary.

The American Society for Clinical Nutrition recently called together a group of distinguished scientists and consultants. The purpose was to gather and present research regarding nutritionally caused illnesses. Obesity was ranked fifth in importance, because it was felt that physical inactivity (especially in children) contributed as much to obesity, if not more, than overeating. It is a vicious cycle: you are heavy because you are inactive, and inactive because you are heavy. However, the cycle can be broken if you are in reasonable good health and sincerely motivated.

Some people are naturally active; it's an easy matter to get them to exercise, as they are miserable when confined. Others have just the opposite inclination, and will look for any excuse to stay seated. These traits appear to be inborn. I heard a European doctor in a symposium on health and aging at the National Institutes of Health state that exercise should begin prenatally. Since the fetus gains fat cells during the last trimester of pregnancy, this may be important. Having been a fat baby is no excuse to throw in the towel now; you just have to make activity a habit, and empty out those cells.

Through the years I have heard all kinds of reasons for not exercising, and watched all kinds of phony exercise activity. You can stroll reading a novel, and tell yourself you have walked for an hour. You can wade and float and believe you are swimming. You can't do anything at all today because you are menstruating, or it's your birthday, or you have a headache, or a mosquito bite. The same excuses a sedentary person will have for **not** exercising will be used by an active person **TO** exercise. The sedentary person will blind herself to the difference in activity intensity, and wonder why Fate made her fat!

MOST IMPORTANT ARE AWARENESS AND MOTIVATION. Through being aware of what you are doing, and being motivated to change, you will succeed.

Motivation, like everything else that has to do with the human mind and body, is an individual matter. I have been reading lately that men are more successful at losing weight than women because maintaining health is their prime motivation, whereas women are more concerned about cosmetic benefits. Don't believe everything you read! One writer commented that this assertion was debatable, and I agree.

If men maintain a weight loss more easily than women, it is because of their physiology. They have a lower percentage of fat and a greater muscle mass to begin with. I have known too many men with hypertension who smoked and ate salty foods, to believe that men are more concerned about their health than women. Some men are even able to keep off weight they lost on the dangerous Atkins or Stillman diets. I have never known a woman who has not regained all of the lost weight and then some.

You lose weight for YOURSELF, not your husband, your doctor, your boss or your friends. In fact, other people in your life may, at one time or another, attempt to undermine your endeavor. Your husband may bring home candy, saying he loves you fat. You'll feel guilty when you throw it away, but that's what you'll have to do. Your "good" friends may inquire if you are sick, and the overweight ones will offer buffet luncheons. They have THEIR insecurities, but don't let them lay them on YOU.

To do good things for you, you must first place value on yourself. Make a list of the things you like about yourself. Make another one of your successes and achievements, even small ones. This may include awards and praise you have received, things you have done well, and times you looked especially good. Keep these where you can meditate upon them often. Whenever you hear a negative or self-derogatory inner monologue, replace it with a complimentary one. There is a tendency to dwell on our mistakes and failures. Don't! YOU ARE IMPORTANT! YOU ARE SUCCESSFUL!

Visualize yourself looking the way you would IDEALLY—**your** "ideal" figure, posture, clothing. Keep goals realistic, however, or you are doomed to failure and disappointment. If you are five-foot-two, you will never be a six foot ectomorph, but **you can become what is best for you.** When working towards your goal, take ONE DAY AT A TIME. Some days will be better than others. If you go off your diet one day, don't think you blew it, and give up. Start again the next day.

Goals should be flexible. They should be short and long term, and may have to be revised periodically. Remember, it took over forty years for you to get where you are!

If you have trouble visualizing yourself the way you want to be, try putting up an old, slimmer picture of yourself in strategic places: bathroom and bedroom mirror, the refrigerator. If you don't like your own picture, find bodies in magazines you admire, adding your own head. Hold the picture of the IDEAL YOU in your mind the last thing before falling asleep, and first thing upon arising. Gradually, your self image and your body will change.

Make another list, one showing all the reasons YOU want to lose weight. It may include increased energy, better health, a new job, prevention of diabetes, admiration of friends, strangers, men, or any other PERSONAL reason. Keep this list handy also, and refer to it when you get depressed or discouraged. It too, is subject to modification—add or subtract when the need arises. We all have times when we are down; it is part of the cycle of life. When this happens, instead of giving up, or reaching for a candy bar, do some kind of "fun" exercise. Exercise raises your blood sugar and is an upper. Go inside your head and fantasize. See yourself looking terrific, and doing some wonderful, crazy, thing!

Be aware that life's situations can either support or demoralize you. For instance, your own scale can show no weight loss, even though you have been dieting and exercising faithfully. There are reasons for this. You may be replacing fat with muscle, and muscle weighs more, but takes up less space. Unless you are trying to build muscle mass, your measurements will be smaller. The goal is to lose fat, not necessarily weight.

Another reason has to do with fluid retention. At times during your diet you will show no weight loss even though you are actually losing fat. This is a natural occurrence. I know of a woman who lost no weight for three weeks. On the fourth week she lost thirty pounds! Her doctor found nothing wrong; she had simply lost the water she had been retaining. Cut back, or eliminate the salt you use in cooking and on the table, and eat no foods that taste "salty." We get enough sodium naturally in the foods we eat. Even if you add no salt at all, you are probably getting between two to six grams of sodium per day, enough to meet your needs. Use a pepper mill with fresh peppercorns, and experiment with herbs. Once your taste buds adjust, you will find you are now really tasting food, and you will never go back to salting again.

Even with restricted sodium, our body fluid levels vary from day to day. For this reason it is better to weigh on a weekly basis when losing weight. Once you have reached your goal, daily weighing (at the same time each day) will help you keep it there.

The encouragement and support of family and friends is extremely helpful, and if they share your diet and exercise programs, ideal! However, this is not always the case. And just as you are not always aware of what you are doing, others may not be aware of the effect they have on you. For instance, men tend to feel they automatically know more about exercise than women. Your husband may be destroying his back and knees with the exercises he learned in the Army thirty years ago, yet laugh at your attempts to do a sit-up. I have known men to go behind locked doors to do my exercises, unwilling to admit to their wives that they can be both strenuous and beneficial.

You may have to do yours in private, although if a friend joins you it will be more fun. It may mean preparing two meals, one for your family, and one for yourself. This is unfortunate, because the whole family will benefit from less sugar, salt and fat. It helps to join a group such as Diet Workshop, as they will give you support, and help you work out a diet suited to your lifestyle. Eventually, you may find you no longer need a group, but in the beginning it can be helpful to have the encouragement of people with similar goals. Remember, YOU ARE WORTHWHILE, and you are doing this for YOU.

The feeling of being important connotes self-esteem and self-love. This doesn't mean you must be self-centered or lose perspective on the larger scheme of existence. When you respect yourself you are able to love others, and accept (and love) them without making conditions and demands. Your goals will be clearer and more easily achieved, because they are YOURS.

Sometimes we receive negative or hostile reactions to our lifestyle or appearance. Remember, others have problems we are not aware of, and they may be unconsciously venting frustrations on us.

One Saturday as I sat in the sun, my neighbor felt compelled to stop his car and shout angrily "How dare you sit while I have to work like a dog?" His outburst was so vitriolic, he was embarrassed. He has his problems about which I can do nothing, and I have no reason to feel guilty. Guilt leads to feelings of depression, worthlessness and failure. How do we react to these feelings? By eating! Don't burden yourself with feelings of guilt, if you decide to go off your diet on occasion. Accept your decision, enjoy, and go right back on your diet!

Being AWARE is part of being ALIVE, living in, and enjoying the Here And Now. My mother was an example of lack of Awareness. She seldom sat at the table to eat, but nibbled constantly while cooking, and was a garbage pail afterwards. She believed she would lose weight if she never ate bread, but of course, she didn't.

It's important to know when, why, and where we eat, what CUES trigger eating, and the caloric and nutritive values of food. Regarding the latter, the first step is to eliminate junk foods, as they are loaded with salt, sugar, fat and empty calories. "Junk Foods" have minimal nutritive value, containing less than 5% of the USRDA for protein, calcium, iron, vitamins A and C, and the B vitamins riboflavin, thiamin and niacin. There are many good calorie counters around. Two of the best, Handbook Number 8, and the Nutritive Value of Foods, are put out by the USDA, or, refer to the charts in this book.

You will find that some foods have nutritional value, but an inordinately high calorie count. Fast foods are an example, as they are extremely high in fat. Those snack packs filled with raisins, seeds and nuts are also nutritious, and may be good to eat on the trail in cold weather because they have high energy value, in other words, calories! Because of some of the fad diets that have been around, people have the misconception that it's carbohydrates that make them fat. Fat in all of its forms—margarine, vegetable oils, butter or chicken fat—has twice the number of calories as protein or carbohydrates. Although carbohydrates can cause fluid retention, they are a necessary part of our diet. I have a friend who thinks he is removing half of the calories in a Big Mac by taking off the top half of the roll. Wrong! The fattening goodies are right in the middle!

Before we become aware of what's happening between our hands and mouth, let's look at what's going on in our heads. Do you eat because you are hungry, or are you automatically responding to some external stimulus? Are you obsessively thinking about your favorite food, and then bingeing on it? Much of our lives is spent in our heads. We are remembering, projecting, imagining, worrying, hating, fearing and experiencing a host of other thoughts and emotions that may have little to do with reality. We tend to attract to us the things we fear the most and act out some of our internal scripts.

The first step is to get and keep your favorite foods out of the house. Don't kid yourself by thinking you are buying them for the kids. They're really for you, and if they're there you'll eat them. If food is inaccessible, you are less likely to go after it. That means there will be no more dishes of candy and nuts around, and no cheesecake in the front of the refrigerator. If it's not there, you won't worry all day about it going to waste if you don't eat it.

ACTIVITIES AND DISTRACTIONS THAT CAUSE OVEREATING

A. Situations at home:
1. Preparing meals
2. Clearing the table
3. Eating leftovers from other's plates
4. Snacks with children, or when they return from school
5. Snacks and drinks before dinner
6. Watching TV

B. Situations away from home:
1. Coffee break
2. Cocktail at lunch
3. Movies
4. Shopping
5. Restaurants

C. Emotional feeling occurring in conjunction with overeating:
1. Anxiety
2. Anger
3. Sadness
4. Loneliness
5. Fatigue
6. Boredom

The next step is to replace food fantasies with others even more pleasant. Saying "I won't think about food" doesn't work. Obviously, you are thinking about it. Instead, when the thought of food enters your mind, dwell on something that gives even more pleasure. The brain is only able to concentrate on one thing at a time, and if the thought evokes a pleasant emotion, we are likely to want to continue thinking it. I return often to a little lake, apple blossoms, a favorite person. In fact, even when I am truly hungry while hiking in the mountains, I can forget about it while I lose myself in the natural beauty of the surroundings.

When I am tired, I tend to respond by eating. Hunger is the false message that is reaching my brain. It's smarter to go to bed or take even a brief nap. You are seldom hungry when you first awaken; and you needed rest, not food, in any case. Depression, anxiety, anger and other emotions also trigger eating responses. My response to these emotions is being unable to eat, and often I will lose weight quickly. However, when I start eating again the weight returns immediately, as it always does with any weight loss that is too rapid.

The most accurate way to find out about your eating habits is to keep a record. It must be accurate, because if you are false you will learn nothing, and you will be cheating only yourself. Everything that goes in your mouth must be written on your chart, even snacks, nibbles and tastes. Your chart will show the following:

- Food (And Amount): A scale is important. There is a huge caloric difference between one ounce and three ounces. Be accurate.
- Eating Time: Many obese people eat so fast that they barely taste their

food. The food is not properly masticated, and the brain has not had time to register "full" before large amounts of food have been ingested. These habits contribute to a faulty "appestat," that control in the pituitary that says you've eaten enough!

- Calories: Record the caloric values as shown in your book, and become familiar with the number of calories found in your favorite foods.
- Location: Where did you eat, kitchen, bedroom, car, den, patio or in between.
- Social Conditions: Were you at home, at work, or in a restaurant? Were you with a friend, or alone, or whatever?
- Time: Twelve noon or midnight? Write it down!
- Feelings: Were you happy, depressed, bored, angry, anxious, or neutral? Get in touch with your feelings, and write them down.

EATING BEHAVIOR CHART	

Eating Time
  began
  ended	

Food (and amount consumed)	
Calories	
Eating location and social condition	
Time of day	
Feeling	
Comments and alternate behavior	

Save room on your chart for any comments you may wish to make, and if an alternate behavior comes to mind, write that in.

You have scrupulously written it down, it's there in black and white, so you can't say "But I only ate a bite of cottage cheese all day, and I can't understand why I don't lose weight!"

Now that you have taken a hard look at your behavior, see how it can be changed. Remember, habits were learned. They can be unlearned and replaced by others!

Perhaps you learned from your chart that you ran to the refrigerator during TV commercials. Did you know that commercials are louder for this reason? What are some alternatives? First of all, don't waste your time with stupid, boring programs. Tube watching is also a habit that can be broken. You would be far better off reading an interesting book, or better yet, replacing a sedentary activity with an active one such as dancing, bowling, walking, tennis or swimming. Don't use fatigue as an excuse to keep you glued to your chair. Unless you are tired from an activity such as digging ditches all day, the exercise will give you energy, and you will have fun. A less active alternative to television would be a concert, movie, art show, theater, or other group program. If there is no one to accompany you, go alone. You will soon enjoy the feeling of independence.

What to do when you choose to stay home with the tube? You can have your mending with you, or your correspondence. You can be working on a picture or a poem, or glance through the paper during commercials. You can do chair exercises, standing stretches, barre exercises, or even jog in place.

Give yourself a manicure or a pedicure, or work on zone therapy. Instead of eating while watching television, you can do many of the little things you didn't get to during the day. The commercial can be a stimulus to sew the hole in your sweater instead of filling the hole in your face! Your new behavior will be reinforced by repetition and will become a habit.

Mealtime can be a problem that can be resolved by careful planning and awareness. It helps to plan your meals a week in advance so that you don't throw in a lot of extras to compensate for a poorly planned meal. Never shop when you are hungry, always have a list, and make sure it includes the necessary condiments such as lemons, yogurt or herbs. If possible, buy only the amounts you need, which may mean having the butcher prepare your meat or poultry for you. The FDA has finally officially agreed with nutritionists that the American diet is overloaded with salt, fat and sugar; so it would be a wise decision to make fewer trips to the butcher shop and more to the fish market. You will be cutting not only calories, but saturated fat and sodium as well. Don't be afraid to try fish with strange-sounding names. They may taste better than your usual flounder, be just as low-fat, and cost a lot less. Experimenting with new foods and recipes takes the boredom out of dieting as well.

You could be putting more on the table than should be eaten, and eating it because it is there. If you habitually get up from the dinner table "stuffed" you have eaten too much. If you are still hungry, you have not eaten enough and will start nibbling soon. If you feel satisfied at the end of a meal, good; if not quite satisfied, wait fifteen minutes and you will be.

There are several ways to eat less at meals. If you are on a diet plan that calls for 1,200 calories daily (such as Diet Workshop's), follow the recommended amounts and you will be within the ball park. You can eat a piece of fruit and an eight ounce glass of non-caloric liquid (coffee, tea, water, herb tea) twenty to thirty minutes before a meal, and this will take the edge off before you begin. My favorite beforemeal fill-up is a mixture of raw miller's bran, brewer's yeast and lecithin granules in juice or water. These foods are all high in phosphorus; so I am careful to balance my diet with calcium.

You can eat less at meals by cutting portions in half. If you are in the habit of taking seconds, don't. Get up from the table, remove and rinse your plate,

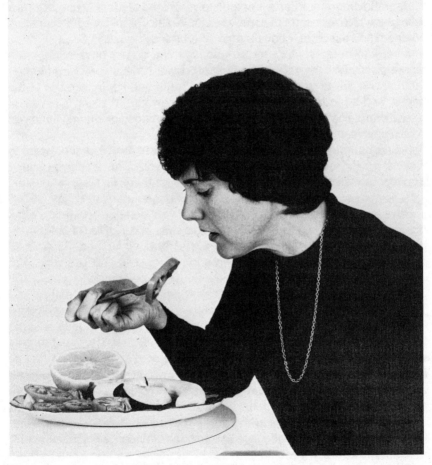

You can eat less at meals by cutting portions in half.

and don't sit back down. If you want to talk to others still eating, talk from the sink as you clean up, or bring something to occupy your hands, such as knitting, if you return to the table. Try sipping a cup of mint or other herb tea to give you that feeling of satisfaction.

If you feel deprived if you don't see a full plate in front of you, try using a smaller plate, and fill the spaces attractively with low calorie cucumber slices, parsley, celery, watercress, raw broccoli or cauliflower. Try eating your main course before your salad. The protein and fat it contains will cause your stomach to register full, and salad can be your dessert. Dressing should have no more than six calories per tablespoon.

Get leftovers off the table immediately. Wrap and store them, or throw them away. Never eat off of someone else's plate, or take his leftovers and put them on your plate. Food storage in your body equals FAT!

When the meal is over, get up and walk the dog or have some other planned activity. If the activity is pleasant you will be less likely to remember that cake in the back of the refrigerator. Better yet, keep cake out of the house, and let your family eat their sweets elsewhere. Walking is excellent after a meal. The fats you ate will be circulating instead of forming lumps on your hips and in your arteries.

Dining out may be one of the pleasures in your life. You don't want to eliminate it and feel sorry for yourself. What can you do to avoid overeating? You may be taking in extra calories; so allow for them. Eat less than usual for a day or two in advance, but don't go to the restaurant starving!

Have a cup of fill-up liquid before you go. If your companion wants a drink before dinner, have a glass of Perrier with a twist, a cup of tea or cofffee, or, as a treat, allow yourself one glass of dry wine with your meal. There's 75 calories in three ounces of dry wine such as chablis and sauterne, 125 calories in dessert wines, (i.e., port or sherry), 125 calories in a jigger of 100 proof whiskey, and 250 calories in a pina colada. They add up fast!

Know what the restaurant serves before you go. Many are now offering low calorie, nutritious "diet" foods as well as the usual fatty foods covered with sauce and gravy. Be assertive in ordering your meal. Many restaurants will gladly leave the gravy off the turkey or the corn starch out of Chinese food. If the bread appears before the meal, and that is a problem for you, ask them to remove it. Know that you can eat 1,000 calories at the salad bar alone if you load up on chick peas, salads filled with mayonnaise or whipped cream, and heavy dressings. Bring a small container of diet dressing, using it on the low calorie salad offerings like spinach, lettuce, celery, cucumbers, broccoli, or other raw vegetables.

Eat from your own plate only, put the fork down between each bite, and when you are satisfied, ask the waitress to remove the plates. You have control over food; so leave something on your plate. If it is sitting there tempting you, even though you know you have had enough to eat, pour salt or pepper over it. Repulsive!

Don't kid yourself by thinking that if your food is low-or reduced-calorie you can eat all you want. It is just as easy to get fat eating a lot of low calorie foods as it is by eating a little high calorie food. It just takes a little longer. In any case, never eat the whole thing, even if it is a head of lettuce. You can say you'll eat the goodie tonight and eliminate a corresponding number of calories tomorrow, but are you really going to want to live on 600 calories when the new day dawns?

So what to do instead of dessert? Coffee (or tea) and conversation. I like mint "tea." Bring your own to a restaurant. It's easier, of course, if your dining companion also forgoes dessert. If not, perhaps he could convince you it really is a little stale, and you are not going to eat from his plate to find out!

Parties may be a problem. If you are hostess, you can include raw vegetables and a dip made of yogurt and herbs or low calorie dressing along with other foods, and you stick with these. Don't even fix your favorites! If you are a guest, and there is one thing you really love, don't try everything else first, because you're going to get to what you like eventually. Instead take a small amount so you don't feel deprived, eat SLOWLY, and keep mingling.

What about ball games and movies where you always ate popcorn, candy, and hot dogs, and where everyone else **still** eats popcorn, candy and hot dogs? The ideal behavior change is to eat in one place only, ALWAYS. This would most likely be your kitchen or dining room. If you stick to this principle it will eliminate all the in-between and other place eating you do. If you decide you ARE going to eat at the movies, don't be the victim of the candy stand. First, you're not going in hungry. Secondly, you will decide in advance what you will eat. It may be a low calorie snack such as a peach or even sugarless mints or gum. If you choose popcorn, eat it without butter or salt. You may eat only half your dinner and bring the other half with you. Pace yourself, so that your allotted snack lasts through the whole movie.

What about coffee breaks? Eat a piece of fruit, or better yet, go into the lounge and do some standing exercises. Have a piece of fruit and low-fat cheese for lunch, and walk or exercise on your lunch hour.

All of these things are easier with a little help from your friends. If they join in your program, so much the better. If not, ask them to refrain from eating fattening foods in front of you. It helps if they compliment you on your good behavior and new appearance. Ask them for encouragement when your motivation wanes, and it may when your diet has been strict, but your weight loss nil. Remember that setbacks are only temporary, and keep going. Don't even weigh yourself if you feel heavy on a particular day; wait until you feel thinner; the chances are you will be.

What happens when you crave something sweet? Eat a piece of fruit! If you eat candy you will be temporarily raising your blood sugar, only to have it drop lower than it was before. Along with the drop in blood sugar comes a drop in energy, so you reach for another sweet. Certain B vitamins are burned in the metabolism of sugar, again contributing to a lack of energy. Even soft drinks have about a teaspoon of sugar per ounce. That, added to all the sugar found in almost everything we consume, adds up to produce a nation of sugar junkies, suffering from obesity, fatigue and depression.

What about snacks? Snacks are fine, provided you are not snacking all day. Whether you eat three regular meals a day or five small ones depends on your preference and lifestyle. There is evidence that the body utilizes more calories when the meals are small, and that the excess from one large meal will be stored as fat. I find this works well for me; I seldom eat a lot at one time and am not overly hungry for the next meal.

When eating snacks, be aware of foods you have already eaten and those you will eat later in the day. Your snack could consist of a low calorie liquid, a piece of fruit and skim milk cheese. All of the raw vegetables are good for snacking, as are a few whole wheat or rye crackers with a glass of skim milk. Try plain yogurt or low fat cottage cheese with fresh fruit sprinkled with raw wheat germ, or instead of the fruit, unsweetened apple butter. You may have your sugarless cereal as a mid-afternoon snack instead of for breakfast. Raw sunflower seeds and fresh nuts in the shell are nutritious but loaded with calories because of the fat content. Remember, just because it's good for you does not mean it is not fattening!

Eating before going to bed is another "fat habit." In fact, many never stop eating from dinner until bedtime. That momentum needs to be halted!

One way of avoiding actual hunger in the evening is to make sure you eat enough during the day. This means eating breakfast and lunch. If you save all of your calories for the evening, you will store as fat what you don't use.

Most people don't eat out of hunger, but out of habit. You can postpone your dinner hour so there is less time to be tempted afterwards, acknowledge the habit, and substitute some of the other activities we mentioned.

Suppose you ate a light dinner at six, and by eleven you are actually hungry. A cup of herb tea or a glass of skim milk is all that is needed to keep your stomach from digesting itself during the night. You DO NOT need a piece of cake or bread to go with it! That habit is well broken at any time of day! Another way to discourage further eating in the evening is to do your evening dental routine, such as brushing, flossing, or waterpicking right after dinner. You won't want to do it all over again, which you must if you continue to eat. Make dinner a pleasant ritual, one with a beginning and an end, and spend the rest of the evening enjoying other activities.

We have looked at behavior changes regarding eating. You have kept a record, and are AWARE of habits that contributed to your weight problem. You should realize how much you are eating, how fast, and what feelings make you want to eat. You may, by now, have substituted alternate behavior and begun to see a weight loss.

Reinforce your new patterns by rewarding yourself. Rewarding begins in the mind. Simply feeling good about your choices and taking control over your life is the big first step. You may be starting to enjoy the way you look and feel, and the way others are looking at you. Don't forget your own importance, and the fact that what you are doing is for yourself. Keep up your positive fantasies and inner monologues, even during periods of feeling down. Stick with your supportive friends, and stay away from the others, for now.

Reward yourself by giving yourself time to do something you really enjoy. That could be going to the theater, or taking a walk alone. It could mean taking a sunbath, or leaving the phone off the hook, so you can watch your favorite program. Treat yourself to a new outfit or makeup; but if money is a problem, keep your expenditure low, as extravagance can lead to guilt, and guilt is an emotion that can lead to overeating. If you can't handle it, don't do what makes you feel guilty. If you choose to do it anyway, forget the guilt, and enjoy! You'll do better next time. Rewards can cost nothing, but be worth everything! Concerts, art, nature, or even your favorite record can fill your senses far more than food can ever do.

Just as eating can become a habit, or compulsion, so can exercising. I've heard women complain that their husbands were compulsive exercisers, yet those same women were compulsive eaters. Guess who looked and felt the best? Complusion may be too strong; let's just say GET INTO THE HABIT OF MOVING. How you do it is up to you. You could put on disco or rock music and clean the house to a brisk beat (sneaking in a few dance steps). Walk up and down the stairs at work if it's only a few flights—walk to the store—clean the kitchen while you talk on the phone—go up and down stairs instead of asking the kids to go for you—make many trips—carry your own groceries—join a club or a class—form a group and exercise in your home—use your scale to do exercises with a light weight, or your towel. When you can, stand instead of sitting. When you can, walk instead of standing. When you can, run instead of walking.

Do not sprint to the corner if your only other exercise has been a walk to the refrigerator. Gradually change your way of thinking and acting so that you don't experience unnecessary fatigue or injury. You will find that energy begets energy, and your body will tell you to do more, not less. Your mind and body need time to adapt to the new, more active person you've become. Once the adaptation is made, you will never want to go back to your old habits.

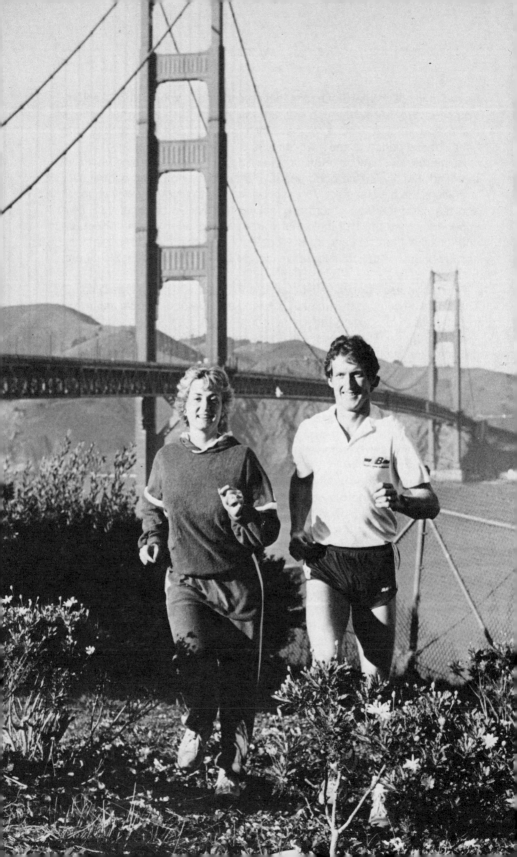

4
BE FIT, STAY FIT: EXERCISE!

Exercise! Does the word dredge up horrible memories of dreaded gym classes? Of being forced to play baseball, and other types of torture? Forget all that. There's hope for the most confirmed sitter: read on.

I hated gym, especially during my early teens. I had chronic tonsilitis, and undiagnosed illnesses, such as rheumatic fever, that kept me weak for years, and I especially hated baseball, probably because I was never very good at it. Today we recognize that that particular sport, although requiring skill, is virtually worthless as far as fitness is concerned. Furthermore, it is not a lifetime activity, the kind we like to promote in young people today.

Fortunately, there were other things going for me. I have always been "naturally" active, preferring moving to sitting; our family recreation was walking and hiking, things I still love to do and have since expanded into running.

If it makes you feel more motivated, replace the word "exercise" with one like "activity" everytime you see or use it. We cannot escape the fact that our bodies were intended to move, even at given intervals during sleep. Young healthy children are naturally active, and a total lack of movement is a condition known as "death." We all fall into the broad range in between, perhaps closer to one end of the spectrum than the other.

Most of us no longer live and work on farms, and many things we once did by hand are now done by machines. We live like rats in cages, trapped in our houses, cars, offices and in front of our television sets. It amazes me to see how people adapt to this kind of life. Many live entirely "in their heads," and have no awareness of the rest of their bodies.

Physical activity can prevent and cure hypokinetic diseases. It improves the quality and perhaps the quantity of life. It will add life to your years, or in other words, help you to be alive as long as you live—certainly, a worthwhile goal! What kinds of diseases do we refer to as "hypokinetic?" Some that fall into this category are coronary artery disease, hypertension, obesity, anxiety and depression, and musculoskeletal diseases and disability.

Recently a new phenomenon has been observed. Many sedentary office workers are in better condition than their counterparts working in construction or other active fields. It seems that white collar workers are making a conscious effort to get in shape, jogging being one of the most popular. Many corporations are offering exercise classes at noon, exercise equipment, and shower facilities. People who are active on their jobs often don't feel like running when they come home, even though their work may not provide the kind of activity that is beneficial.

Just what does exercise do that is helpful? We are looking at the benefits of exercise as it effects our strength, endurance, flexibility, balance and coordination. These are all attributes that decline naturally as we age; yet much deterioration we see in older people is due not only to aging and disease, but to inactivity. These same symptoms can be produced in young people if they are bedridden or extremely inactive. The old tale about using it or losing it is truer than ever.

What are some of the benefits of exercise? First let's look at some of the "symptoms of aging" that are amenable to exercise. Depression, aches and pains in the muscles and joints, osteoporosis, fatigue, loss of coordination and balance, even sexual disinterest are all conditions that **may** be corrected by exercise. As far as I am concerned, I refuse to consider any of these as normal until I have done all that is possible to prevent and/or correct them. I absolutely refuse to age gracefully, and will fight it all the way down the line!

Even if you haven't experienced any of the above "symptoms," exercise is beneficial in numerous ways. First of all, you will gain confidence by knowing that you have taken your life into your own hands by doing something that is not only good for you but is pleasurable.

Women who are divorced or widowed at our age especially need this, but so do married women who may find themselves fat, passive and unfulfilled because they have taken a secondary role for years. Running that first mile can truly be a milestone and bring a great deal of pride and gratification. I might inject a word of caution here. Husbands and marriages may be threatened by a wife who attempts to shed a passive-submissive role. Men can be easily intimidated, especially in the area of fitness. They may admire svelte figures on other women, but a wife who can outrun them can damage a macho image. If your husband is "old fashioned" and falls into this category, it may be difficult or impossible for him to change. It appears to be less marriage-threatening for a husband to take up a sport that brings him pleasure and fitness than for his wife to do so. That old kitchen-church-and-

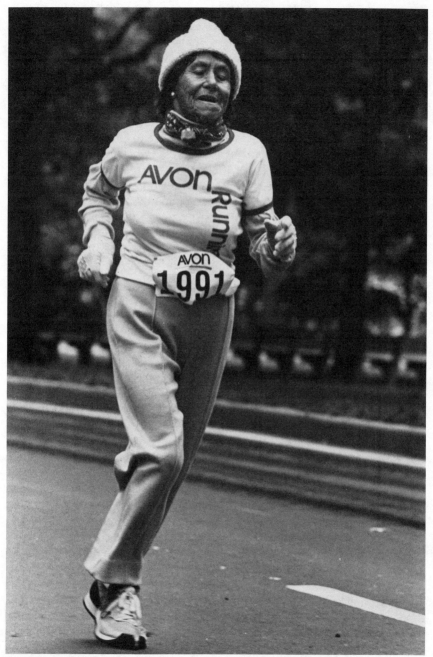

Physical exercise improves the quality and perhaps the quantity of life.

children mentality still abounds; believe me, I have seen it! Even in the areas of diet, many husbands will bring home "treats" of cakes and candy to wives who are seriously trying to lose weight. And they do a real guilt-trip number on them if they don't eat it!

Ideally, couples will find a recreational sport to do together. Fast dancing is fun, but to be effective you must dance at least two or three times a week. Once a month won't do. Second choice would be for the wife to exercise on her own or with a group, and for her husband to promote and encourage her. If this is difficult or impossible for him, she will have to go out on her own with or without his knowledge or consent. If she is also working, and her exercise time is after work or in the evening, this may pose a real problem. If she truly wants to do something for herself, it is in this situation that she will have to make choices and decisions. If the lines of communication are open, her needs can be discussed and the situation resolved so that neither husband nor wife ends up feeling a "victim."

Unfortunately, some couples lose or never had the ability to speak openly with each other, or to reveal their true needs and feelings. Many find counseling helpful, but it is most often the husband who refuses to go, preferring the status-quo. It is at this point that a woman can be faced with the decision of seeing herself as a "person" and perhaps breaking up her marriage; remaining the way she is; or changing, and inviting dissention. Often, if the change is gradual it is more acceptable and less threatening. Choices or changes are never easy.

Look at your life and assess how happy and healthy you are the way it is. Don't overlook the possibility that your husband may be happier if you get in condition so that you can join him in some of his favorite sports! You may find that your marriage is better, not worse, when you take control of your own life.

There is an unfortunate tendency in our society to be overly competitive. Competition can cause a spouse or friend to feel inadequate, the competitor to train to the point of injury, and a beginner to feel frustrated and quit. You are not competing with anyone but yourself, and don't be overly challenging there, either! Trying to squeeze out an extra mile may lead to an injury that can cause you to give up running (or any other sport) altogether.

Exercising to the point of pleasure is the rule, especially for people who are untrained and over forty. If you feel unhappy because you are not doing as well as your neighbor, you will be undoing all of the good psychological benefits that can be derived just from doing something more than you were doing! For this reason it may be well to exercise alone in the beginning, until you feel comfortable with your achievements and with yourself.

Psychological benefits from exercise include an immediate feeling of relaxation or stimulation. There is usually a sense of well-being and a relief from depression, which may or may not be permanent. There is no question about the fact that exercise is addictive, both psychologically and psychologically. Most authorities consider the addiction "positive"; however, many agree that it becomes "negative" when you exercise to the point of damaging your health, or losing your job and family. It all boils down to using good sense. I am a firm believer in the ancient Greek's "Golden Mean."

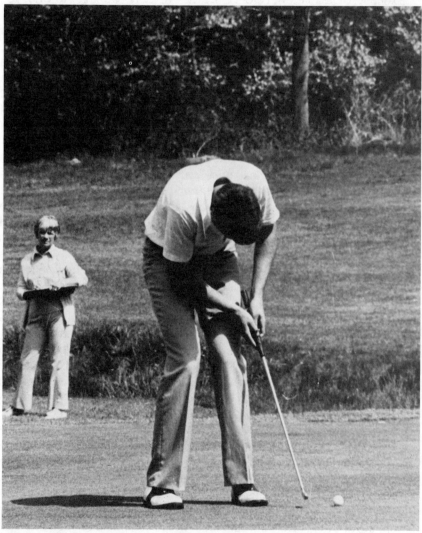

Ideally, a couple will find a recreational sport to do together.

Exercise also helps in very direct ways to relieve some of the ravages of stress. Not only do you release emotional tensions through the use of large muscle masses, but aerobic exercise has a direct effect on the heart itself by removing excess adrenalin which may be deposited there as a result of tension. Exercise can help you to relax and see problems from a new perspective, resulting in a more positive attitude towards your work and life in general.

Exercise DOES HELP YOU TO LOSE WEIGHT! Contrary to what you may have been told, exercise will not increase your appetite. In fact, it usually has the other effect, especially if it is vigorous enough before a meal. It is difficult to lose weight through diet alone and still get enough nutrients. Exercise, like calories, is cumulative. If you expend an extra 100 calories a day and do not change your diet in any way, in 35 days you will have lost one pound of fat. That does not sound like much, but it adds up to about 10 pounds a year. It is at that insidious rate that many women put on weight. Of course, the ideal way to lose weight is to cut down on your caloric intake at the same time you increase your energy expenditure.

Exercise does more than just use a given number of calories for a given activity. Strenuous exercise can raise your basal metabolic rate anywhere from 4 to 24 hours. This means that you will be burning more calories, even at rest. Furthermore, as you replace your fat with lean muscle, you will also be utilizing more calories at rest, as muscle has a higher BMR (Basal Metabolic Rate) than fat, which is relatively inert. The main reason we gain weight as we get older is because our basal metabolic rate slows down. This is due in part to our more sedentary lifestyle, and because muscle loss is part of the aging process. The muscle that is lost is being replaced by fat, which means that we are going to have to eat less just to maintain the status quo. It is far preferable to replace some of that lost muscle through exercise using light resistance. Muscles use fat for energy; fat we don't need.

Exercise has other, unexpected health benefits. It can help normalize your glucose tolerance, and is especially useful in adult-onset diabetes. If you have hypoglycemia or diabetes, you will need to include diet as part of your treatment, and consult with your doctor before exercising. If you are on insulin, you may find that your medication needs to be adjusted once an exercise program is begun.

Exercise may make childbirth and recovery easier. Pass this information on to your daughter, but again, have her check with her doctor. It is to be hoped that she will have a doctor who is informed and interested in exercise.

Proper exercise reduces the frquency of low back pain. It aids in the digestion, absorption and utilization of food. It is a cure for constipation, and lowers the uric acid levels in your blood, which contribute to gout. Exercise lessens the chance of blood cotting, thus reducing your risk of having phlebitis, stroke or heart attack. Through regular exercise, you will find that all your tasks are easier, and it will take you longer to become breathless upon exertion. Exercise improves your neuromuscular coordination. This has a direct effect on your self confidence!

AEROBICS

What does the word "aerobic" mean? How are we benefited by aerobic exercise? Literally, aerobic means "with oxygen." During exercise, oxygen intake is increased, allowing more to be available to the working muscles. Eventually, through aerobic training, the cardiovascular system becomes more efficient, so that the muscles require less oxygen to perform the same task. Bicycling, running, swimming, fast dancing, racquetball, fast singles tennis (if there is continuous movement) and cross-country skiing are all aerobic activities.

To get aerobic benefits, or an aerobic training effect, one must continue the activity for a minimum of 12 to 20 minutes, 3 or 4 times a week, at 60 to 80 percent of your maximum heart rate, beginners working at the lower heart rate. Remember, increase gradually! Before we learn how to go about this, let's look at some of the changes that take place with aerobic conditioning.

First, there are changes in the heart itself, relieving the risk of heart disease and increasing the chance of recovery if you do have a heart attack. One of the reasons for this is that active people have corollary arteries in the heart which can be called into use if a main artery is damaged. In sedentary people, these arteries are entirely closed.

The heart becomes stronger and somewhat larger like any other muscle that is exercised, enabling it to have a larger capacity and stroke volume. With training, the heart does not have to beat as frequently, resulting in a lower heart rate at rest. Activities that once were difficult now come easily. Exercise lowers blood pressure, and coupled with other measures such as sodium restriction, relaxation and weight control, **may** eliminate the need for medication for hypertension.

As the heart becomes more efficient it pumps more fuel and oxygen to the working muscles, allowing them to reach higher levels of performance. Changes in the blood lipids take place. Triglyceride levels are reduced, and beneficial high density lipoproteins that remove excess fat from the body are increased. There is evidence that exercise slows the aging process. You may see an immediate improvement in the color and clarity of your skin.

Aerobic exercise is the most beneficial for weight control. If you want to lose weight, it is better to exercise at a lower heart rate for a longer period of time, than at a higher intensity (jumping rope, for instance) for less time. The heart works very hard during rope jumping, at a level that cannot be maintained. Jumping rope also puts a great deal of stress on the joints, especially the knees. I do not recommend it for anyone who is obese, or has joint disease. If you do choose jumping rope as your aerobic activity, jump slowly, wear cushioned shoes, jump on a soft surface, and intersperse intervals of brisk walking with jumping.

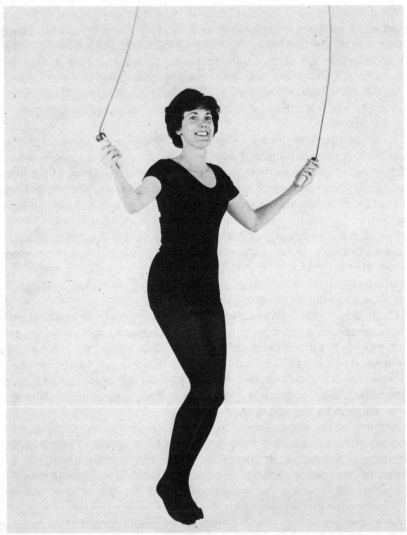

Through aerobic training, your cardiovascular system becomes more efficient, so that your muscles require less oxygen to perform the same task.

There may be a period of two or more weeks before you see a training effect from aerobic exercise. You will know, because you will have to work harder to bring your heart rate up to "training." The nervous system, however, responds immediately to exercise, making the second time you exercise (assuming there is not a long time span in between) easier than the first, as indicated by a reduction in the secretion of norinepinepherin in response to the stress of exercise.

If you are fortunate enough to have a sports medicine clinic near you, get tested on a treadmill and have your training heart rate established according to your oxygen intake. In any case, it is important to check with your doctor before you begin, especially if you have been sedentary, a smoker, overweight, not in "perfect" health, and there is a family history of heart disease.

Let's take a look at what your exercise heart rate should be, according to your age and ability. Beginners and older people are benefited by a heart rate of 120 beats per minute. You may keep your training at that level for 20-30 minutes per session. If you are a beginner, then choose aerobic activities such as brisk walking, **slow jogging,** gardening, cycling, golfing on a hilly course (no cart), dancing, skating, doubles tennis or badminton. Begin with at least 10 minutes or so, and work up to an hour. You may take your pulse for 6 seconds, and multiply by 10 (add a zero to the figure you get) or 10 seconds and multiply by 6. The better condition you are in, the faster your heart rate returns to normal. For this reason it is necessary to take your pulse immediately after exercising, and not wait a minute or two, as there will be a large error. **Do not stop and stand while you take your pulse: KEEP MOVING.** Use a watch with a sweep second hand, or a digital that reads out the seconds. If you use a second hand, start when it reaches a numeral, and say "zero." Practice finding your heart rate by taking your pulse after climbing a flight of stairs, or jogging easily for a minute.

Locate your pulse in the carotid artery in the neck by feeling for it directly beneath your chin or in the identation between the muscle at the side of your neck and the front of your throat. **Press lightly, on one side only.** Never take your pulse with your thumb, as you will get a double reading. After exercising, the carotid pulse is throbbing and easy to find. There is some question, however, that the count may not be entirely accurate, as pressure on this artery tends to slow it down. For this reason, one must press gently. If you prefer, or if you have any problems with your heart, count your heart rate in the radial artery beneath your thumb. To do this, wear your watch on the underside of your wrist so that you may see it easily as you count. Spread apart the thumb of your right hand so that there is a wide notch between thumb and forefinger. Place the inside of the wrist of your left hand in this notch, and reach the first two fingers of the right hand around the wrist of the left hand so they are resting gently beneath the thumb of the left hand, where you will feel your pulse.

Your resting heart rate is an indication of general fitness; usually it will be between 60 and 90 for women. As a rule, well conditioned people have a slower pulse, this being one of the benefits one gets from training. However, some medications also slow the heart, and an older person with a very low pulse may be suffering from cardiac disease.

Find your true resting heart rate by taking your pulse for a full minute immediately after arising. For your own interest, take it at several other "resting" times during the day, and note how it changes. Caffein and cigarettes will speed up your heart, as will stress, activity, and food allergies. Eliminate these factors when taking your pulse.

Once you "know your body," counting your pulse will no longer be necessary, as you will be able to tell how rapidly your heart is beating by the way you feel. For instance, if you perceive that you are barely exerting yourself, your pulse will probably be under 90. Very light exertion will produce a rate around 90, and light will make it about 100. A little more exertion will raise your pulse to 110, and moderate will be about 120. Heavier will be 130, heavy 140, very heavy 150, and extremely heavy 160. Most women our age should not elevate the heart rate to that extreme, although it may happen — especially if you are overweight and out of condition. This is why it is important for a beginner to take a reading immediately after exercising to determine the exercise heart rate; at rest, to get an indication of your general condition; and 5 and 15 minutes after exercising to see how quickly you recover (another indication of fitness). If your pulse is not **close** to normal 15 minutes after exercising, you have worked too hard.

How can one determine what the exercise heart rate should be? There are sophisticated methods involving your resting heart rate or the stress test we mentioned, but the simplest is the formula:

220-your age = maximum heart rate. NEVER EXERCISE AT THIS LEVEL! For beginners, 60% of this figure will provide excellent training. Use it for 6 weeks. After that, 70% for another 6 weeks or longer. 80% is for those who are well trained; however, many do not like to exceed 75% of their maximum heart rate, which is fine. At any level, the heart rate will not be the same every day. There will be days you will feel like flying, and other days you will barely be able to move. Listen to your body. If you are running, be able to carry on a conversation and still smile. Here are figures to follow if you are a beginner:

AGE	LOWER LIMIT		UPPER LIMIT	# OF BEATS IN 10 SECONDS
41-50	approx. 96	to	126 beats/min.	approx. 16-21
51-60	approx. 90	to	114 beats/min.	approx. 15-19

For those over 60, an increase of approximately 20 beats over the resting heart rate will bring about a training effect. Beginners should keep the exercise rate around 100, not exceeding 110 beats per minute. Work up gadually to 120-125 taking as long as you need to do so comfortably.

If you are already actively exercising routinely two to four times a week, you may start at a higher level. Your activities could be singles tennis or badminton, basketball or raquetball, jogging, cross-country skiing, and mountain trail hiking.

Heart rates based on a 10 second count for **trained** women are:

AGE	LOWER LIMIT		UPPER LIMIT	# OF BEATS IN 10 SECONDS
41-50	approx. 120	to	150 beats/min.	approx. 20-25
51-60	approx. 108	to	138 beats/min.	approx. 18-23

If you are over 60, do not exceed 120 unless you are already well conditioned. Remember, the above figures are for those who have exercised 3 to 5 times per week for 6 weeks at a lower level. No matter what your degree of fitness, if you can't talk while exercising, you are pushing too hard! On the other hand, if your pulse indicates you are not at a training level, then work a little harder. A slow stroll may be romantic after dinner, but it has no exercise value.

Here are some general rules for everyone to follow, no matter what her abilities:

- **Begin slowly.** Sudden bursts of exercise after years of inactivity can result in injured joints and muscles, severely sore muscles, and discouragement.
- Be able to talk. If you are alone, talk or sing to yourself.
- Although a certain amount of breathlessness indicates you are exercising, loud wheezing means you are pushing to hard.
- Get the correct shoes. They are your most important piece of equipment. Don't wear tennis shoes for jogging. To protect your joints, make certain the heel is well protected, the sole cushioned, and there is space in the toe for the foot to expand as you exercise.
- Use common sense regarding the weather. Exercise in the coolest time of day in the summer, the warmest in the winter, and dress accordingly in removable layers. Drink plenty of fluids especially in warm weather. It's o.k. to drink while you are exercising, as long as the drink is not icy cold and you don't overload. In summer, wear as little as possible, and a hat that is ventilated if you are in the sun. In the winter, especially if you are jogging, wear several light layers that can be removed and tied around your waist. If you finish with a walk, you will

probably want to put them back on again. Exercising in winter (especially shoveling snow) increases your risk of heart attack. Wearing a face mask is one precaution, and avoiding excess fatigue is another.

- Don't get challenged into being overly competitive. I emphasize this many times; even competing with yourself can be dangerous! Push yourself to the point of training, not straining, a place that is different for everyone, and varies from day to day. The pulse is a good indicator until you get used to reading your own body signals.

- It's a good idea, especially if untrained and/or overweight, to alternate bone-jarring activity days (tennis, jogging) with days that put less stress on the joints. Your "off" days could include swimming, bicycling, or walking. Some sports medicine experts suggest taking two aspirin before or after sports that stress your joints. Taking aspirin before exercising in hot weather can cause serious side-effects; so it would be wise to take it after, if your joints hurt. Also, alternate "hard" days with "easy" days, as it can take up to 48 hours for your muscles to recover from a strenuous workout. There was a time in my life when I was teaching (and doing) four or more strenuous exercise classes every day. My muscles hurt all the time, and I was constantly in a state of heavy fatigue. I finally became ill, and never returned to this type of health-destroying regimen again.

- Do something every day, even on your light days, as it is easier to stick to a routine. Weather can be a deterrent; so here are some fun activities to do at home:

AEROBICS EXERCISES

Walking, especially for beginners. If you live in an apartment building, walk up and down the halls, and intersperse that with a flight or two of stairs. It's more fun if you do it with a friend or group. Many of the older people in my classes do this on days the weather keeps them indoors. Sometimes they walk and talk for hours, making it into a pleasurable social event. **Remember, walk briskly, swinging your arms freely!** Do the same if you live in a house, going up and down the stairs. Try to keep moving for a half hour.

If you are a runner, jog around your house, again, adding the stairs. Remember, your heart rate will increase going upstairs, and drop going down, so keep your level of fitness in mind. You may want to run in place in front of the TV, or buy one of those trampoline-like joggers, that take some of the stress off your joints. Cool down with a walk, and finish with stretching the back, hamstring, calf and thigh muscles.

When you lift your body weight against gravity, your heart works harder, making activities such as stair climbing, jumping and jumping rope difficult. **Jumping routines are not for beginners.** Keep in mind that THE HIGHER YOU JUMP, THE HARDER YOU WORK. Try the following routines, changing movements frequently and stopping to walk when you get tired. Begin with 3-5 minutes, working up to a total of 12 minutes jumping, and 20 or more minutes walking. Put on some lively music and:

- Jump lightly forwards, backwards, and to the sides.
- Lift your left knee as high as you can as you hop on your right foot. Keep alternating feet.
- Hop on your left foot as you kick your right leg as high as you can to the side. Alternate legs.
- Hop 5 times on the right foot, 5 times on the left.
- Hop on your right foot as you kick your left leg as high as you can in front of you. Alternate legs, then try kicking your legs across your body, from left to right and right to left.
- Invent any of your own hopping and jumping movements.

Jump on a soft surface, such as a thick carpet, and wear tennis shoes that are well cushioned. Be sure to warm up with walking and slow jogging, and cool down in the same way, finishing with stretches. Running shoes are usually not good for this, as they are designed to move you forward, not to the side. In addition to aerobic benefits, such as weight control, these movements are superb for toning and strengthening the thighs and hips.

TIPS TO KEEP YOU MOVING AND MOTIVATED

The larger the muscle mass used, the greater the energy expenditure. This means activities involving the legs are more beneficial for weight control, especially when moving the body weight against gravity. Walking would be better than bicycling, unless you have joint problems.

Enjoy your exercise, do it on a regular basis, and increase the intensity so there is progression in training.

Make it convenient, and suitable to your lifestyle. Running on an indoor track at the Y is a good idea for bad weather, but not if it takes you two hours to get there.

Since we seem to be creatures of habit, set a special time for exercising. Of course, you will need to vary it according to weather and other commitments.

Allow an hour after eating before strenuous exercise.

Don't exercise when you are sick or injured; however, you don't need to let your whole body fall apart if one part is out of commission. If, for instance, you have a sprained ankle, you can still work all the other parts of your body. Swimming or bicycling in a chair would be a good aerobic activity.

If you are not a self-starter, join a group or exercise with a friend.

If one of your goals is reshaping your body, take measurements on a regular basis to reinforce this. You will not see any difference if you exercise only once a week. **You could get larger if you use heavy weights.**

Become educated. Read books, and attend lectures and discussions on exercise and other health related subjects.

Finally, if you miss a day or more because of illness or other good reasons, don't feel that you have become a jellied mass. It's true that once you are hooked into regular exercise, you will become restless and irritable when forced to discontinue, and you will be anxious to get back. If you stop for a week or more, especially if due to sickness, you will need to start at a lower level when resuming exercise. Don't panic! Most of the time the return to your former level of fitness is swift. Be aware that if you try to push yourself to your former level too quickly you could suffer injury or a relapse of your illness, both of which will knock you right out again.

I cannot stress enough that the human body was designed for movement, and that sedentary living contributes greatly to all kinds of physical deficiencies and abnormalities. If health is of no particular concern to you, then think of the way you look and feel. Exercise will relieve tension, give you increased energy and vitality, improve your posture and contribute to a more youthful appearance. All are excellent reasons to move!

The following summary of how different sports rate in promoting physical fitness was in **Medical Times**, May, 1976, (pp 65-72), written by Carson Conrad, Executive Director of the President's Council on Physical Fitness and Sports. To arrive at these ratings he asked 7 experts for their opinions. These authorities were: **Samuel Fox**, M.D., (Professor of Medicine, Cardiologist, Georgetown University); **Evelyn Gendel**, M.D., (Asst. Dir., Bureau of Maternal and Child Health, Kansas State); **Warren Child**, M.D., (Past President of the American College of Sports Medicine); **Theodore Klumpp**, M.D., (Medical Consultant to the President's Council on Physical Fitness and Sports); **Hans Kraus**, M.D., (Clinical Professor of Physical Medicine and Rehabilitation, N.Y.U. Medical School); **Lawrence Lamb**, M.D., (Cardiologist, former Professor of Medicine, Baylor Medical School); and **Allan Ryan**, M.D., (Professor of Physical Education and Rehabilitation Medicine, University of Wisconsin).

The sports and exercises were rated on a point system according to the various benefits of physical fitness. The criteria were: CARDIORESPIRATORY ENDURANCE (STAMINA), MUSCULAR ENDURANCE, MUSCULAR STRENGTH, FLEXIBILITY, and BALANCE. Under the heading of "General Well Being," the criteria were: WEIGHT CONTROL, MUSCLE DEFINITION,

DIGESTION, and SLEEP. Jogging received the most points. In descending order were: bicycling, swimming, skating (ice or roller), handball/squash, skiing-Nordic, skiing-Alpine, basketball, tennis, calisthenics, walking, golf, softball, and bowling. The golf ratings were based on the fact that most Americans use a golf cart. If a golfer walks, the values go up appreciably. The sports were rated on the basis of regularity, (a minimum of four times per week), and a duration of 30 minutes to 1 hour per session.

The article concluded with the following statement made by Dr. Guild:

"A minimum of 30 minutes, 4-5 times a week is ideal, and not unreasonable because minimal benefits toward endurance or stamina are "prompters" of cardiovascular reserve. There are 4 S's in sports: Speed, Skill, Strength, and Stamina. The first 3 are of importance to the young. The last (Stamina) adds to longevity, to vigor, to 'joie de vivre', to one's ability to do a day's work effectively, and yet to have enough pep left over to enjoy leisure time."

WALKING

This is one sport I cannot mention often enough, partly because it is one I have always especially enjoyed. We can walk almost anywhere and almost everyone can do it. Walking is especially good for those over forty and "out of shape." Some say walking is a science, others, an art. Actually, it can be

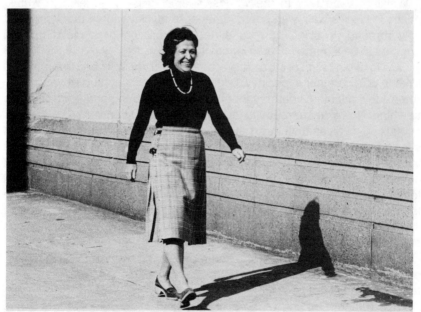

"Walking is an idea whose time has come."

either or both. According to C. Carson Conrad, executive director of the President's Physical Fitness and Sports, "Walking is an idea whose time has come."

It's truly a shame that we have to rediscover walking, for after all, it's what we were naturally intended to do. Our muscles stretch, turn and knead with every step, and cardiovascular fitness is promoted. Cardiologists refer to our legs as our "second hearts," and walking is most often recommended as a preventative and curative for heart disease. Certainly it is relaxing and an anti-depressant. You can walk to think, or not-think, and you can be blessedly away from your phone and other physical stressors. Walking improves your circulation, skin tone, mental abilities, and personality. Walking can help you lose weight (about 300 calories per hour), and reduce your hip measurements. (The adult hip width has been increasing an inch a generation since the advent of the automobile.)

Many famous people advocate walking as a way of life. President Harry Truman began because he had cardiovascular disease. Walking enabled him to live to the age of 88. Senator William Proxmire (D, WI) walks the 5 miles from his office to his home every day, and Justice Douglas walked the entire length of the C and O Canal, 180 miles. Henry David Thoreau was one of the most famous of American pedestrians; the poets Wordsworth and Shelley walked 14 miles a day or more, and Abraham Lincoln, for hours.

Walking, especially in the woods, seems to be conducive to writing poetry. I always walk with pen and paper to quickly record the words that flow through. Walking can be either tranquilizing or stimulating, and appears to be a prime factor in longevity.

How to begin? First of all, as in any other sport, you will need to warm up a little. In cold weather especially, begin a circulatory warm up slow-walking. After a few minutes, you may then do some stretching and bent-knee toe touching. Now you are ready to increase your pace, and WALK!

Walking involves rhythmic, natural, effortless movement. Walking is not strolling, waddling, or shuffling. Maintain correct posture so that your chest is lifted, head up, back neither arched nor rounded. The feet point straight ahead, not in or out, and you land on your whole foot, rocking from the heel to the balls of the foot. Don't walk on your toes, as this will cause pain in the feet, ankles and calves. Don't worry about your breathing. Your rate of respiration will increase naturally. If you wish, you may add specific yoga breathing exercises during a couple of minutes of your walk. To do so, exhale completely to the count of 6 (more or less) steps, hold the air OUT for one pace, then inhale completely to the count of 5 (more or less) paces. Try this only once at first, and increase to three breaths.

Walk without carrying purse or parcel, and allow your arms to swing freely. Relax your hip muscles, so there is a sensual swinging movement of the hips over the legs. This is far more relaxing to your lower back, and allows you effortlessly to lengthen your stride. Don't try to change your stride abnormally, as you waste energy and inhibit free movement. Look around you, and enjoy!

Like any other exercise, the more you do, the more efficient you become. You will soon be able to go faster and farther. Depending on your age and ability, eventually increase your pace to three and a half, or even four and a half miles an hour. Walking five miles is not an unreasonable goal; however, if you can't do it all at once, go for two, three, or more walks a day.

The one piece of equipment you will need is shoes. If you are just taking a short walk on your lunch hour, low or medium heels will do. But for serious walking the Footwear Council offers the following advice:

- Avoid high platforms, high heels, and flat sneakers. I have known several women who have fallen off high heels and broken bones. High heels throw off your center of gravity, put strain on your back, and weaken the muscles in the front of the body.
- There should be at least a quarter inch of room in the front of the shoe, and the toe-box high enough so there is no rubbing.
- Look for cushioned heels and soles, for bounce on hard surfaces and traction on slippery ones.
- For support, have a rigid shank between the heel and the ball of the foot, or a solid wedge.
- Get special "walking" shoes for long walks. These should tie snugly, but should not rub or irritate any part of the foot or heel. I have found that blisters occur in a direct reverse ratio to the cost of the shoe.

Walking should refresh and revive you. If you find you are overly fatigued, then you have gone too far for your current level of fitness. Like any other sport, pleasure is the key.

A final work about muscle cramps, or spasms, that can ruin any exercise. Some of the most common causes are unnatural use of under-exercised muscles or a deficiency in the electrolytes*, calcium or magnesium. Some people get cramps when they over stretch or contract a muscle.

We instinctively massage the area that's hurting. Exercise physiologist Dr. Herbert DeVries recommends a passive stretch to relieve the spasm, holding the stretch for at least 20 seconds. A technique I have seen work many times is to cup your hands over your mouth and nose, and breathe into your cupped hands. I am not sure why this works, other than the fact that it alters the blood chemistry. Now there is "acupinch" from China, which may be a practical joke, but I have seen it work, too. Take your upper lip between thumb and forefinger, and press hard for 20 to 30 seconds. The pain in your lip makes you forget the pain in your leg.

*water, sodium, chloride and potassium

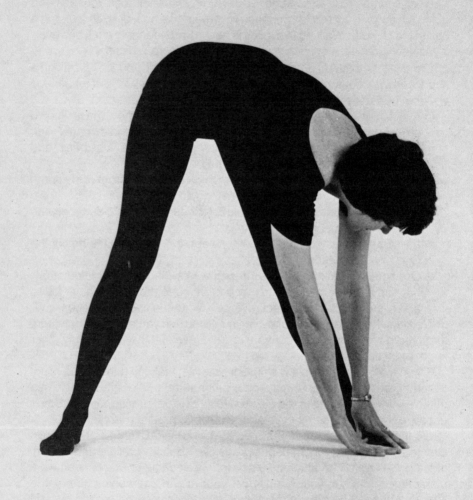

5
DYNAMOTION EXERCISES

The DYNAMOTION EXERCISE program consists of one hour of movement, at varying levels and paces. The same format can be used beginning with twenty minutes or even less, and increased according to your own progress.

Several elements apply to everyone. The first is body awareness. Awareness of what you are doing and feeling is important if you are to see results, and not inefficiently waste energy. I tell my students what muscles they are using, how to use them and how to "feel" the movement. Body awareness is extremely important in the maintenance of correct body alignment, or posture.

One way to get to know your body is to exercise nude in front of a mirror. Watch the muscles as they are working, and concentrate on them. You can even use imaginary weights to increase muscular strength.

Move continuously during the allotted time. Alternate the top half of the body with the bottom, and fast with slow. When you get tired, move at a slower pace. Walk, take some deep breaths and exhale hard, shake, stretch, or massage your muscles, but don't sit down or just stand. Keep moving!

Allow time for warming up, the main body of exercise which should bring your heart rate up to at least 120, and a cool down. Warm-ups consist of circulatory exercises done while walking at a fast pace, flexing (bending), range of motion movements, and stretching. Flexing is always done before stretching, as muscles can be injured if they are stretched too soon, especially if they are tight, cold, or tense.

Cool-downs consist of walking or moving at a slower pace until your breathing and heart rate are close to normal. Cooling down helps rid the muscles of pain and fatigue-causing waste materials, and returns the venous blood to the heart and away from the extremities where a clot may form if it is allowed to pool. Stretching is important at the end of your exercise routine. Not only is it relaxing, but when the muscles are warm, permanent lengthening takes place. Muscles that are not stretched properly will become larger and bulkier. This happens to women as well as men, although usually to a much lesser degree. I have seen hundreds of women who went to health clubs to reduce their thighs, and achieved just the opposite. We want long, strong, flexible muscles, although there is nothing wrong with muscle definition on women, up to a point.

TAKE PRECAUTIONS TO PROTECT YOUR KNEES AND BACK

● Numerous, fast deep knee bends can damage your knees. One or two fold downs are fine as a warm up, and to relax and stretch your back.

● If you do any jumping with your knees bent, quarter or half knee bends or plies, your knees should go directly over your feet. You should be able to see only the big toe on the inside of your knees.

● If you already have damaged knees, be extremely cautious with any knee bends or lunges. Don't let your knees go any further than the end of your toes.

● Always keep your body perpendicular to the floor, with the center of gravity directly beneath you. Never lunge with your weight going into your knees.

● **If you have a bad back, check with your doctor before any exercise**, avoiding those he forbids. Do all forward bending very slowly with your knees bent, avoid twisting, and roll up through the pelvic tilt. Lateral movements should always be straight to the side. You may want to do only the exercises in the "back" chapter.

● If yours is the typical tight, under-exercised back, or even if you are just out of condition, keep your knees bent when doing forward and lateral movements. This is a good rule for everyone. **When you twist to the left, lift the right heel, to the right, the left heel.** ALWAYS TWIST SLOWLY. You can strain your lower back if you do a fast twist with both heels planted firmly.

● Do the exercises from easy to hard, using the easy ones as a warm up. Don't attempt a difficult exercise until you can comfortably do ten in the sequence. If you are quite out of condition, or overweight, do the easier versions only. TRAIN, DON'T STRAIN. You are not competing with anyone, even yourself.

- The exercises are fun. Put on some lively enjoyable music, and get a friend to join you.
- **If it hurts, don't do it.** You may be doing the exercise incorrectly, or you may be especially tired or tense. Listen to your body. We are all different, and some of the exercises may not be for you. If you are very tired, cut your routine short. Often you start tired and feel "raring to go" by the time you finish. If you can do more, do so. I feel that large numbers of repetitions of a single exercise are counterproductive. Unless you are training for a sport, it is better to do a variety of exercises, working the muscles in many ways, to prevent fatigue and excessive muscular tension and pain.

Create your own movements. Ignore exercises you hate, as you won't continue in any case, and your motivation will be undermined. Instead, do others that work the same area. Exercise, like sports and other activities, is enjoyable. Let the music and the movements turn you on!

Vary fast with slow, top with bottom, but keep moving. Using the instructions, take your pulse after aerobics while you are walking. Enjoy!

WARMUPS

Increase your warm-up time and number of repetitions if the weather is cold or damp, or if you are especially tight or tense. A warm (not hot) 15 minute tub or shower before exercising helps limber tight joints and muscles. Begin the movements slowly, gradually increasing the pace. The older you are, the more time you need to spend with flexibility and warm up exercises.

- Fold downs flex almost **every joint in the body**. From a standing position, take a deep breath, exhaling as you tuck your chin to your chest and lower to a squatting position, hugging your knees. Get your fanny down,

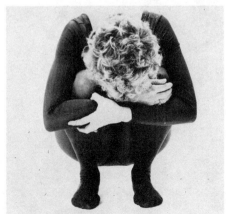

Fold downs.

even if your heels come off the floor. Stand near a support if you feel you will tip over. Your knees should be hip-width apart, and your feet directly under your knees. Hold for a few seconds, then roll up slowly, one vertebra at a time, head coming last, and knees staying slightly bent until you are upright. Repeat twice, slowly.

- **For the neck:** With your shoulders still, slowly turn your head left and right, as though you are trying to look over your shoulders. Next, make a circle in front of you with your nose, both clockwise and counter clockwise. Pause for a second when your chin comes to your chest, but **don't tilt your head back so that you are looking at the ceiling.** Do this two times each direction.

- **For the back and waist:** With your head and neck loose and relaxed, slowly reach down alternately one leg and then the other. Pretend you are reaching straight down an imaginary seam on the outside of your leg. Keep your knees slightly bent.

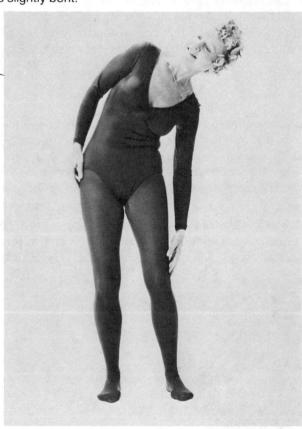

● Vigorously shake and wobble your **arms, legs, and whole body** to warm up and relax muscles and connective tissues. Keep it loose, free, and relaxed.

● **Hip joints:** Standing with your feet slightly apart, moving from the hip, roll your entire leg so the knee is pointing alternately in and out. Repeat three times with each leg.

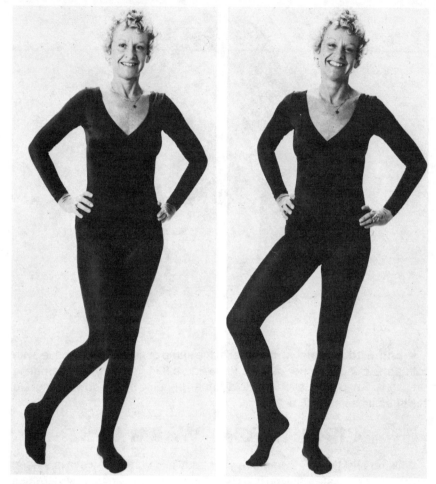

Hip joints: knee in.   **Hip joints: knee out.**

● **Knees:** With your thigh parallel to the floor, circle each knee three times in both directions.

WHOLE BODY WARM UPS

• Stand with your feet about 8 inches apart. Stretch your arms overhead as you inhale, then swing them through your legs with the knees bent as you exhale. The movement should be free and fluid throughout, eyes following your hands.

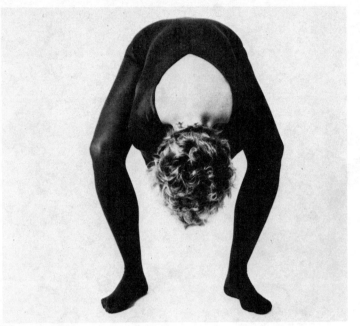

Exercise #7.

• **Entire body, waist and spine:** In the same position as the above, with both arms close together make a large figure 8 in front of you, alternating directions. Keep the movement fluid, knees bending on the downswing. Do this three times each direction.

CIRCULATORY WARM UPS

Walking briskly while you move your body in a variety of ways is a good way to warm up safely as you burn additional calories. Circulatory warmups are especially important for older people and in cold weather, when even stretching can cause injury. We walk in a large circle in my classes, but you can walk from room to room or down a hall. To add variety, increase your pace, skip, or do some dance steps as you move along. Do these after you spend a few minutes limbering with the previous exercises.

ALL OF THESE ARE DONE WHILE WALKING BRISKLY

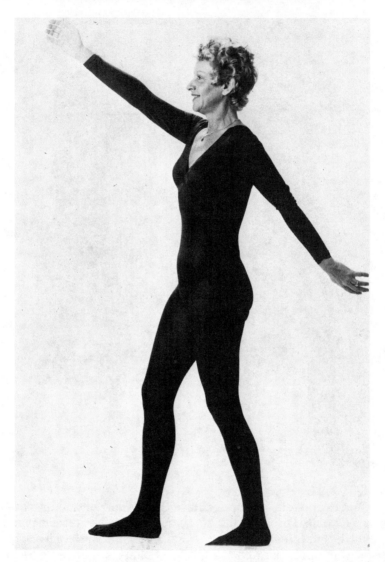

● **To strengthen the upper back and triceps:** Swinging as far as you can, swing your right arm up as your left one goes back. Keep alternating, then hold for five seconds with the right arm up as high as it will go, left arm behind you as far as it will go. Change arms and repeat.

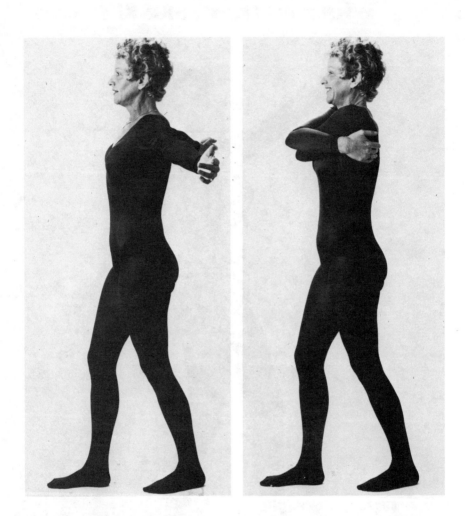

• **Stretch and relax the upper back:** Swing your arms out as far as they will go. Alternate with swinging them across your chest, reaching around as though hugging yourself. Repeat several times, and finish with a tight hug, rocking your upper back back and forth. Feel your muscles moving and stretching under your fingers.

- **Upper arms and waist:** Stretch your arm above your head in a straight line with the side of your body, palm facing the ceiling. Hold the stretch a few seconds, then change arms. Imagine you are lifting and lowering a weight.

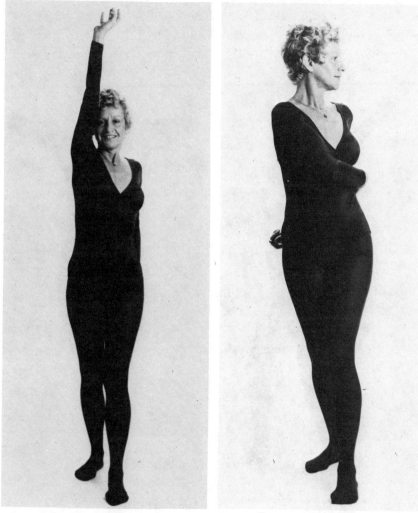

Upper arms and waist exercise.   **Waist and arms exercise.**

- **Waist and arms:** Swing both arms together at waist level so they wrap around your body. Maintain the movement from side to side, free and relaxed, knees slightly bent.

● **Whole body stretch:** Stretch your right arm towards the ceiling, palm facing up, then twist your upper body to the right, and press your arm down against imaginary resistance until it returns to your side. You should feel this in your waist and arm. Do this twice on each side.

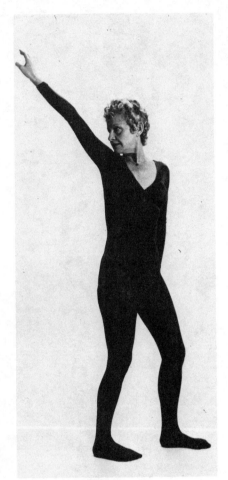 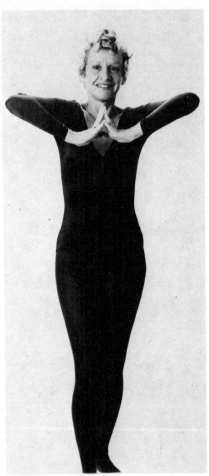

Whole body stretch.   Tension reliever.

● **Shoulders, upper back, and to relieve tension:** Place your palms together, and lift your elbows towards the ceiling. Hold for a few seconds, lower, and repeat several times.

STRETCHES FOR LENGTHENING MUSCLES, FLEXIBILITY AND TO PREVENT INJURY

Do BEFORE and AFTER aerobics, and after circulatory warmups.

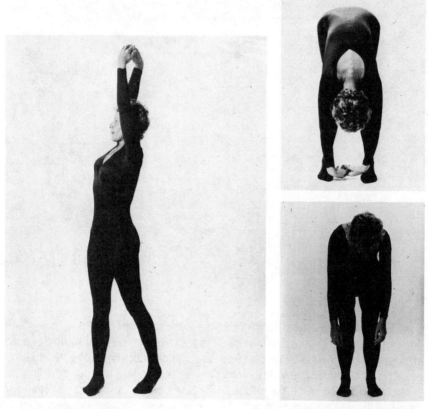

• **Waist and spine:** Stretch your arms overhead, fingertips touching. Lift your chest, and lengthen your waist, as you slowly turn to the right, lifting your left heel as you do so. Do this two times in each direction, then roll down in a bent-knee toe touch, with the top of the head pointing towards the floor. In this position, bend your right knee as you straighten your left. Hold. Do this twice with each leg. Now bend both knees, and roll up through the pelvic tilt, one vertebra at a time. Be sure to keep your chin tucked on your chest until you are all the way up. Repeat the sequence two or three times.

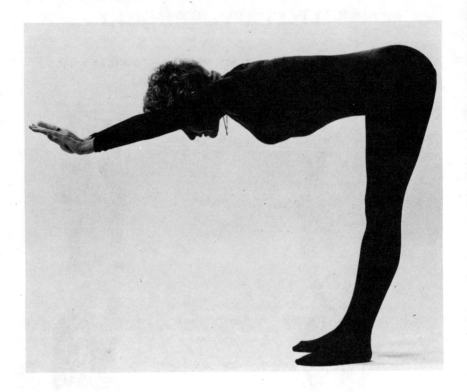

● **Hamstrings and back:** With your hands clasped behind you, bend forward from the hips, with your back in a straight line. (Your head does not drop as it does in the toe touch.) Feel the stretch in the back of your legs, not your back. If there is any discomfort in your back, you are either doing the exercise incorrectly, or it is one you shouldn't do. Once you have mastered bending from your hips, stretch your arms in a straight line even with your head and shoulders. Alternate reaching in a long stretch with one arm and then the other, feeling the stretch in the back and legs. Do this twice, and follow with a toe touch, being sure to drop your head first, and roll up.

● **Front and inner thigh:** Stand with your feet about 3 feet apart. Lunge to the right, making certain your knee goes directly over your foot, and your body remains perpendicular to the floor, with your weight directly beneath you. Hold the lunge position 10 seconds or more, and change sides. When you are lunging to the right, flex your left foot. Do this 3 times in each direction, followed by a toe touch with your legs apart. Bend your knees, and roll up, head last.

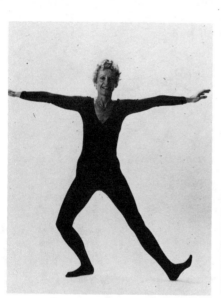 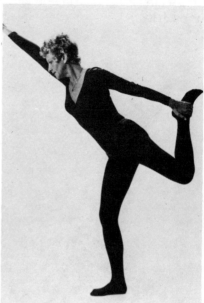

Front and inner thigh stretch.   **Front of thigh stretch.**

● **Front of the thigh:** Hold on to something for balance if you need to. Stand with your weight on your left foot. Clasp your right ankle (or foot, if you can reach), and stretch your right thigh up behind you. Lift your head and feel the stretch all the way through your abdominals, but do not arch your back. It is easier on your knees if you keep a space between your calf and the back of your thigh, instead of pressing your heel into your buttocks. Hold the stretch for at least 20 seconds, and do this twice on each side. Once this becomes easy, work on improving your balance at the same time by stretching your right arm out in a straight line with your torso as you hold the stretch on your left thigh.

● **Calf and achilles tendon:** Stand with your right foot about 2 feet in front of your left, BOTH FEET POINTING FORWARD. Keeping **both** heels on the floor, bend your right knee as you stretch your arms up in a straight line with your torso. Keep your chest lifted, and your abdominals and spine lengthened. The more you lunge, the more stretch you feel in your calf. If it is too painful, decrease your lunge, and slightly bend your rear knee, still keeping the heel on the floor. Calf muscles can become shortened, tight and bulkȳ from wearing heels, or from dancing, running and jumping without proper stretching. Hold the stretch for at least 20 seconds, and do this twice on each leg.

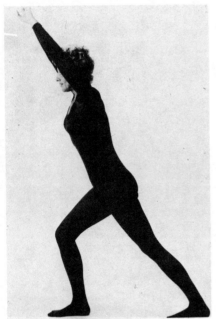
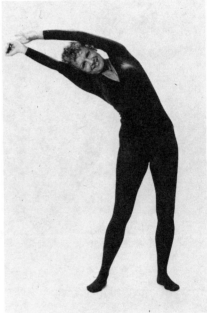

Calf and achilles tendon stretch.   **Waist and spine stretch.**

● **Waist and spine:** Stand with the legs about 6 inches apart. Stretch both arms straight up from the shoulders, keeping them close and parallel, chest and waist lifted. **Slowly** bend straight to the right, making certain you do not twist. Return **slowly**, and repeat to the left. Do 3 in each direction, then hold the side bend position for a few seconds. Work up to 8 in each direction.

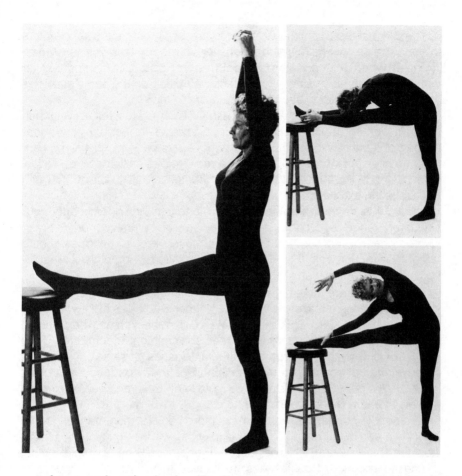

● **Legs and entire body:** (Don't do this one if you have lower back trouble, or exceptionally tight hamstrings and lower back muscles.) Stand with your left leg in normal step position, and your right foot resting on the back of a chair at about waist level. Inhale as you stretch your arms over-head, lengthening your spine and abdominals. Exhale as you slowly stretch over your extended leg, bending from your hips. If your knee insists on bending slightly, let it. When you have reached as far as you can, relax your whole torso, letting your head come towards your knee. Clasp your leg, gently coaxing your body closer. NEVER FORCE A STRETCH! Roll up slowly to the standing position. Do once on each side, then once again with the foot flexed. Now turn your standing foot so it is parallel to the chair. With your right foot on the chair, circle your left arm overhead next to your left ear, and slide your right arm down your right leg, as you bend to the right, with your right ear comng towards the right knee. Do this once on each side.

You can include any of the stretches in the "back" or "sexercise" chapters in your stretch routine. Stretch whenever your body tells you to, **under-doing it when the muscles are cold and/or tense.** It is important for women to finish exercising with stretches. You can do the same stretches you began with, holding each for 20 seconds or more.

BREATHING AND RELAXATION ARE CRUCIAL. Muscles won't stretch if the movement is filled with tension and haste. In fact, they may tear instead of stretch. When you think you have stretched as far as you can, hold the position, inhale deeply, and as you exhale slowly, relax, and allow your stretch to increase. Do this several times, increasing the stretch with each relaxing exhalation.

The time to do your aerobic and specific toning exercises is after your circulatory range of motion and flexibility warmups. Work your entire body, with emphasis on areas that need it the most. Aerobic exercises should adapt to what you enjoy, time and space limitations, and physical restrictions. (See aerobics.)

Often women are more interested in the cosmetic benefits than in all the other good things exercise does for them. Improved looks are a valid goal. We all want to LOOK, FEEL, and BE WELL. Trouble comes when women think they can diet and spot reduce themselves into perfect health. They can't. Looking good is only part of it. Fatal diseases can also cause you to lose weight, but you are far from healthy. One of my pet peeves is being asked: "Why are you exercising? You're so thin!" Everyone needs exercise —men, women, children and older adults.

Cosmetically speaking, women have more body fat than men, and more specific areas of fatty depots. Aerobic exercise will indiscriminately use fat from the entire system, which is good, but certain areas need special toning.

The most common trouble areas are the hips, thigh, back of the upper arm (triceps), upper back and abdomen. Unfairly, it seems that women's muscles do not seem to age as well as men's. This may be because women are (traditionally) less active, and because we have less muscle and are influenced by hormonal changes. It does seem unfair that a man who may do nothing more strenuous than push a pencil will retain firm upper arms while his wife who does the gardening and housework, sags. Part of the problem is that most activities involve the biceps at the front of the arm, and the tricep muscle itself actually separates away from the bone. Despite this, it is necessary to keep the muscle toned, and that is best done with light weights or some other resistance.

Men and women accumulate fat around the middle as they age. Much is subcutaneous fat, but part is due to fat filling the omentum, a sac beneath the muscle that surrounds and protects the organs. Many studies show that firming the abdominal muscles by doing many sit-ups will not remove the fat that sits between the muscle and skin. I agree to a point. It is certainly possible to have very firm, strong abdominal muscles and still have fat on them. This is especially true if you are over forty. The Italians have a saying: "If you want a flat stomach over 40, you must have sunken cheeks."

Despite this, I think that certain yoga exercises, and correct posture will discourage fat from forming on the abdomen, and help eliminate what is there.

Women tend to store fat around the hips, thighs and buttocks. Often this begins at puberty and increases with age. We see this dimply fat on thin women. The French call it cellulite, claiming it is fat that has degraded, hardened, and mixed with fluid and waste materials. In this country, most "experts" say it is just pure, simple, fat.

The French have been going to aestheticians routinely for treatments that include special massages, creams and diets. They claim that cellulite is influenced by the hormones, and I don't think this is entirely wrong.

I think you can reduce this type of fat with exercises that cause a general weight loss, and specific exercises that tone and stretch the areas. Diet is also important.

A "cellulite" diet would include at least eight glasses of water between meals, apples, grapefruit and asparagus, which are mildly diuretic, the elimination of salt and salty foods, and a balanced B complex vitamin that contained B6 (to eliminate fluid retention and normalize estrogen), and niacin (a vasodialator).

The following exercises are designed to tone common problem areas. To be beneficial, you need to go beyond the point where it is easy, but stop short of straining or injury. Remember the rule, IF IT HURTS, DON'T DO IT. I am not talking about the aches that come from the buildup of lactic acid and other waste materials formed during exercise. You get rid of those by deep breathing (exhaling completely), shaking and massaging the muscle, and cool down stretches. Stop short of injury by working within a range that is fun. Put on some lively music, and do it!

Women tend to store fat around the hips, thighs, and buttocks.

TRICEPS FIRMERS

The first exercise works the upperarm, forearm, and latissimus dorsi at the side of the upper back. In my classes we use rubber strips cut from inner tubes as an aid in stretching and as resistance for the waist, thighs, arms and back. You may use one or two pound weights to begin with, working up to 5 pounds. Rocks or soup cans may be used as weight. If your muscles become sore, use lighter weights and fewer repetitions.

● Holding a weight in each hand, lean forward slightly from the hips, keeping your tummy in and back straight. Pull your elbows up past your rib cage, keeping your upper arms close to your body. Flex your biceps by bringing your fists towards your shoulders, then your triceps by extending your arms straight up behind you. (Make sure you keep your upper arms close to your ribs throughout.)

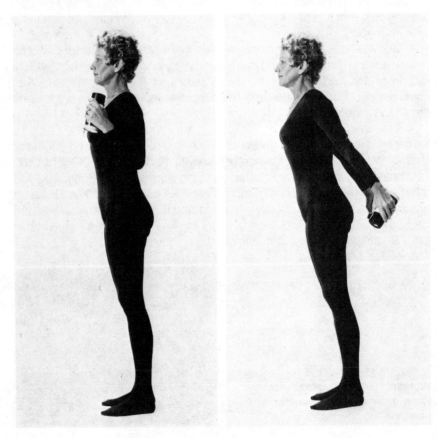

• Stand about 3 feet from a wall, hands on the wall at shoulder level. SLOWLY press your forearms towards the wall until they touch. Hold for a count of 5, and repeat 4 times. You should feel a strong stretch and contraction in the back of the upper arm. Do these any time you pass a convenient wall.

• With weights clasped firmly in your hands, and upper arms next to your ears, lower your hands behind your neck. SLOWLY straighten your arms overhead, keeping them parallel and close to your head. Build up to 2 sets of 5.

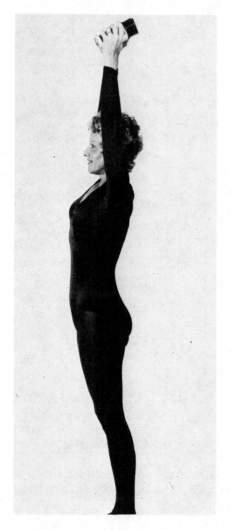 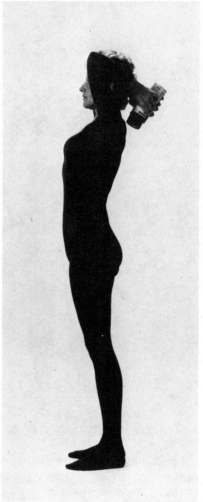

WAIST AND MIDRIFF

The most important thing you can do for this area and for your general health is to improve your posture. (See Chapter 14: "Oh, My Aching Back.") Lifting your rib cage with your shoulders relaxed will automatically reduce your waist an inch or more. Hold this lifted and lengthened feeling at all times; walking, sitting and standing. **It is necessary to keep lifted while you are exercising, even though you are simultaneously bending,** to maintain correct alignment, to reduce fat on the abdomen, waist and midriff, and to keep new fat from settling there. Make sure that you do not arch your back when you lift your ribs. Breathe deeply.

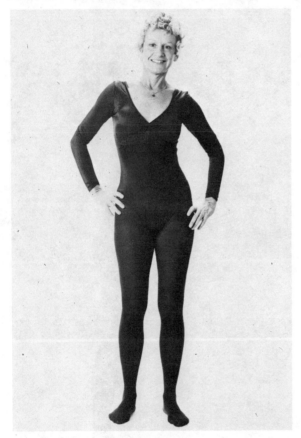

Exercise #1

#1. Isolate your ribs and lift them as high as you can. Push them slowly to the right and left without moving your hips. Put your hands on your waist and feel the muscles working.

#2. Side bends are listed below from easy to hard. If you are out of condition, or have a tight lower back, stick with the easiest ones.

- With knees slightly flexed, reach slowly down the right and then the left leg, making certain the movement is straight towards the floor.

- Standing with your legs apart, circle your left arm overhead, close to your ear. Lift your ribs on the left side of your body as you bend to the right. Do several repetitions on each side, then try with your wrist flexed so that you are reaching with your palm. Finish with a 20 second hold in each direction, reaching as far down the side of your leg as you can. **Keep your neck relaxed throughout.**

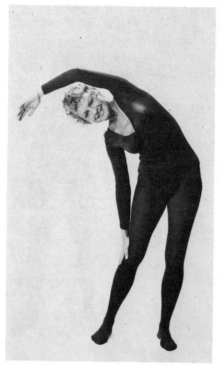 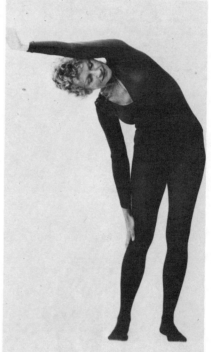

Side bends   **Side bends**

- Stand with your feet about 6 inches apart, ribs lifted, arms next to your ears, hands clasped overhead. Bend straight to the right SLOWLY, hold for a few seconds, slowly return to the center position, and repeat to the left. Three in each direction. (Left photo.)

- Stand with feet apart, arms straight to the side at shoulder level, palms facing forward. Without moving your hips or right arm, try to touch your right palm with your left hand. Return to center, and do 3 in each direction slowly. (Center photo.)

- Start with your left arm overhead, next to your left ear, fingers pointing to the right and your right arm behind your back at waist level, fingers pointing to the left. Keeping your head and neck relaxed, pull your left arm to the right, and your right arm to the left as you bend to the right. Go as far as you can 10 times in each direction, feeling the stretch in your waist. (Right photo.)

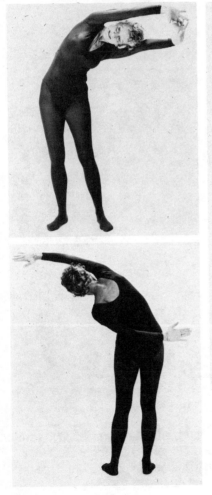

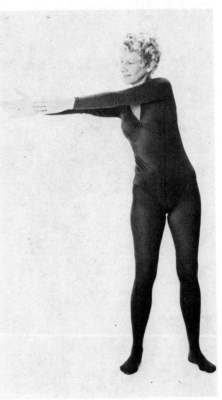

Side bend exercises.

The following waist exercises are done while lying on your side on a carpet or mat. Again, they range from easy to hard. Beginners should stick with #1 only, and so should those with back problems. Do not advance before your muscles are ready. If you do these every day, you should see improvement within 2 weeks.

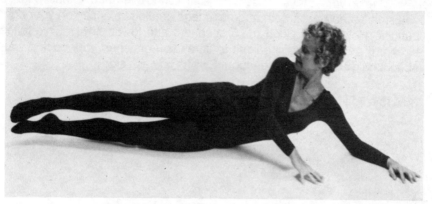

#1. Lie on your right side with your right arm stretched overhead beneath you, your left arm resting on your left leg. Slowly lift your torso and legs simultaneously so that you are balancing on your right hip and supported by your right arm. Look over your left shoulder at your left heel. Hold for 5 seconds. Lower slowly. Begin with 3 on each side, working up to 8.

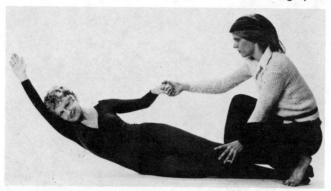

#2. Lie on your right side with your right arm stretched in a line straight with your body overhead, head resting on your arm. Have someone hold down your legs by either sitting astraddle or stepping lightly on your calves. If your legs are not held down firmly, you won't be able to do the exercise. It is not necessary (but helps for balance) if your assistant holds your left hand. However, don't let her pull you up! Keeping your head and arm together, lift your torso straight up from the floor without twisting. This is a

97

difficult exercise, and if you do it correctly, you won't move very far. Begin with 2 slow lifts, and work up to 5 on each side. It is one of the best for strengthening both the internal and external oblique muscles.

#3. Lie on your right side, both arms stretched overhead. Exhale hard as you simultaneously lift both torso and legs, ending balanced on your right buttock. Hold this position for 5 seconds, and lower slowly. This takes strength; so beginners shouldn't try it, as you may hurt your back if your abdominals are not strong enough. Six lifts on each side.

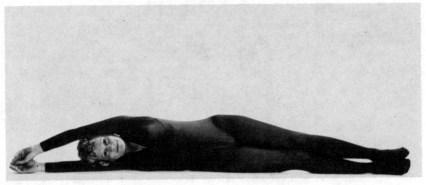

Exercise 3: starting position.

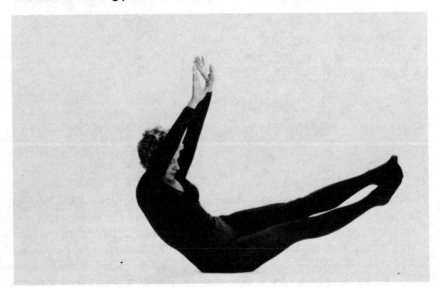

Exercise 3: mid-range position.

WAIST, ABDOMEN AND HIP FLEXORS

These exercises, including the sit-ups and curl-downs, are done in, or moving through, the pelvic tilt position. This takes the strain off the lower back and strengthens the abdominal muscles. The LOWER part of the pelvis is slightly forward, upper pelvis and abdomen in, back round.

All the many variations of sit-ups and roll-backs, or curl-downs, are done with a round, never arched back. The chin is always tucked on the chest, and you move one vertebra at a time, if you can. Beginners may find the exercises easier if they tighten the abdominals first. DO NOT ATTEMPT THE NEXT EXERCISE IN THE SEQUENCE UNTIL YOU CAN DO 10 OR 15 OF THE PREVIOUS ONES EASILY. ALWAYS DO A FEW EASY VARIATIONS AS A WARM-UP. If a sit-up is too difficult, most women can do a curl-down, or partial curl-down. Advance slowly to avoid straining muscles. You did not get out of shape overnight, and at the age of 40 plus, it will take you longer to restore lost muscle tone.

The first exercise takes you to where the abdominals start to work when you are rolling back, and gets you in the correct position. If your muscles are extremely weak, or if you have lower back trouble, do only this one for the first 2 or 3 weeks. Once a week doesn't count! Do abdominal exercises every day if you expect to see results.

BASIC CURL-DOWN POSITION

#1. Sit with your knees bent, feet flat on the floor, hands resting on your knees, chin tucked on your chest. Roll back slowly, starting with the base of your spine, until your arms are straight. This is where your abdominals begin working as you roll back, and stop working as you sit up. Hold this position for 5 seconds, and roll up slowly. Don't hold your breath, but either breathe normally or exhale. Do this 5 times, twice a day. If it is easy, continue rolling down, one vertebra at a time, keeping your arms parallel and close to the floor, head coming last.

#2. If you found it easy to roll slowly all the way back, try holding in several positions on the way down. Keeping your neck relaxed and your chin tucked on your chest, starting in the basic curl-down position, roll back a few inches. Hold for 4 seconds, and continue doing this until you are in the position with just your head, neck and shoulders lifted. Exhale as you lower down, and keep your arms relaxed and low, palms facing up.

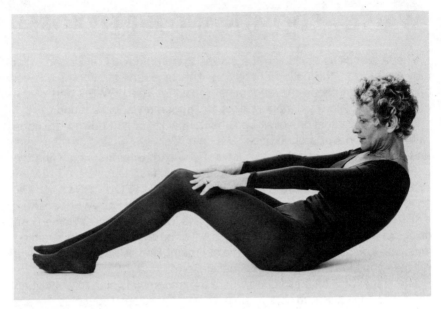

Exercise #1: basic curl-down—back off the floor.

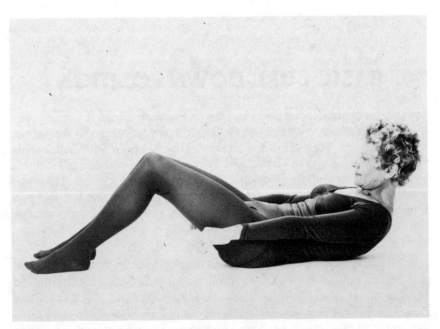

Exercise #2: basic curl-down—roll down till back rests on floor.

#3. Assume the basic curl-down position with your hands resting on the floor behind you for support, your abdominals contracted. Tap your right heel about 2 feet in front of you as the left comes in close to your body. Alternate legs as you tap forward and back in a continuous rhythmic movement. When this becomes easy, try tapping both heels in and out together, keeping knees slightly bent as the legs are extended. You should feel the contraction in your thighs and abdominals, not your back. Those with tight or weak lower backs should do only one leg at a time.

#4. Start in the basic position, arms behind you for support, left knee bent with the foot flat on the floor. Make large circles with your right leg, both clockwise and counterclockwise. Repeat several times with each leg. Always keep your back round, chin tucked on your chest.

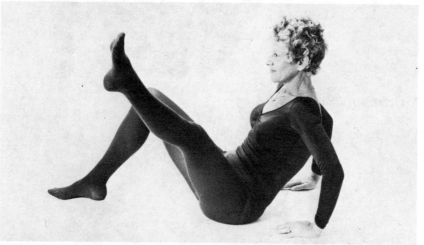

Exercise #4: basic position—making circles with the left leg.

THE NEXT THREE EXERCISES ARE ADVANCED AND SHOULD NOT BE ATTEMPTED BY BEGINNERS OR THOSE WITH WEAK LOWER BACK AND/OR ABDOMINAL MUSCLES.

#5. Start in the basic position, arms behind you for support. With both legs at the same time, make large slow circles going **outward**. The feet should touch as you come through the center position at about a foot off the floor. When you become good at this exercise, try holding for three seconds when the feet touch. Now try it with the legs circling in. Always keep your knees slightly bent. Work up to 10 repetitions in each direction.

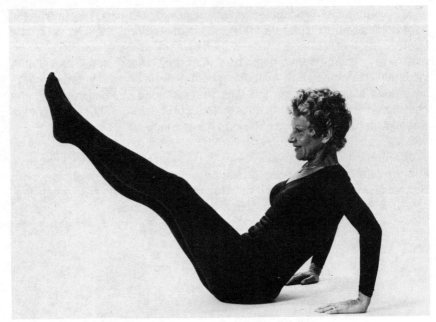

Exercise #5: starting position.

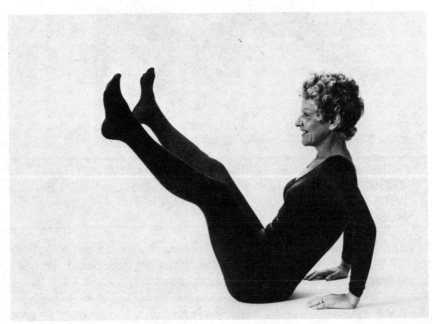

Exercise #5: mid-range position.

#6. Maintaining the basic curl-down position, try 3 or 4 slow circles in each direction with both legs together.

#7. In the basic position and balanced on your buttocks, go through rowing motions, starting with your knees to your chest and your arms straight in front of you. Bend your elbows, bringing them behind your ribs, and lean your upper body back as you simultaneously extend your legs forward, knees slightly bent. Go through a smooth rowing motion several times, or until you are tired.

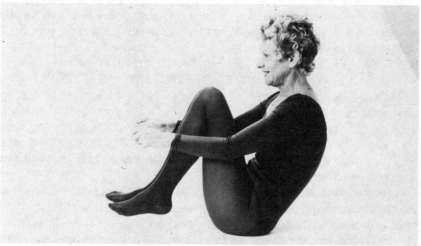

Exercise #7: starting position.

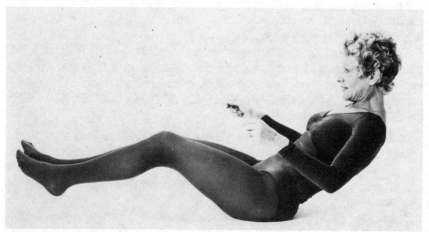

Exercise #8: mid-range position.

SIT-UPS

One of the most common problems people have with both sit-ups and curl-downs is that they try to pull up with their arms, neck and shoulders, or push forward with their back muscles. This is usually because they have weak abdominals and tense neck, back and shoulder muscles.

If you are having trouble, remember it is not important that you sit all the way up or roll all the way back. **The purpose is to strengthen your abdominal muscles without straining your neck or back.**

Sometimes just tucking your chin on your chest is all it takes to get the strain off the neck muscles. If your neck and shoulders are still tense and straining, try shaking your shoulders as you sit up, and rolling your neck from side to side after you have tucked your chin down. As with all exercise, KEEP RELAXED THE MUSCLES THAT ARE NOT ACTIVELY INVOLVED IN THE MOVEMENT, AND MOVE AS EFFICIENTLY AS POSSIBLE.

There are many variations of sit-ups, but certain rules apply to all. Roll up one vertebra at a time, head coming first, chin tucked on your chest. Keep your knees flexed, and exhale as you roll up. To make sit-ups harder, bend your knees more, so you are eliminating the iliapsoas muscle. Roll back through the curl-down position even more slowly than you sat up, one vertebra at a time, head coming last.

Sit-ups and curl-downs should always be done slowly, with awareness of the abdominal muscles. Have your feet held down with a heavy object if you need to, working up to the point where it is no longer necessary. (Some people with heavy or short torsos and thin legs always need to have their feet held down, even when their abdominals are strong.)

The sequence is given from easy to hard. Remember, don't try a hard variation until you can do at least 10 of the previous ones in the series, and warm up by doing easy exercises first.

The degree of bend in the knee and arm positions are two variables that affect the difficulty. Sit-ups and curl-downs done on a diagonal work the waist. Beginners, stick with the easy ones until you see a noticeable improvement. BEGINNERS SHOULD NOT ATTEMPT LARGE NUMBERS OF SIT-UPS.

- To bring you to the point at which the abdominals begin to work: Lie on your back, knees bent, feet flat on the floor, arms resting at your sides. Roll up head, neck and shoulders. Hold for 5 seconds, then roll back slowly. Work up to 10 repetitions, then go on to the next exercise if you are able.
- On your back, feet flat on the floor, knees bent, hands on your thighs. Tighten your abdominals, put your chin on your chest, and roll three-fourths of the way up to a sitting position. Your hands should be almost

up to your knees. Hold for 5 seconds, and roll down slowly. If you can't roll up that far, go as far as you can, and hold there. Repeat 5 times, working up to 10.

- This time roll all the way up if you can do so **without jerking or straining.** Exhale as you come up, and remember, the object is to strengthen abdominal muscles, not to sit up! If there is a tough spot you can't get past in trying to sit up, hold on to your thighs for a little help, or stick with the previous exercise. When you can do at least 10 of these easily, go on to the next exercise.

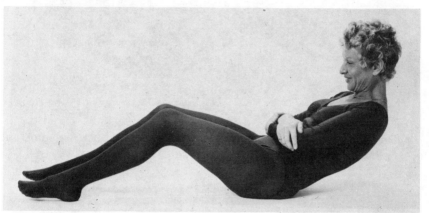

- Roll up, head coming first, with your arms crossed on your abdomen. Roll back slowly, arms straight, parallel and close to the floor. Work up to 10 before progressing to the next arm position. (Photo above.)

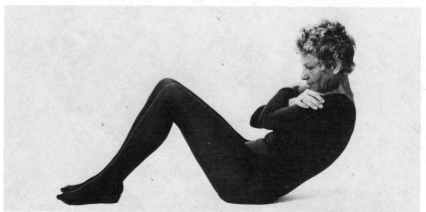

- This time roll up with your arms crossed on your chest. Come down the same as before. Keep your back round so you are rolling up and down through the pelvic tilt. Do 10. (Photo above.)

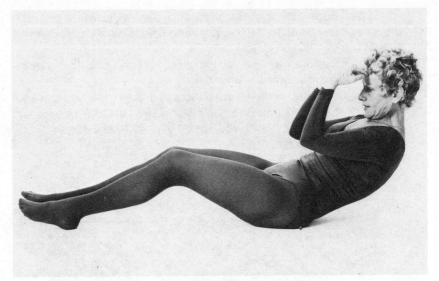

- Roll up with your fingertips on your forehead. Roll back the same as before. Work up to 10 before you progress. (Photo above.)

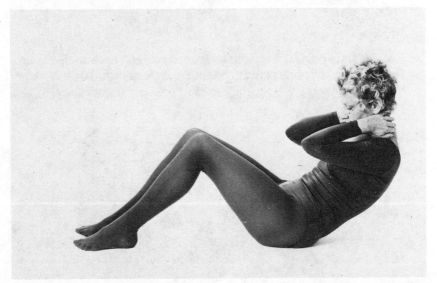

- Roll up with your fingers laced behind your neck, elbows forward. Be sure the back is round, abdominals working, head coming forward first as you sit up, and last as you roll back. This may be as far as you can safely go in the series. Do 2 sets of 15 after warming up with easier sit-ups. (Photo above.)

THE FOLLOWING EXERCISES ARE ADVANCED, ONLY FOR THOSE WITH EXCEPTIONALLY STRONG ABDOMINAL MUSCLES AND A HEALTHY BACK. NEVER TRY THEM WHEN YOU ARE TENSE OR HURRIED. WARM UP FIRST WITH FLEXIBILITY EXERCISES AND EASIER SIT-UPS. YOU SHOULD BE ABLE TO DO 2 SETS OF 15 OF THE PREVIOUS EXERCISES FIRST. ALWAYS TUCK YOUR CHIN ON YOUR CHEST, ROLL UP AND BACK THROUGH THE PELVIC TILT.

- Roll up with your knees bent, thighs perpendicular to the floor, calves level and parallel to the floor. Arms straight overhead. Arms crossed on your chest. Five times.
- Legs straight overhead, ankles crossed, arms overhead. Exhale hard as you roll up and back slowly.

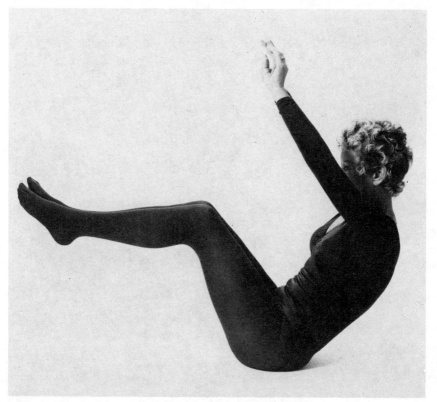

Roll up exercise with your arms straight overhead.

SIT-UPS FOR THE WAIST: In a sequence from easy to difficult.

- Lie on your back, knees bent, feet flat on the floor, and about a foot apart, arms at your sides. Place your right hand on your left thigh, and slowly roll up, from right to left, head coming first, until your hand reaches your knee. Hold for a count of 4, and roll back from left to right, head coming last. Maintain the diagonal movement both up and back, 5 times in each direction.

- Lie on your back, knees bent, feet flat on the floor, arms overhead. Imagine you are reaching over a large barrel as you lengthen your waist and abdominal muscles while you roll up from right to left, right hand going towards your left foot. Roll back from left to right, five times in each direction.

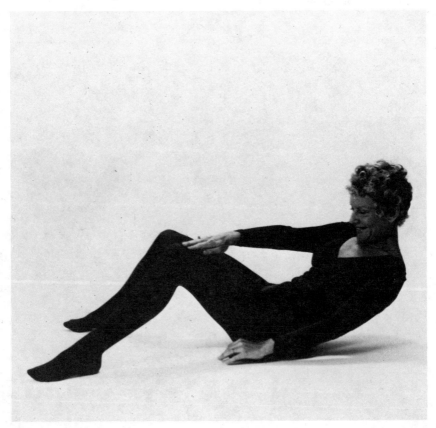

Sit-ups: arms at your sides.

● Same starting position, with your hands laced behind your neck, elbows forward. Try to touch your right elbow to your left knee. Bring your knee simultaneously towards your elbow as you roll up. Don't forget to keep your chin tucked and exhale as you roll up. Do five times each direction.

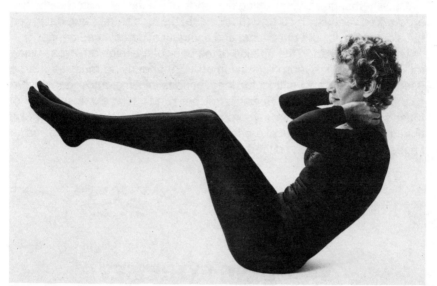

Sit-ups: starting position (hands behind the neck.)

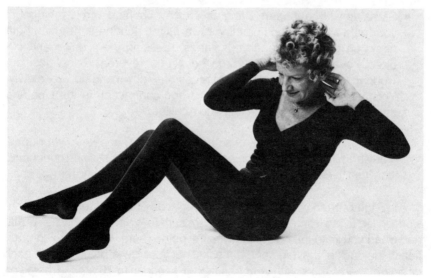

Sit-ups: action (twist and touch right elbow to left knee.)

HIPS AND THIGHS

Many exercises for the hips and thighs also work the lower abdomen and waist. Whether done lying, sitting or standing, the thighs, buttocks and hips are worked variously by **lifting** (not kicking) the legs to the front, back, center, side, circling, both directions, and a variety of partial knee bends.

The inner thigh, and the outside of the back of the thigh are areas where fat deposits form, even on thin women. The underlying muscles are not used frequently, and sitting for long periods of time and poor posture contribute to the problem. Special stretching and toning exercises work on these specific places. Take inventory: Is your back straight, or is your pelvis tipped forward? Do you express your tension by standing with locked knees? This will make you tired, and your thighs larger.

STANDING EXERCISES

● Standing with feet apart. Bring your left foot behind and to the right of your right foot, left toes pointing towards the right heel. Keeping both heels on the floor, bend your knees, pressing them down and out directly over your toes. Slowly do 3 or 4, then reverse the foot position, working up to 6. It is important to press both down and up very slowly. You needn't go very far to feel a strong contraction in the hips and thighs, and a stretch in the calf and Achilles.

● Hold lightly onto the back of a chair for support, and keep your upper body from moving, as all the action is done with control and concentration from the waist on down. Always use the leg that is away from the chair.

#1. Slightly bend your support leg throughout. Slowly lift (don't kick) your working leg to the front, side, and back. Be sure to lower as slowly as you lift, and when you lift to the rear, lift only to the point where you feel the contraction in the back of the thigh and buttocks, not your lower back. Do 4 in each direction, then 4 more with your foot flexed. Work up to 10 reps. (Photos on page 111.)

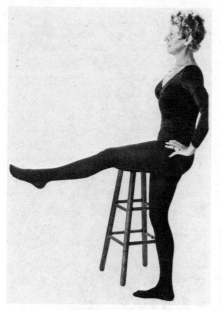

Step 1—Exercise #1: lift leg to the front.

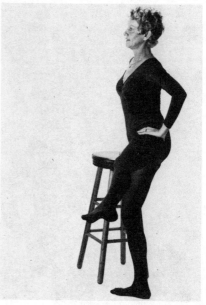

Step 2—Exercise #1: move leg to the side.

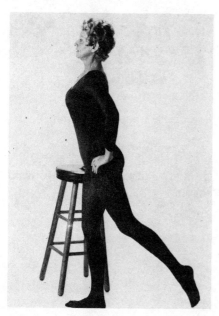

Step 3—Exercise #1: slowly move the leg from the side to the back.

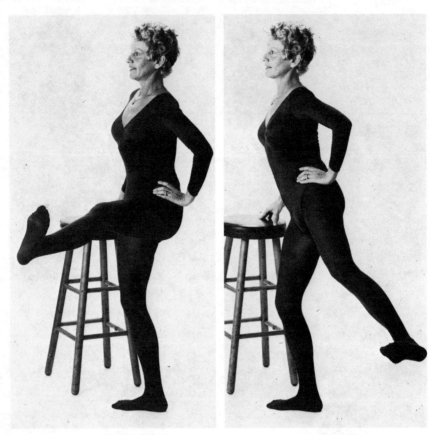

Exercise #2: starting position.   **Exercise #2: mid-range position.**

#2. With your foot flexed, make a large figure 8 at your side, both forward and back. Do this three times each direction.

SIDE-LYING

All of these exercises are done lying directly on your side, leg beneath you bent, head resting on your hand, palm of the hand in front of you and resting on the floor for support. If your leg gets tired, shake it briskly, and change sides.

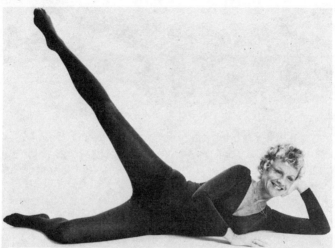

#1. With your leg going straight towards the ceiling, lift and lower rapidly 10 times. Do the same with the heel going first. Now try the same thing **very slowly**, stopping in several positions on the way **up or down**. Once is enough.

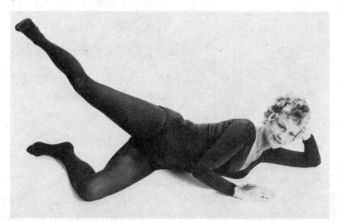

#2. With foot flexed, lift the leg behind you at a 45 degree angle. (Halfway between straight up and straight back.) Do 6 slowly, working up to 10.

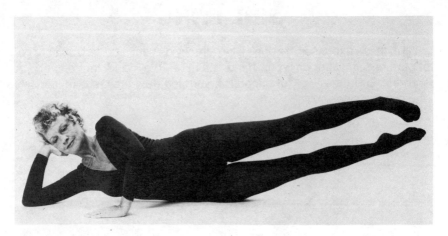

#3. Push against the floor with your hand as you lift both legs together and simultaneously. Do 3 or 4 slowly. You will feel the contraction all the way to the waist. Now hold the position and clap your feet together, as though you clap hands.

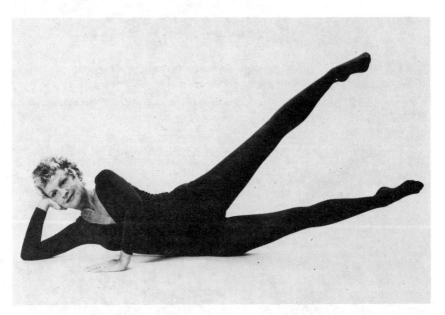

#4. More difficult: With both legs lifted off the floor, weight resting on your hips and supported by your hand: keep your bottom leg off the floor as you slowly lift and lower your upper leg 4 times. Lower both legs slowly to the floor, and relax.

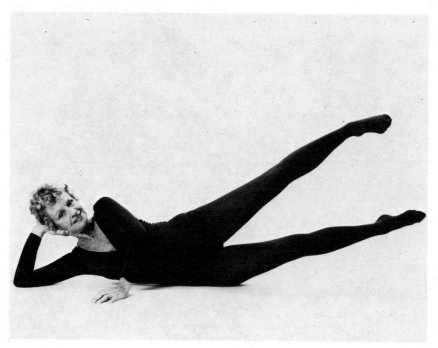

Exercise #5.

#5. In the same position, lift your upper leg as high as you can. Slowly try to touch it with your lower leg, lifting and lowering it slowly, as the upper leg remains stationary. You should feel this in the hip and outer thigh of the upper leg, inner thigh of the lower leg. Do 4 times.

#6. This works the inside and outside of your thighs, arms, chest and shoulders as a bonus. Sit on the floor with your knees bent, soles of your feet touching about 10 inches in front of you. Put the palm of your right hand on the inside of your left knee, left hand on the inside of your right knee. Resist with your hands as you slowly push your knees together and apart. You should feel resistance as your knees move in both directions. Now try it with your hands on the outside of your knees (right hand on right knee, left on the left). Push OUT against the resistance of your hands. The more you resist, the harder the exercise. Begin with 4, working up to 8 in each direction.

#7. Specifically for the inner thigh. Lying on your left side, put your right foot on the floor in front of your left leg. Flex your left foot, and slowly push the inner thigh straight towards the ceiling. Do 5 slowly with each leg.

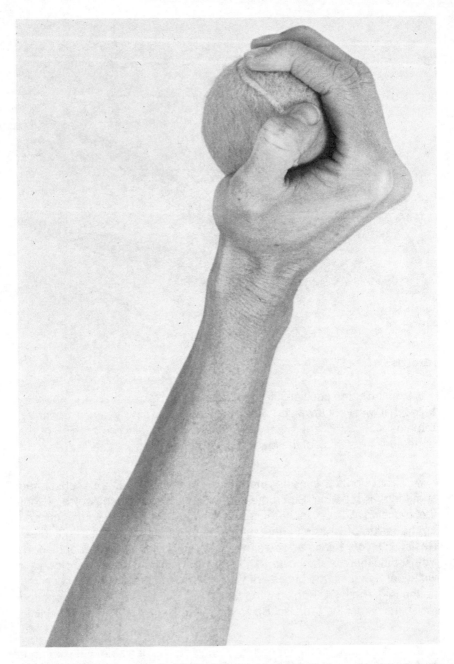

One exercise that may be helpful is to keep a tennis ball around and squeeze it whenever possible to strengthen your hands, wrists, and forearms.

Get a soft rubber ball, about 8 inches in diameter. Put it between your knees, and press your knees together, holding for 5 seconds. Do 3 or 4 times. Try holding the ball between your knees and walking with it. Keep the ball handy so you can do these inner thigh firmers whenever you have an odd moment. Keep an old tennis ball around, and squeeze it to strengthen your hands, wrists and forearms.

Stretch and move whenever you find the opportunity. Better yet, make the opportunity! Walk from room to room with your knees bent to strengthen your thighs, or on your heels to stretch your calves. Walk barefoot to strengthen your feet, go upstairs two at a time. When you feel stiff and aching, move, bend and stretch, and take some deep breaths of fresh air. Your work and your spirits will improve.

According to some experts, you can get aerobic training benefits from spot toning and weight training. The secret is to keep moving for at least 20 minutes. (The minimum energy expenditure for a training effect is about 300 calories, so 20 minutes is a bare minimum.) In my classes, we move continuously for an hour, and we are walking WHILE DOING ARM AND UPPER BODY MOVEMENTS.

For most people, aerobic exercises, such as walking, jogging, slow jumping or chair stepping, need to be done additionally in order to achieve a training effect. Find one that brings you the most pleasure, and best fits your lifestyle. You will feel and look better, and have energy left over for fun.

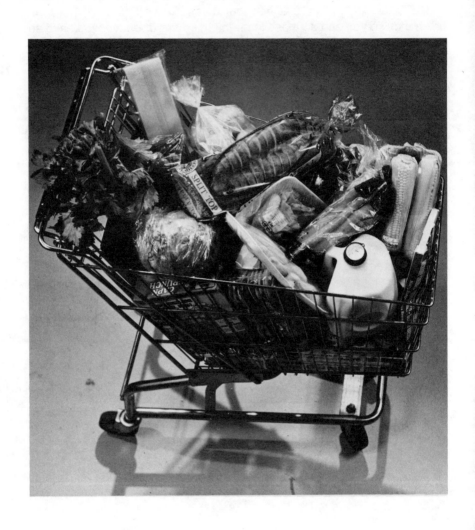

6
NUTRITION— AND DIETS

Almost every woman you meet is on a diet or thinks she should be. It's our national pastime. Even my friend Michelle who is 5'4"—and miserably unhappy because she went from 92 to 98 when she stopped smoking —diets. (She was fat as a teenager, and never changed that image of herself.) My friends from less affluent countries tell me that it is only here that we have this real or imagined fear of fatness. In other parts of the world, the problem is getting enough to eat and the concept of "dieting" is unknown. And, as is exemplified in both cases, whatever is scarce, or difficult to obtain, is idealized or sought after. Here, we seek to be lean. I have combined diet and nutrition, because nutrition cannot be separated from any part of our being, whether it be our ability to withstand stress, to run, or to lose weight. I firmly believe that for most people, weight loss must include both exercise and diet, although the proportion may vary, depending on physiology and lifestyle.

I wish I could say to you "I have the ultimate diet; one that will help you to lose weight, and is nutritionally complete." I can't. There are thousands of diets, all of which work for some, and not for others.

As far as weight loss goes, the ultimate diet is starvation; however, even that has proven unsuccessful because, if we want to live, at some point it is necessary to eat. We are then faced with the questions of "how, when, and what". People regain more fat than what was lost on extreme diets, and destroyed muscle tissue may never be regained.

The same ambivalence holds true regarding nutrition. Even though there are published "minimum daily requirements," below which we may suffer from deficiency diseases, and "recommended daily allowances," which supposedly provide the proper amounts of known nutrients, obviously, the same diet cannot guarantee optimal health for everyone. Within the scientific community itself there are many disputes. Also, theories change; as soon as you read that something is "gospel," it has been invalidated. Certain claims that were once made within the domain of "health nuts" are now being espoused by standard nutritionists, even the slow-acting federal government. Take, for example, the new Department of Agriculture publication, **FOOD**, a free booklet containing tips on nutrition and recipes. The section on fiber suggests eating whole grains, seeds and nuts. It is only a couple of years ago that I attended a conference on aging at the National Institute of Health and engaged in an argument with one of the guest speakers as we stood in line at the cafeteria. He maintained that white bread was nutritionally as beneficial as whole grain, and, since he taught at a prestigious medical college, he knew all the answers. Today the "official" publications acknowledge that thirteen or more nutrients are refined out of white flour (in addition to the bran and some germ) and only three are added back. (Add this to the fact that white bread tastes something like facial tissues, and it's amazing that anyone eats it at all!)

Let's return to the question of obesity. Friend Michelle notwithstanding, the fact remains that we are heavier than we were twenty years ago, and two-thirds of the cases of severe overweight in this country are women. Medically, 20 percent above ideal weight is considered overweight. Those few pounds you gain over the holidays are not important in themselves, but if left unchallenged, may easily compound into ten or more pounds of additional weight per year. This happens much more easily as we get older and our body composition changes. This is especially true for women, as we have a higher percentage of fat than men to begin with.

This extra fat is not all bad; it's why we have curves instead of angles. Furthermore, when we become too thin (around 14 to 15 percent body fat, or less), the brain stops releasing a hormone that signals the pituitary to stimulate the ovaries, and we stop menstruating. It seems to be nature's way of preventing pregnancy during times of famine. Amenorrhea is becoming more common now that women are getting into such demanding sports as running. However, it is not a problem for the woman who is out there running for pleasure, health and weight control. If you are over forty and run or starve yourself to the point of 14 percent body fat, you are definitely not in this category!

True obesity can cause health problems. The most common is a lack of energy. Often this is accompanied by pain in the weight-bearing joints, especially the back, hips, and knees. The risk of diabetes and hypertension are increased. Often these conditions can be reversed simply by losing weight. Heavier women may have difficult childbirths, and are more likely to

122

have spontaneous abortions once they do become pregnant. They may have a greater risk of uterine and breast cancer, and there is a strong correlation between gallstones and gallbladder disease and obesity. Overweight people are more prone to falling and accidents, and are more likely to hurt themselves when they fall.

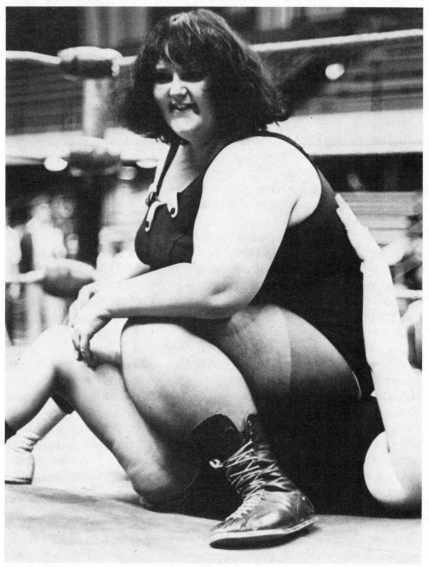

True obesity can cause health problems.

Despite all of the possibilities of adverse health situations, most women will admit they want to lose weight for cosmetic reasons. In their desire to take a magic pill and lose weight quickly, they are willing to go on fad diets that may be more damaging than their real or imagined obesity.

Although men may diet to become more attractive, more commonly they wait until they feel their health is threatened by such things as hypertension, diabetes or cardiovascular disease. The old double standard still exists; a woman is judged first by her appearance, whereas a man is more likely to be judged (and accepted) by his accomplishments, position and wealth. Furthermore, women of normal weight often feel overweight because our standards for women are thin, thin, thin! In fact, being thin is associated (in this country) with being rich; obesity is seven times more common in low income women.

Being overweight, or perceiving yourself as overweight, leads to emotional as well as physical difficulties. The woman who is only a few pounds over what she considers to be her ideal may suffer as much as one who is very overweight. Maintaining underweight is much more difficult than losing weight when you are obese (for most), so there is constant struggle and frustration. Very few are lucky enough to be able to "eat anything" and not gain weight, and I am certainly not one! Often this very frustration leads to depression and overeating. There is no question about the fact that food brings comfort, pleasure and solace, even though we may not even be aware of the fact as we are eating, and the penalty is self-destruction and a furthering of guilt feelings.

Often women who are very heavy feel unloved, isolated and rejected, whether or not this is, in fact, true. If they cannot, or will not, do anything about their obesity, it is important that they learn to accept themselves, because out of acceptance may come a true desire to lose weight. Desire, motivation and awareness are the keys, all the way down the line.

Sometimes being overweight is a cop-out. It can be used as a reason to be dependent and sick; to stay home and not look for that good job or get an education; to go without clothes or dates. It can be used to cause rejection of a husband, or total dependence on him.

The causes of obesity vary widely. They may be psychological, physiological, behavioral or chemical. How many times have I heard women say to me that I'm so lucky to be thin? Believe me, it's not luck, other than the fact that I have always been active by nature. The thought of sitting or lying around all day drives me up a wall!

For instance, I was recently called for jury duty. I knew that most of the day would be spent waiting in the jury room, so I brought an apple and cheese for lunch, and planned to take a long walk on my lunch hour. I did not feel in any way deprived because of my limited lunch, and was looking forward to the walk. While we were waiting for orientation, a woman came and plopped herself down on the closest chair. She looked to be at least 30 pounds overweight. We later struck up a conversation. She bragged about how she found a parking place in the adjacent public lot, instead of the place designated for jurors which she complained was too far away, and a real "hike." (It was half a block.) She also invited me to join her for lunch, as she had located a pizza parlor that served large hoagies. I declined. Enough said!

Part of the reason "thin is in" today is that many women are fulfilling themselves in roles other than wives, mothers and homemakers. These roles often demand that they look and feel well, and be active, vigorous and independent. Obesity does not fit well into this image; in fact, employers often discriminate against a fat person. Part of this is prejudice, and part is justified. Certainly a woman who is happy with the way she looks is more self-confident, and better able to sell herself. The fact is, most fat people are unhappy with themselves. An employer may also feel that a fat person is more likely to become sick, and less likely to withstand stress.

It is necessary to understand why we are overweight (see the chapter on behavior modification), and do something about it sensibly. This means recognizing emotional factors and habits, increasing activity and eating a healthful, low calorie diet. Do not look at the destructive "magic" of intestinal or gastric bypass operations, diuretics, amphetamines, tranquilizers or extremely unbalanced or starvation diets. What you may lose is your health, or even your life!

The truth of the matter is that much more needs to be learned about both nutrition and weight control. We are not sure why some people not only survive but thrive on what is considered a poor diet, while others become sick and develop "deficiency" diseases — why some need an extremely low calorie diet to lose weight, while others with approximately the same physiology can eat more.

What I have found most commonly is that people are truly not AWARE of the amount of food they eat and drink, or of the amount of activity in their lives. (See the chapter on behavior modification.) They come to my spa and swear they eat no more than 600 calories per day and spend all their spare time exercising, yet cannot lose a pound. Invariably they lose weight in the 5 days they are with us, and on an 800 to 1,200 calorie diet. The only way they can become cognizant of the amount that is going into their stomachs at home is to write it down. This means every bit, and every drop of fluid, including bites off other people's plates, "little bits," and nibbling while standing, watching TV, etc. Of course, they are encouraged to break these diet-destroying habits.

You may read this and say "I know I eat very little, and exercise every day, and STILL have trouble losing." You may be absolutely right, and are a victim of those partially understood bioichemicals, some of which create an opiate-like addiction. One, Beta-endorphin, according to Dr. David Margules of Temple University, is called upon in special circumstances, such as stress, hunger and starvation. Apparently, eating in response to these circumstances triggers the hormone, which is addictive, causing one to want to continue eating.

Also implicated in obesity, according to Dr. Jeffery S. Flier of Beth Israel Hospital in Boston, is the enzyme ATP-ase. In a recent study, overweight subjects were found to have significantly lower levels in their red blood cells than a comparison group. According to Dr. Flier, who headed the study, "It is possible this defect predisposes these people to being overweight by causing fewer calories to be burned up as heat, and more to be stored as fat." ATP-ase performs a number of functions in all body cells, including the transport of minerals across cell membranes. Its activity generates 20 to 40 percent of the body's heat energy, and overweight people were found to be 22 per cent less efficient in cellular transport activity, as measured by levels of ATP-ase.

What we can do to "normalize" our biochemicals is not clear. As you may have gathered, I am a strong advocate of exercise. It has been shown that overweight people of all ages move slower in everything they do. Whether they move slowly because they are overweight, or are overweight because they have always moved more slowly is not certain. Chemicals and diet notwithstanding, we burn fat as well as carbohydrates for energy, so move, Move, MOVE!

The Harvard Medical School Health Letter, (December, 1980, Vol. VI, no. 2) had weight control as its primary topic. They state that an estimated 20 million Americans are seriously dieting at any given time; yet on the average, we are reported to be gaining weight. (I have read elsewhere that according to food that is consumed, our calories are down but weight is up.) One possible reason may be our addiction to television, and dependence on the automobile. The Health Letter contains a warning against quick weight-loss diets, products and gimmicks.

The Letter admits that there is no satisfactory definition of obesity, and although there are illnesses associated with overweight, most women want to be thin for cosmetic reasons. They reaffirm the fact that ultra-thin is neither a realistic nor a healthy goal. Some of my very thin students have asked me to help them put on curves in selected places. This is difficult, and requires a lot of time and the judicious use of weights.

The Harvard Letter concludes by listing the following common "myths," which led to many fallacies regarding weight control:

- **"It's better to smoke than be fat."** This is untrue, because cigarettes are deadly, and the few pounds they MAY keep off are insignificant.
- **"Calories Don't Count."** Not true. The only thing that **does** count is

the balance of calories you eat versus the number you use up every day. The kind of food the calories come from doesn't matter. Remember, calories are expended in the metabolic processes, as well as activity, and 3,500 calories equals one pound of fat. That means you will gain a pound of real body fat if you eat that many more calories than you burn. The reverse is true for weight loss. It's difficult to estimate accurately a day's calories within 2 or 3 hundred calories. Counting is useful for losing, but less effective for maintaining weight.

- **"Some foods, such as boiled eggs or grapefruit burn up more calories than they contain."** Wrong. Digestion of food does consume energy, (specific dynamic action), but, claims Harvard, no food costs so much energy that it favors weight loss. Some (not all) people do burn more energy when they eat pure protein, but it is impossible and dangerous to live on this type of diet.

A Yale study confirms the dangers of following a pure protein diet, showing side effects of low blood pressure, problems in the nervous system, and a loss of sodium. The findings confirmed the danger of the possibility of abnormal heart rhythm that may lead to death. The Yale study showed the additional weight loss on this diet was due to the loss of sodium and fluids. WHAT WE WANT TO LOSE IS FAT!

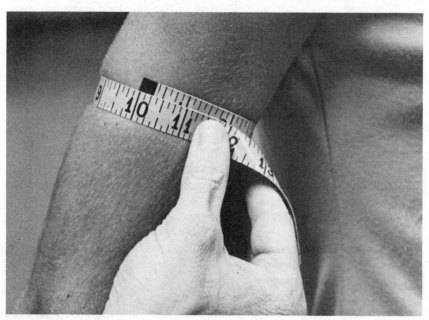

Authorities confirm the fact that "ultra thin" is neither a realistic nor a healthy goal.

Harvard says that **food should be selected for the maximum nutritional value (vitamins, minerals, and other esential substances) for the minimum amount of calories.** This is one of the most important statements regarding nutrition and weight control, and is central to my philosophy. Vegetables, whole-grain products and fruit are desirable; 3 ounces of roast beef, on the other hand, contain 270 calories.

- **"A crash diet is a good way to begin a weight loss program."** Bad, because most of the initial weight lost is fluid. Most crash diets are soon abandoned, and if continued, protein as well as fat and fluid is lost. You may be losing muscle that you need, and when the diet is discontinued, weight will be regained as fat, and you can end up fatter than you started. This will make losing weight in the future even more difficult, as muscle has a higher metabolic rate than fat, which is relatively inert. A person with more muscle can, at rest, burn more calories than a fat person moving about. Yes, women need muscle!

- **"Exercise is unimportant in a weight loss program."** False! In fact, exercise may be the one factor that means success over failure. It not only burns up extra calories that may be added as fat, but it helps regulate the appetite and increase the metabolic rate. It can also lower blood pressure, improve cholesterol, and lower blood sugar.

- **"If you eat more in the morning, you won't get fat as easily."** There may be a slight difference between the way the body handles food between morning and night, but Harvard feels the difference is insignificant.

- **"Everyone gains weight with equal ease."** No! There are differences in the way people gain and lose weight and these are not clearly understood. To return to chemistry, it seems that often an obese person gains weight after one "feast", whereas a thin person will not. This may have something to do with the chemical composition and type of fat each has.

The letter concludes with the following RECOMMENDATIONS:

- **High pressure dieting can lead to compulsive binge eating;** so eat enough low calorie foods to be comfortable, and don't limit yourself to grapefruit, coffee and lettuce. It won't work in the long run, and that's what counts. Losing weight when you are over forty is not the same as it may have been when you were younger. You will probably have to be on some form of maintenance diet for the rest of your life, and it should be sensible and nutritious.

- **Behavioral modification programs,** although not "the answer" they were once thought to be, do seem to help, along with group support. Changing **the way** people eat does work better than simple dieting.

- **Exercise** is a valuable part of any weight loss program. Heroics aren't necessary or desirable, but it should feel like exercise and cause you to perspire and breathe faster. (See the chapter on exercise.)

- **Prevention of weight gain** is ideal, as, once gained, pounds are hard to lose. They mention keeping up with activity and cutting back on desserts when you notice those few extra pounds. This may be enough for some, but not enough for others. Desserts may have to be eliminated altogether, along with making other changes in your diet.

  The significance of weight gain in children is not as clear as it was a few years ago. Although very fat children tend to be fat adults, putting infants on a strict diet may be impractical or even harmful.

- **People suffering from massive, uncontrollable obesity** are likely to seek drastic forms of therapy.

  This includes the protein-sparing modified fast which, as we have seen, can be dangerous and cannot guarantee long-term weight loss. Various types of surgery have been tried. One, the intestinal by-pass, has led to serious complications and is not recommended anymore. A newer technique, which makes the stomach smaller, seems safer; however, all the answers are not in.

Harvard authorities conclude that much needs to be learned about weight control and appetite. They warn against the charlatans that are happy to exploit people's ignorance and unhappiness by selling them worthless and dangerous "miracles." To which I'd like to add that we'd all like to find a fast, miraculous easy answer to all of our problems, but there just isn't any. The pounds that have slowly accumulated through the years will have to be removed the same way.

Fortunately, the fat we put on quickly, say over the holidays, does tend to come off quickly, as those fat cells are "active," the fat is soft, and it comes off first where it last went on. Other than that, the ideal way to lose weight and keep it off is to do it slowly, no more than around 2 pounds a week. The initial weight loss is mostly fluid, and the plateaus that people reach when they are religiously following a diet are caused by fluid retention. Don't panic when this happens, as you may still be losing fat at the same time. If there's one thing that bears repeating, it's COMPOSITION. We are not overweight, but overfat!

People who take diuretics to lose weight are not only kidding themselves, but seriously endangering their health. My friend who borrowed her neighbor's diuretic was thrilled when she lost 5 or 6 pounds. She was not so happy when her entire arm and hand went into an excruciating, painful spasm that lasted 24 hours, as a result of the loss of minerals. She had lost weight, but not a drop of fat. There may be times when diuretics are useful drugs, such as in the case of hypertension or excess fluid retention. They should be taken only under a doctor's direction, and careful attention must be paid to replace potassium, magnesium and calcium through the diet. As far as a natural diuretic is concerned, water is the best. Drink one or two glasses at a time BETWEEN meals, and you will notice the diuretic effect almost immediately.

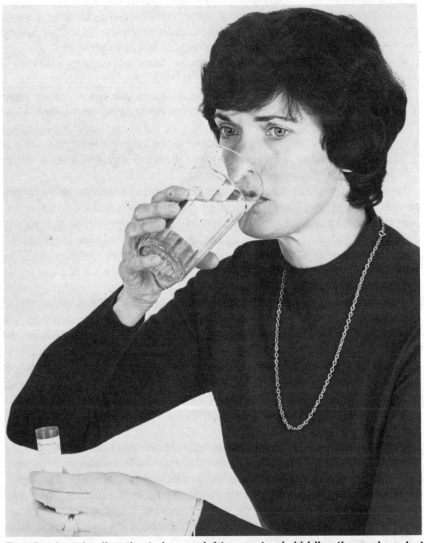

People who take diuretics to lose weight are not only kidding themselves, but seriously endangering their health.

What is an "average" percent of body fat for women over forty, and what is the ideal? According to figures compiled in 1975, the American female in this age category averaged 35% body fat. At that time they felt a realistic ideal would be 30%. Certainly, this is an attainable goal for most. Today some experts would like to see that figure lowered to 25%, or even slightly less. Women should never go below 14% body fat, as they will not only stop menstruation, but will lose essential body fat which is found in the bone marrow, glands, heart, brain and other organs. It is storage fat we want to lose, and if there's lots of it, it must come off slowly.

It is of greater importance for women who are very obese to lose weight slowly. This helps to avoid the "yo-yo" syndrome that is so common, resulting in regaining more fat than what was lost.

To understand this better, we must realize that there are differences between the obese and non-obese person in both the size and number of fat cells. Fat cells in the obese are enlarged (hypertrophy) and increased in number (hyperplasia). It appears that there is an upper limit regarding the size of fat cells, and after this is reached the number of cells determines the extent of obesity. For example, the average person has 25 to 30 billion fat cells, someone moderately overweight about 50 billion, and the very obese may have as many as 237 billion. Weight loss reduces the size of the fat cells, but not the number.

Since the number of fat cells remains constant, the chance of regaining weight remains. This is why we emphasize the necessity of making permanent lifestyle changes regarding exercise and diet. There is absolutely no way you can go on a crash diet, lose a lot of weight, and return to your old lifestyle and not regain the weight—and as we said—a higher percentage of fat. Furthermore, when weight is lost too quickly, those "hungry" fat cells will just gobble up whatever they can as soon as a normal diet is begun.

Although much is to be learned about human fat cells, it appears that the number and size are determined during the last trimester of pregancy, the first year of life, and the adolescent growth spurt. Harvard, however, felt there is danger in putting a young baby on a severely restricted diet. The American Heart Association officially recommends skim milk products, but not for babies under a year, because they need the fat for development of the brain and glands. It seems that once we become adults there is little we can do to alter the number of fat cells. Getting back to the subject of exercise: it can alter both the number and size of fat cells early in life. At our age we can increase the size of muscles, which will replace fat. Do not be afraid of adding a little muscle; unless you use heavy weights and do not stretch properly, you will not gain massive muscles. And I think that today most men would rather touch "firm" than "fat."

Let's look at the different categories we fall into regarding dieting. First there are the massively obese. These women may be carrying around 100-plus pounds of excess weight. They will ALWAYS have to CARE-FULLY monitor their food intake, both during the weight loss period and during maintenance. They should also maintain a lifetime habit of moderate exercise. Brisk walking, flexibility and abdominal exercises are excellent, with concentration on other spots as desired.

The same is true for women who are 30 or more pounds overweight. However, as the weight comes off they will be able to increase the intensity of their exercise, health permitting. They, too, will have to stay on a mainte-nance diet forever; however, they will be able to go off on special occasions as long as they **don't feel guilty about it**, and return to the maintenance or weight loss diet.

I must mention here that the heavier you are the more (food) energy is required to meet the needs of the body, therefore a heavy person will lose more weight on the same diet than a lighter person. You can get an idea how this works by the following formula: If you want to maintain your present weight, multiply your weight by the number 14 to determine the approximate number of calories you must eat daily. Of course, to lose weight, the number changes.

If you are 15 to 30 pounds overweight, it probably came on slowly (although I have known some to gain that much in less than a year). Forget the ads that say you can lose it in a week. You can, with your doctor's permission, engage in vigorous exercise 3 times a week, and increase all of your general activity levels. It will help if you can identify the habits that helped you put the weight on such as wine and cheese before dinner, and television afterwards.

If you have been from 5 to 15 pounds overweight for years, or if you are not actually overweight, but would like to take that much off, you may have to work harder than the others. You have probably reached a comfortable equilibrium where the energy intake is balanced with the energy expended, and you are not carrying around a great deal of excess fat. You will have to monitor your diet carefully, and strive for daily exercise of a half hour or more in duration. Remember, that half hour of exercise, no matter how vigorous it may be, does not take you out of the category of sedentary. Add a daily fast walk in addition to your exercise program, and have active recreational activities. Even with the additional exercise, you will have to make permanent changes in your eating habits.

Now let's look at the woman who put on a few pounds over the holidays. Because it came on quickly, if you are careful, it should go off the same way. Don't depend on diuretics, however. Although some of the weight may be fluid due to eating salty snacks, most of it is soft fat. Go on a 1,200 calorie diet, eliminate salt and make sure you don't miss a day of exercise. You, too, should increase your energy expenditure, even if it's just an extra walk per day.

Those of us who are able to maintain our weight fairly consistently over the years fall into two categories. The first is where I am. We lead a physically active life and, although are not actually "on a diet," are watching our diets, and are always aware of what we eat. We can indulge on occasion, but return to a low calorie diet immediately. We are also aware of the times we get more or less exercise than usual, and adjust our diet accordingly. I will explain how this is done easily.

Finally, there are those lucky few who can eat all they want and never gain an ounce. Believe me, they are in the minority, and many who were always able to do so often find they no longer can when they reach 40. They should concentrate on eating nutritious foods rather than counting calories. For instance, they should choose dried fruit or raw nuts as a snack, rather than candy. They still need to exercise, but for the fun and health of it.

At the end of this chapter will be an approximately 1200 calorie diet. First, let's look at general rules regarding nutrition and weight loss, and see where they coincide.

We must start with the understanding that food consists of proteins, fats, carbohydrates, vitamins, minerals and enzymes, all of which are needed in the diet. Proteins and carbohydrates each contain 4 calories per gram, while fat contains 9. Although fat has more than twice the number of calories that carbohydrates have, excess carbohydrates do tend to cause fluid retention. This is one of the reasons you lose weight on a low carbohydrate diet, however, as I said before, it is fat we want to lose, and this kind of diet can be very dangerous, causing interference with the electrolyte balance. The fats, carbohydrates and proteins come in different forms, which we will look at further.

First, let me throw out a general statement. One way to cut your caloric intake in half is simply to cut your food intake in half, all the way down the line. Of course, first you must be aware of how much you usually eat, and this means keeping a record. For instance, if you usually have 2 eggs, have one, and one piece of toast, instead of your usual 2. If you take seconds, eliminate them; eat half a potato, half an apple, and half your normal amount of fish, chicken or beef. If you find you can live with this and lose weight, fine. It is not for everyone.

Another way that works (for those who are not very overweight, and in good health) is to have a diet of either juice or just one fruit, one day a week. The best fruits are pineapple, grapes or watermelon, and the best day is Monday. You are allowed 3 meals a day, or 5 small meals, and nothing else except coffee, tea (or herbal tea). The amount is not unlimited. If you eat a whole watermelon, or 5 pounds of grapes, you are defeating your purpose. You may lose 2 to 3 pounds on your fruit fast day, but remember, MOST of it is water. Also your fast day should be one of "easy" exercise, such as yoga and walking.

You need an idea of the number of calories that are found in your usual foods. There are a number of good calorie counters available. One, "Calories and Weight," made available by the U. S. Department of Agriculture, contains diet information and a weight range chart for adults. (To purchase, write: Superintendent of Documents, U. S. Govt. Printing Office, Washington, D. C. 20402; ask for 1976 0-205-760, Price, $1.00.)

Other publications are available from the Government Printing Office. They are: "Food and Your Weight" (20¢, G-74), "Food for Fitness" (15¢, L-424), "Nutritive Value of Foods" (75¢, G-72), and "Composition of Foods," Ag. Handbook No. 8, ($3.60 Catalog #AL1/6:38/963). The last 2 publications are excellent references for those of you who are seriously interested in nutrition. They not only show the amount of food energy (calories) found in a wide variety of common foods, but also many of the nutrients, including protein, fat, carbohydrates, calcium, potassium, some of the B vitamins, vitamin C and others. Handbook #8 also shows the sodium content. This manual is currently being revised; so make certain you get the latest information available.

Most Americans eat too much fat, sugar and salt. These are found in large amounts in processed and canned foods, usually along with chemical additives, some of which have not been adequately tested. It has been estimated that most Americans eat about 140 pounds of sugar a year, most of it hidden in unlikely sources such as ketchup and mayonnaise. (Mayonnaise happens to be one of the most fattening foods, containing about 100 calories per tablespoon. Use mustard instead!)

The easiest way to avoid eating these foods is always to eat foods in their simplest, most natural forms. That is, you would eat a baked potato instead of potato chips. If you ate half of a medium-sized potato with the skin you would be getting about 60 calories as opposed to 115 in just 10 potato chips. And who can eat only 10 chips? The fact that they're salty makes you crave more. The baked potato would also provide some calcium, phosphorous, vitamin C and quite a bit of potassium if you ate the skin. Boiled potatoes are even lower in calories. To retain mineral content, boil them in a small amount of water in their skins. You can later jerk the skin off if you want to, but the yellow layer that contains the minerals will be there. It's the butter and sour cream that make potatoes so fattening. Use low fat yogurt and cottage cheese instead, even as a low calorie spread on toast. (Place the yogurt in a coffee filter in the frigerator and let the fluid drain out overnight.)

Some of the lowest calorie foods are also highest in vitamins and minerals. You can eat freely of lettuce, celery, kale, watercress and other greens, as well as green peppers, raw onions, raw mushrooms, sprouts, cauliflower and broccoli. Notice I said eat freely, but not all you want and can hold. Pigging out on nutritious food is still pigging out: poor behavior! When selecting raw vegetables, look for the freshest and those with the darkest green color.

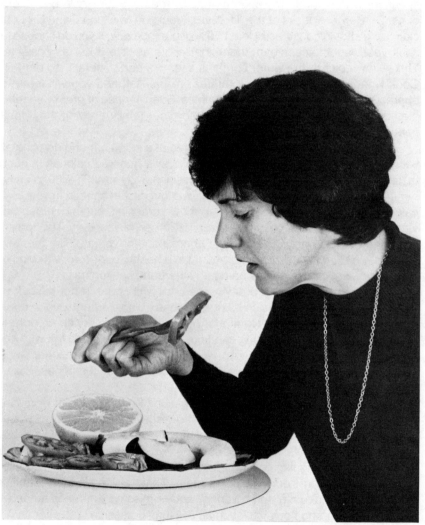

Some of the lowest calorie foods are also highest in vitamins and minerals.

These have the highest amounts of vitamin A, magnesium and other vitamins and minerals. Keep them stored in the crisper in your refrigerator so they retain nutrients. I mentioned raw vegetables for a reason: first of all, we are likely to eat fewer raw than cooked vegetables; and all of the speakers who come to my spa emphasize the need for RAW food in our diets. Dr. Berger speaks of the "lifebonds" found in raw foods, and Dr. Lutz claims we should consume at least 50% of our food raw. If you do choose to cook your vegetables, steam them lightly with as little water as possible. The yellow color in the water contains vitamins and minerals, so drink it! Cook with herbs instead of salt, butter or other fat, and you will learn to appreciate the true flavor of the vegetables. Soon canned or greasy vegetables become repulsive. Cook this way for your family as well; they don't need the sodium or fat either.

Often I see people loading up their plates at a salad bar and dousing all with lots of dressing. You can be getting over a hundred calories in each tablespoon of dressing. Reduced calorie dressings may have 25 or 30 calories, but there are some on the market made without oil that contain as few as 6 calories. (Bunker Hill is one.) Make your own dressing, but remember that vinegar has almost no calories, and oil 120 per tablespoon. Try herbed vinegar, or herbs with a little cottage cheese and/or yogurt. I like the new low-sodium "Vegit," which can be bought in a health food store. It's good in dips and dressings, as well as being an all-around seasoning.

Once we are aware of the differences, we will find it is not difficult to choose whole, natural foods. We would choose a whole orange over orange drink or even orange juice. No matter how much food is enriched, or how many vitamins we take, nothing can take the place of the food the way nature intended. It is possible to live on food, but not vitamin pills alone. Since we do not know all of the factors found in "live" foods, it is impossible to duplicate them.

Why would we choose an orange over juice? For one thing, it would be guaranteed fresh, with no nutrients lost to oxidation. Secondly, we would eat the pulp, which contains fibre and bioflavinoids (see the section on fibre and supplements). We would not consider wasting our time, money and health on something like orange drink. Although it has been fortified with ascorbic acid (which is only one component of natural vitamin C), it contains sugar, artificial flavoring and coloring, and is missing the other nutrients found in a real orange or juice, such as calcium, potassium and vitamin A.

The same philosophy can be carried over to almost everything we eat. Most dry cereals have lost nutrients and fiber, and contain sugar, some to the extent they should be considered candy (see chart). Grape nuts and shredded wheat are two that are made without sugar, but when you have time, make your own oatmeal and cook your wheat whole. I have a supply of whole wheat (not ground, processed, or anything). I soak the amount needed for the following day's breakfast overnight in a small amount of water or papaya juice, then steam it slowly in that same liquid in the morning (or use a double boiler). You will find that with enough fluid in a covered pan you can do other things while your cereal cooks for about 15 to 20 minutes. Do not discard excess liquid, as it contains nutrients. The cereal will be firm, but not hard, and very tasty and satisfying. It contains ALL of the value found in whole wheat, including the germ and bran, and has a natural sweetish, nutty taste. I like to add half a banana, a few raw almonds and sunflower seeds.

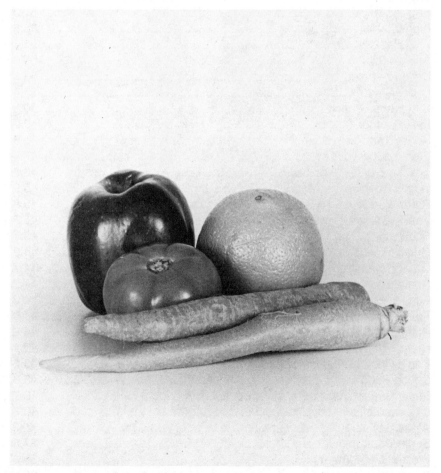

No matter how much food is enriched or how many vitamins you take, nothing can take the place of food the way nature intended.

% Sugar in Breakfast Cereals
from
JOURNAL OF DENTISTRY FOR CHILDREN
Sept.-Oct. 1974

While Keebler's Deluxe Graham Crackers are 48.4% sugar, Nabisco's Fig Newton Cakes are 22.3% and Chocolate Chip Snaps are 45%, Breakfast Cereals are rated in the following way:

BRAND	PERCENT SUGAR (Sucrose Content)
Super Orange Crisp	68.0
Sugar Smacks	61.3
King Vitamin	58.5
Fruit Pebbles	55.1
Apple Jacks	55.0
Cocoa Pebbles	53.5
Lucky Charms	50.4
Cinnamon Crunch	50.3
Pink Panther	49.2
Honeycomb	48.8
Froot Loops	47.4
Trix	46.6
Cocoa Krispies	45.9
Baron Von Redberry	45.8
Vanilly Crunch	45.8
BooBerry	45.7
Quisp	44.9
Orange Quangaroos	44.7
Count Chocula	44.2
Frosted Flakes	44.0
Frankenberry	44.0
Kaboom	43.8
Crunch Berries	43.4
Cap'n Crunch	43.3
Cocoa Puffs	43.0
Super Sugar Crisp	40.7
Sir Grapefellow	40.7
Alpha Bits	40.3
Sugar Pops	37.8
Frosted Mini Wheats	33.6
Sugar Sparkled Corn Flakes	32.2
Bran Buds	30.2
Sugar Frosted Flakes	29.0

BRAND	PERCENT SUGAR (Sucrose Content)
Super Sugar Chex	24.5
Heartland	23.1
Fortified Oat Flakes	22.2
Granola (with almonds and filberts)	21.4
All Bran	20.0
100% Bran	18.4
Granola	16.6
40% Bran Flakes (Kellogg)	16.2
Brown Sugar-Cinnamon Frosted Mini-Wheats	16.0
Team	15.9
40% Bran Flakes (Post)	15.8
Sugar Frosted Corn Flakes	15.6
Granola (with dates and/or raisins)	14.5
Life	14.5
Buck Wheat	13.6
Heartland (with raisins)	13.5
Raisin Bran	10.6
Rice Krispies	10.0
Concentrate	9.9
Crisp Rice	8.8
Rice Chex	8.5
Total	8.1
Corn Flakes (Kellogg)	7.8
Grape Nuts	6.6
Peanut Butter	5.1
Corn Flakes	5.1
Wheaties	4.7
Special K	4.4
Corn Total	4.4
Product 19	4.1
Post Toasties	4.1
Alpen	3.8
Puffed Wheat	3.5
Grape Nut Flakes	3.3
Wheat Chex	2.6
Uncle Sam Cereal	2.4
Puffed Rice	2.4
Cheerios	2.2
Shredded Wheat (spoon size)	1.3
Shredded Wheat (large biscuit)	1.0

Raw seeds and nuts are a delicious way of adding raw foods to your diet, but THEY ARE FATTENING because of the fat content. If you are on a low calorie diet you will have to save them for special occasions or when you are on "maintenance." The best way to eat nuts is from the shell. Then you know they're fresh, and you can't pick them up by the handful and gobble them down.

Dried fruits, such as raisins, apricots and figs are good sources of iron, but are "high energy" foods, which means fattening! They are excellent foods if you are maintaining your weight through exercise alone, or are not overweight, and are nutritious snacks for your children instead of candy; however, children should brush their teeth afterwards.

A word about peanuts, that favorite all-American food. They are nutritious, like other legumes such as soybeans, and seeds and nuts. They are a good source of magnesium (794 mg. in 1 pound shelled) and essential fatty acids (which is why they are so fattening!) The least fattening way to eat them is roasted without oil or salt. This way they contain the most fiber, which helps prevent some of the fat from being absorbed. The most fattening is in the form of pure oil, (120C/TB) and peanut butter contains 95 calories in one tablespoon. I seldom buy peanut butter because it is one of my weaknesses. When I do, I get either fresh ground without salt, or the "natural kind" made from only peanuts and salt. (The others contain sugar and hydrogenated vegetable oils.) Peanut butter on whole grain bread, perhaps sprinkled with sunflower seeds, is an excellent, although fattening, source of complete protein. One thing I do to cut down on some of the calories is to drain off the oil that may separate to the top.

Animal products such as beef, fish, chicken, eggs and dairy products have been the traditional sources of complete protein. Today, for reasons of health and economy, many people are modifying their diets by eliminating beef, or going vegetarian all the way. If you are eating no animal products, you must be careful to balance your proteins and get adequate iron and B-12. My own preference has been to eliminate red meat and most chicken, concentrating on fish, eggs and dairy products, as well as seeds, nuts and whole grains as sources of protein.

Because it is the fat content that has the greatest effect on calories, remove the skin from the chicken before cooking, and buy water-packed tuna. Also, look for lean turkeys and beef, and trim off all visible fat. Some fish contain more fat than others. (See chart.) Cook all meats by broiling, baking or poaching, rather than frying. Season with garlic, mushrooms, onions and herbs, rather than butter or margarine.

Not all fruits have the same caloric or food values. Some of the low calorie ones to choose (these figures are for fresh fruit) would be strawberries (30C per half cup), raspberries (35C per half cup), a quarter cantaloupe (40C), and a peach (40C). Half a grapefruit has 45 calories, and if it is pink or red, 50. However, those 5 calories are a small price to pay for the additional vitamin A. Grapes have only 35 calories per half cup, but the problem is, the quantity is hard to control. Apples, pears and bananas each contain about 100 calories apiece, so always cut a large apple or banana in half. If you eat the skin of the apple you are getting fiber and pectin, a nutrient that aids digestion and has been said to lower cholesterol. The banana will contain high amounts of vitamin B-6 and potassium, the citrus, vitamin C. The best way to keep your diet interesting and to assure that you are getting the maximum amount of nutrients is to eat a wide variety of foods. When choosing fruit, concentrate on the ones in season, and get them tree-ripened if possible. Bananas, this country's most popular fruit, can be purchased all year round. Despite what Chiquita says, if they are getting too ripe you can put them in the refrigerator. Only the skin will darken.

SUGAR

Fruit should be your dessert. Even if you have eliminated those empty calories found in white flour and sugar, be aware that desserts made of brown sugar and honey are still fattening, and can overload your system with simple carbohydrates. You can over-eat fruit also, which is why we limit it to 3 servings per day.

Dr. Edwin Merrifield, a young chiropractor who often lectures at my spa, says sugar adversely affects the nervous system so there is an immediate neurological response of muscular weakness, even when the sugar gets no further than the tongue. He asks for volunteers, and without telling them what to expect, he tests the strength of the deltoid muscle. He then places some white sugar on the volunteer's tongue, and retests the deltoid. The muscle is always weaker. He tests again at intervals, and some recover quickly, while others take several minutes or longer. In any case, whether we are fat or thin, as we grow older our body loses its ability to tolerate glucose. There are many diseases other than caries that are related to an excess of sugar in the diet. First, of course, there is obesity, then diabetes and hypoglycemia. There are claims that some kidney and heart diseases are also a result of our overindulgence in sugar, as well as elevated triglycerides and mood fluctuations known as "sugar blues." Honey, on the other hand, provides some minerals, aspartic acid, small amounts of other nutrients, as well as food energy. Use small amounts; it has twice the calories of sugar. Sugar requires vitamins B-1 and B-2 to be metabolized, and replaces nothing but empty calories, which may be replacing those found in whole foods. When you are dieting and counting calories, each one should carry its weight in nutrients.

Catherine Elwood, nutritionist author of **Feel Like A Million**, claims she has not had a bit of white sugar or flour in over 20 years. Most of us, however, can't or don't want to take this extreme position. Who can say "no, thank you" to a piece of wedding cake? The point is, don't eat wedding cake every day, and if you do overindulge, diet before and after, and increase your exercise.

In fact, exercise is the one thing that will give you a little leeway so that you can, on occasion, eat some of those healthfully fattening foods such as almonds, raisins and figs. The goal is balance: don't kid yourself by thinking that because you took a walk (that may have burned 100 calories) you can now stuff yourself on 300 calories of raisins. It won't work; you'll still gain.

FATS

Fat is another place where people tend to fool themselves. Because of all the low carbohydrate diets around, people tend to discount fat as a source of calories. Of course, fat has more than twice the calories of carbohydrate and protein, and it doesn't matter what form the fat takes. Butter and margarine both have the same number of calories—100 per tablespoon. That is less than pure vegetable oils, as they are 80% fat and the rest water. Whipped butter and diet margarines contain less calories because they have been whipped with water. Read labels for exact counts. Besides the fact that you are paying for water, there is the tendency to eat more because the label says "diet." Because of the calories and the controversy over which is better (or worse) for you, I am using yogurt as a spread.

How is the lay-person supposed to know what to eat if the experts disagree? I am referring to our sources of fat. A biochemist once told me that someday (and that may be now) we will be able to choose whether we die of cancer or heart disease. Some choice! Yet these two diseases are APPARENTLY linked to the type of fats in our diets. Can we forego the controversy and calories by eliminating fat altogether?

The answer is "no." Although it was once thought that there were three essential fatty acids needed in our diet, (oleic, linoleic, and arachadonic acids), it is now recognized that we need only one: linoleic acid. The others, as well as cholesterol, are synthesized by the body. Linoleic acid comes from vegetable sources, and corn oil is one of the best.

Fats are usually broken into polyunsaturated, unsaturated or mono-saturated, and saturated. The more liquid an oil remains when it is cold, the more polyunsaturated. Animal fats, such as butter and lard, coconut and palm oils are all saturated fats. Olive oil is monounsaturated, and oils such as corn, safflower and soy, are polyunsaturated. Beef has the most saturated fat, while fish and chicken also contain some unsaturated and polyunsaturated. The same is true of seeds and nuts, but they are lower in saturated fats.

We are all aware that the American Heart Association favors replacing dietary saturated fats with polyunsaturates. Nutritionists such as Jean Mayer tell us to buy soft margarine with a ratio of at least 3 to 1, in favor of polyunsaturated fat. Hard margarine is unsaturated, therefore avoided. In the meantime, manufacturers of those artificial creamers are using palm and coconut oil, and many cracker manufacturers are back to using lard. (They use what's cheapest, and most readily available.) All the consumer can do is make choices based on the latest available information, and read labels.

My first choice of bread and crackers are those made from whole grains, with no fats whatsoever. I buy whole wheat Sahara Bread (Pita) and bagels, and when I buy crackers, I read the labels carefully. I love cheese, and buy those made from partially or totally skimmed milk, such as Farmer's cheese. Bear in mind that cheese is extremely high in salt, except for a limited few marketed as "low sodium." The one I tested was terrible, but there are new ones on the market that are supposed to taste better.

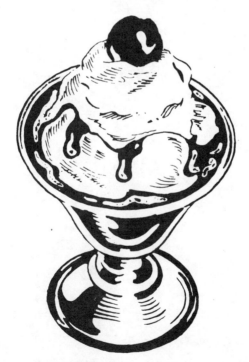

Fats have more than twice the calories of carbohydrates and proteins.

Fat Content, and Major Fatty acid composition of selected foods, taken from **Fats in Food and Diet,** U.S. Dept. of Agriculture Publication, Ag. Information Bulletin #-361

FOOD	Total Fat percent	Saturated percent	Unsatu- rated Oleic percent	Linoleic percent
Salad and Cooking Oils:				
Safflower	100	10	13	74
Sunflower	100	11	14	70
Soybean	100	14	25	50
Peanut	100	18	47	29
Olive	100	11	76	7
Coconut	100	80	5	1
Veg. Fats, shortening	100	23	23	6-23
Margarine, first ingred. on label:				
Safflower oil (liq.) tub	80	11	18	48
Corn oil (liq.) tub	80	14	26	38
Corn oil (liq.) stick	80	15	33	29
Cottonseed or soybean oil, part. hydrogenated tub	80	16	52	13
Butter	81	46	26	2
Animal Fats:				
Poultry	100	30	40	20
Beef, lamb, pork	100	45	44	2-6
Fish, raw				
Salmon	9	2	2	4
Mackerel	13	5	3	4
Herring, Pacific	13	4	2	3
Tuna	5	2	1	2
Nuts				
Walnuts, English	64	4	10	40
Walnuts, Black	60	4	21	28
Peanuts, or peanut butter	51	9	25	14
Pecans	65	4-6	33-48	9-24
Egg Yolk	31	10	13	2
Avocado	16	3	7	2

If the Heart Association says that polyunsaturates are so good for us, by lowering cholesterol, and hopefully preventing plaques from clogging our arteries, why is there any controversy? First, there is the question of vitamin E. When the diet is high in polyunsaturates, the requirements for vitamin E are increased. (See chapter on aging.) Supposedly, the oils themselves contain enough vitamin E to offset this, but not everyone agrees that they do.

The other part of the debate involves cancer, the disease people fear more than any other. Its incidence is on the increase, particularly cancer of the colon. High consumption of animal fats have been linked to cancer by scientists, the National Cancer Institute, American Cancer Society and the (McGovern) Senate Select Subcommittee of Nutrition and Human Needs. In fact, the Committee links the consumption of animal fats to 6 to 10 leading causes of death and suggests eating as little as possible, using vegetable fats instead.

Not all research validates these conclusions. In fact, there is evidence that the reverse may be true.

One researcher who refutes the theory is Mary Enig, working at the University of Maryland. She claims the correlations between animal fats and colon cancer were based on one man's erroneously calculated data. She, and biochemists Dr. Mark Keeney and Dr. Joseph Sampugna of University of Maryland, analyzed the same data and came up with different findings. They found there was an almost 20% decrease in the amount of animal fats consumed in the last 70 years, and a doubling of the amount of vegetable fats consumed. (Furthermore, in the field of research, data that purports to corroborate the theory of the day is readily accepted.)

Mary Enig is particularly interested in the fact that Jewish people have a higher than average cancer rate, particularly breast and colon cancer. Since the advent of "altered" fats, orthodox Jews have been able to eat food combinations they never could before, simply by using them to replace animal products. To determine exactly how dietary habits may have an effect on cancer, Mary is analyzing three groups. They are a Jewish group, a Seventh-Day Adventist group (because of their low incidence of cancer), and a non-Jewish non Seventh-Day Adventist group.

According to Enig, ingesting the unnatural fats may cause them to change their biological functions and accumulate in body tissues. She is not against pure vegetable oils in their natural state. (The most "natural" would be cold pressed oils.) There is even a way of making margarine that would not alter the fats, but the margarine companies are resisting the change because it would be expensive and would price margarine near the cost of butter.

Enig comments that people ate eggs and dairy products for thousands of years, but heart disease is primarily a disease of the twentieth century. She feels that people should avoid processed foods, and eat the way they used to.

This is an excellent idea in theory, and also she is not the only one who advocates it. Dr. Lutz, Director of the Institute of Preventative Medicine, in Washington, D.C., says the same thing. He feels that milk drinkers should return to the non-homogenized variety, and that vitamins and minerals processed out of our foods are equally to blame for many of our ills.

Then there is the story of a nomadic Israeli tribe that ate large amounts of meat and butter products, but had no heart disease. When they moved to the city, and adopted the ways of civilized living, they had the same rate of cardiovascular disease as the rest of the population within only one generation.

It may be simplistic to say that diet alone is to blame. Certainly there have been many other changes in the 20th century. The two most prominent are television and cars, which, with the many other labor-saving devices, contrive to keep us sedentary. There have been major sociological changes adding to our stresses. Surely a more natural way of living, along with consuming more natural foods, would be in order, but this goal appears to be out of reach for many.

FIBER

Fiber, the magic word today, is being touted as a cure-all for everything from heart disease, cancer and obesity, to constipation. However, if we ate natural foods as has been suggested, we would be getting all we needed, and publicity wouldn't be necessary.

Fiber is part of the cell wall in every plant, and is what holds it together. Cellulose, hemicellulose, gum, pectin and lingin, found in fruits, vegetables, grains and nuts make up the fiber in the American diet, typically, 10 to 30 grams. Vegetarian and high fiber diets contain twice this amount.

The various types of fiber perform distinct functions, and have different health benefits. For instance, finely ground bran, which is found in bran tablets and some breads and cereals, is less useful because it does not hold as much water. The fiber in cabbage provides another benefit altogether. Through the process of fermentation, it promotes the growth of useful bacteria that can alter potentially harmful substances.

Numbers listing amounts of fiber in products are confusing, as they have been measurements of crude fiber, that which is left over after it has been treated with strong hot alkali and acid. Actually, dietary fiber consists of all of the cell wall, not just the lingin and cellulose of crude fiber. Nutritionists are working to set standard measurements; so in the mean time, numbers may be meaningless.

Let's look at some of the health (or supposed health) benefits of fiber. The September, 1980 Harvard Medical School Health Letter addresses just this question.

Some of the history of the bran hypothesis goes back 10 years to Drs.

Painter and Burkitt, who noted the low incidence of diverticulosis of the colon in rural Africa, where the diet is extremely high in fiber. As a contrast, this disease is near epidemic proportions in Western societies that eat mainly refined flours and sugars. Other problems linked to fiber deficiencies that are common here but rare there are cancer of the colon, appendicitis, ulcerative colitis, duodenal ulcers, gallstones, hernias, atherosclerosis, diabetes, varicose veins and hemorrhoids.

Harvard makes the critique that it is impossible to name one single factor as an explanation for the difference in disease rate of two populations, when there are many other variables as well. In fact, when Dr. Lutz discussed this, he said he thought part of the reason for the nonexistence of diverticular disease in the rural Africans was because they were outdoors most of the time, and were not forced to hold back gas, the way we do. (That brought some laughs, but there may be some truth to it.) In any case as in all areas of nutrition, more needs to be learned.

Harvard cites the **CURRENT** medical thinking on fiber's role in the following medical conditions:

● **CONSTIPATION:** Fiber helps by increasing the fluid content of the stool, making it bulkier and softer. It is safe to eat on a long-term basis, but one needs to make certain that the diet contains plenty of fluid.

● **DIVERTICULAR DISEASE:** Although the theory has been challenged, they feel that dietary fiber is useful in the prevention and treatment of diverticular disease. (See your doctor if you suspect you have this.) It may take as long as 2 months to see benefits, during which there may be a brief period of bloating and flatulence.

● **IRRITABLE BOWL SYNDROME:** The benefits of fiber may be based more on theory than observation at this time.

● **BOWEL CANCER:** The hypothesis is that bowel cancer, uncommon in Africa, is due to chemical carcinogens that cause the cells lining the colon to become malignant. The theory is that dietary fiber binds the chemicals to make them inactive and promotes earlier defecation, thus reducing their contact time with the bowel wall. A newer theory is that bowel cancer may be related to the fat and protein found in red meat.

● **INFLAMMATORY BOWEL DISEASE:** Fiber has no advantage, either in the prevention or treatment of these diseases.

● **OTHER DISEASES:** It is still conjecture as to whether high fiber diets really do reduce the occurrence of atherosclerosis, gallstones, diabetes, caries, hernias, hemorrhoids, ulcers and the host of other diseases claimed by advocates, although they may be beneficial for sufferers of hemorrhoids and hernias, as there is less straining on defecation.

Although Harvard does not bring up the subject of weight control, apparently it does help, within limits, in more than one way. First, if you eat something high-fiber such as Bran, with a glass of water about 15 minutes before a meal, the fiber expands, giving you a feeling of fullness. I've tried it and found there is definitely a desire for less food. Secondly, fiber, as found in beans, peas and whole grains, is part of a complex carbohydrate, and as such, releases food energy more slowly, avoiding those blood sugar fluctuations caused by refined carbohydrates. These fluctuations often accompany a feeling of weakness, and desire for foods, especially sugar. Third, there is evidence that fiber does cut down on some fat (and calorie) absorption.

Most Americans don't get enough fiber in their diets, and Harvard says there is "no real" hazard to eating more fiber and that it is a relatively simple way to "have an edge" on any possible risk factors for those who are willing to accept a recommendation that does not make any promises."

There is a fly in the ointment of promise. We tend to go overboard in our good habits as well as our bad ones. True, most people would get only benefits from eating foods high in fiber, but some of you are going to start swallowing bran by the fistfulls, and there **IS** danger in that!

Too much fiber can cause diarrhea, and may result in nutritional deficiencies because some fibers can bind with iron, calcium, zinc and other minerals and make them unavailable to the body. Also, because it speeds the passage of food through the intestines, there is less time for mineral absorption, especially calcium.

How do we know when we are getting too much fiber? In this, as everything else, let moderation be your key. Get your fiber from whole, natural foods, rather than those that have been physically altered, such as wood cellulose and finely ground bran. For example, whole wheat, or graham flour, is better than mixed white and whole wheat. READ LABELS. Ingredients are listed in decreasing order of the amount present.

The following is a list of foods, in decreasing order, that are high in fiber:

BREADS AND CEREALS
shredded bran cereal
shredded wheat
whole wheat bread
rolled oats

FRUITS
Apples (unpeeled)
Apples (peeled)
Peach
Banana

VEGETABLES
beans
peas
broccoli
carrots (cooked)
carrots (raw)
cabbage (cooked)

There is fiber in all fruits, vegetables and grains, so these should be the major part of your diet.

SODIUM

We hear so much about salt today, and the fact that it contributes to hypertension in susceptible people, that we want to shun salt altogether. Of course, this would be virtually impossible, since salt is found in all foods, and, in any case, it would be undesirable. Numbers found in popular magazines can also be confusing: one recently said that all we need is 200 mgs. of sodium per day. One would have to be on an extreme diet to obtain this small amount from normal foods.

Sodium, potassium and chloride are the body's electrolytes, and are vital to our health. Sodium and chloride (found together as sodium chloride, or table salt) are found in the extracellular fluid, whereas potassium is in the intracellular fluid. These minerals maintain the acid-alkalin (base) balance of the body, and keep the fluids under homeostatic control. Normally, extracellular fluid is determined by its sodium content. This is why diuretics that cause a reduction in sodium help us to lose fluid weight, and, as we have seen, other minerals as well.

The kidney helps us to maintain sodium balance through the action of the hormone aldesterone. When we increase the amount of sodium in our diet, we lose more through the urine. The reverse is true when we decrease our sodium intake. It is almost never necessary to take salt tablets during exercise, unless you are under conditions to which your body is not acclimated, such as running long distances on a winter vacation in the south. (Common sense tells us that nature didn't intend for us to go from north to south within a few hours, so allow 4 or 5 days to adjust.)

Chloride, which we get from table salt, is important in maintaining fluid and electrolyte balances, and because it aids in the conservation of potassium, helps maintain the proper sodium-potassium ratio. It is a necessary component of gastric juice, is found in the cerebrospinal fluid, and through a process known as the chloride shift, enhances the ability of the blood to carry large amounts of carbon dioxide to the lungs. It is lost along with sodium during sweating and diarrhea, and large amounts may be lost through vomiting.

Sodium, potassium and chloride are essential elements in our diet. There is evidence that hypertension is linked to the sodium-potassium balance, and most of us get about 10 times the amount of sodium that we need, as about a half teaspoon a day is adequate. We easily get this from our foods, even if we add none during cooking or at the table. The 1978 Recommended Dietary Allowances for adults are:

SODIUM:	1,100-3,300 mgs. per day
POTASSIUM:	1,875-5,625 mgs. per day
CHLORIDE:	1,700-5,100 mgs. per day

Potassium is found in all fruits and vegetables. It is especially high in citrus, bananas, potato skins, broccoli, lima beans, cantaloupe, raisins and prunes.

To eat less salt, use lemon, vinegar, herbs and spices in your cooking,

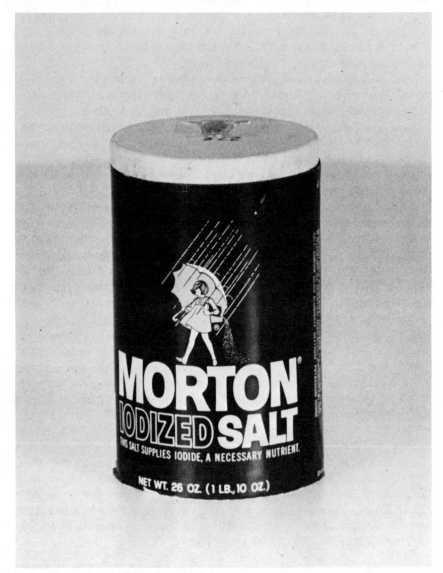

Salt is found in almost all foods. The average American eats about 10 times the amount of sodium (salt) that he/she needs.

and have some on the table as well. Limit foods that are prepared in brine, such as pickles, olives and sauerkraut, as well as salty or smoked meat like chipped beef, hot dogs, lunch meat, ham and smoked tongue. You know that anything that tastes or looks salty is going to contain too much. These foods are potato chips, pretzels, anchovies, caviar, herring, dried and smoked fish. All cheeses are high in salt, especially the processed kinds, and so are canned foods, instant soups, soy and other sauces. You can buy salt-free seasonings. Read the labels. Even things that don't taste salty or have the word "salt" listed as an ingredient may still contain large amounts of sodium. Diet soda is an example. I have known women who habitually drank 3 or 4 a day, lose two or three pounds when they discontinued. True, this is water weight, but it is excess fluid with which you don't need to burden your body.

SEASONING SUGGESTIONS

MEAT AND EGGS:

Beef - dry mustard, marjoram, nutmeg, onion, sage, thyme, pepper, mushroom, bay leaf
Chicken - Paprika, mushroom, thyme, sage, parsley, dill, cranberry sauce
Eggs - Pepper, green pepper, mushrooms, dry mustard, paprika, curry, jelly or pineapple omelet
Fish - dry mustard, paprika, curry, bay leaf, lemon juice, mushrooms
Lamb - mint, garlic, rosemary, curry; with broiled pineapple rings
Pork - onion, garlic, sage; with apple sauce, spiced apples
Veal - bay leaf, ginger, marjoram, curry, currant jelly, spiced apricots

VEGETABLES:

Asparagus - lemon juice
Beans, green - marjoram, lemon juice, nutmeg, unsalted French dressing, dill seed
Broccoli - lemon juice, oregano
Cabbage - dill, savory, caraway seed
Carrots - parsley, mint, nutmeg
Cauliflower - nutmeg, poppy seed
Corn - green pepper, tomatoes, chopped peanuts, chives
Lima beans - minced chives, onion, parsley, marjoram
Peas - mint, mushrooms, parsley, onion
Potatoes - parsley, mace, chopped green pepper, onions
Squash - ginger, mace
Sweet potatoes - candied or glazed with cinnamon or nutmeg; escalloped with apples
Tomatoes - basil, sage, green pepper, onion, oregano

Montgomery County Heart Association
7847 Old Georgetown Rd.
Bethesda, Md. 20014
G57-8678

When reading labels, look for the words salt, sodium bicarbonate (baking soda), monosodium glutamate (MSG), most baking powders, disodium phosphate, sodium alginate, sodium benzoate, sodium hydroxide, sodium propionate, sodium sulfite, and sodium saccharin.

Salt is used in freezing, canning and other processing. If you want to get just the salt found naturally in foods, eat them in their natural, fresh forms.

Some water supplies are high in sodium, including bottled water. Most home water softeners also add sodium to the water. This may not pose a problem for most, however, those with hypertension and on a severe sodium restricted diet need to take this into account when figuring their daily sodium intake. These people should check with their doctors before using salt substitutes, which usually contain potassium salts and may be harmful to certain individuals.

Don't believe the old wives' tale that if you crave something, your body needs it. In the case of salt, it is simply an acquired taste that has become a habit. Let's look at the sodium content of some common foods and their caloric values:

BEVERAGES AND JUICES	SODIUM (mg.)	CALORIES
Apple juice, 6 oz.	2	85
Beer, 8 oz.	15	100
Coffee or tea	0	0
Cranberry juice, 6 oz.	2	120
Grapefruit juice, 6 oz.	2	80
Lemonade, 6 oz.	1	80
Tomato Juice, canned, 6 oz.	360	35
Whiskey, 5 oz.	0	100
BREADS AND CEREALS		
Cornflakes, 1 oz.	250	95
Shredded Wheat, 1 oz.	2	90
French Bread, 1 slice	135	65
Macaroni, cooked, 1 C	1	155
Oatmeal, cooked, 1/2 C	5	65
Rice, cooked, 1/2 C	0	110
Rolls, hard	315	155
Rolls, sweet, 1	215	175
Rye Bread, 1 slice	140	60
Saltines, 4	125	50
Spaghetti, cooked, 1/2 C	1	85
Whole Wheat Bread, 1 slice	120	55
DAIRY		
Buttermilk, 1C	255	80
Cheese, American, 1 oz.	405	105
Cheese, Blue, 1 oz.	395	100
Cheese, Cream, 1 oz.	85	100
Cheese, Cheddar, 1 oz.	175	115
Cheese, Cottage, creamed 1/2 C	455	115
Cheese, Cottage, uncreamed 1/2 C	290	85
Cheese, Cottage, no-salt added, 1/2 C	10	90

	SODIUM (mg.)	CALORIES
Cheese, Parmesan, 1 oz.	530	130
Cheese, Swiss, natural, 1 oz.	75	105
Cheese, Swiss, processed, 1 oz.	390	95
Cream, half/half, 1 T	5	20
Ice Cream, 1 C	115	300
Ice Milk, 1 C	105	185
Milk, whole, 1 C	120	150
Milk, skim	125	85
Sherbet, 1 C	90	270
Yogurt, low-fat, plain, 3 oz.	160	125
FRUITS		
Apple	2	85
Applesauce, unsweetened, 1C	5	100
Applesauce, sweetened, 1C	5	230
Cantaloupe, 1/2	35	85
Grapefruit, 1/2	1	40
Orange	1	75
Raisins, 1/4 C	10	120
VEGETABLES		
Asparagus, 5 spears	2	25
Avocado, medium	10	380
Beans, dried kidney, 1 C, cooked	5	220
Carrots, 1	35	30
Celery, 1 stalk	65	10
Corn, fresh or frozen, 1/2 C	1	70
Corn, creamed, canned, 1/2 C	300	105
Corn, canned, wet-pak drained 1/2 C	195	70
Cucumber, lg.	15	45
Green beans, raw, 1/2 C	3	15
Green beans, canned	150	15
Lettuce, 1C	5	10
Lima beans, raw 1/2 C	1	95
Lima beans, canned 1/2 C	200	80
Peas, raw, 1/2 C	1	55
Peas, canned, 1/2 C	200	75
Potato, medium	5	90
Squash, summer, 1/2 C	1	15
Squash, winter, 1/2 C	1	60
Tomato, madium	5	25
Tomatoes, canned, 1/2 C	155	25
Turnips, raw, 1/2 C	35	20
MEAT, POULTRY, FISH AND EGGS		
Bacon, 2 slices, drained	155	85
Beef, chuck, lean, cooked 4 oz.	55	280
Beef, round, cooked, 4 oz.	85	215
Chicken, light meat, roasted, 4 oz.	75	190
Chicken, dark meat, roasted, 4 oz.	95	200
Egg, 1	70	80

	SODIUM (mg.)	CALORIES
Flounder, raw, 4 oz.	80	90
Haddock, raw	70	90
Ham, baked, 4 oz.	850	330
Lamb, leg, roasted, 4 oz.	70	315
Oysters, raw, 4 oz.	80	75
Pork, roasted, 4 oz.	80	290
Salmon, canned, 4 oz.	590	195
Scallops, steamed, 4 oz.	300	130
Tuna, in water, no-salt pak, 4 oz.	45	145
Tuna, in water, salt added, 4 oz.	250	145
Turkey, dark meat, roasted, 4 oz.	110	230
Turkey, light meat, roasted, 4 oz.	95	200
Veal, cooked, 4 oz.	75	265
FATS, OILS AND DRESSINGS	140	100
Butter (salted) 1 T	140	100
Margarine, (salted) 1 T	140	100
Margarine, (unsalted) 1 T	0	100
Mayonnaise, 1 T	85	100
Oil, 1 T	0	125
Salad Dressings, 1 T each		
Blue Cheese	165	75
French	220	65
Italian	315	85
Russian	130	75
1000 Island	110	80

As you can see from the above charts, foods such as milk, meat, and cheese are high in sodium, and there is a substantial increase with processing. Unless you are subject to hypertension, or have edema or other medical problems, there is no need to buy salt-free products. Reduce your sodium by eliminating free salt, salty snacks, and highly processed foods.

DIETARY GOALS

The Senate Select Committee on Nutrition and Human Needs, originally concerned with programs to eliminate hunger and malnutrition, discovered another kind of problem in this country: bad nutrition. Consumers, scientists, nutritionists and doctors were linking 60% of our killer diseases to diet or obesity.

Some of these diseases, as indicated by epidemiological studies are: certain forms of cancer, such as liver, breast, large and small intestine, and colon; diabetes, hypertension, and cardiovascular diseases. Their recommendations coincided with the advice of 200 scientists from twenty-three countries, that is, to reduce the diet risk factors we should make the following changes in our diets:

- Fewer total calories. Consume only as many as are expended; eat less, and exercise more.
- Less fat, less saturated fat, and less cholesterol. The average American consumes 42% of all daily calories in the form of fat. It is suggested that figure be lowered to 30%, divided equally between saturated, polyunsaturated and monounsaturated. (Pritikin advocates reducing the total fat far below this amount.)
- Reduce the consumption of refined and processed sugar from the existing 45% of our diet to not more than 10% of total caloric intake.
- Increase the consumption of complex carbohydrates and naturally occurring sugars from about 28% of energy intake to about 48%.
- Reduce cholesterol to about 300 mgs. a day.
- Reduce sodium intake to about 5 grams a day.

How do we achieve these goals? It's easier if you stick to the natural, whole foods I have been suggesting. Increase your consumption of fruits, vegetables, and whole grains, and decrease foods high in sugar. Just keep them out of the house altogether. Read labels. If an ingredient listed high on the label ends with "ose" such as glucose, lactose, or fructose, you know it contains lots of sugar.

Decrease your foods that are high in fat. Choose poultry (remove the skin) and fish instead of meat. Except for young children, substitute low-fat or non-fat dairy products for those made with whole milk. The Committee suggests we reduce our cholesterol by eating less of foods that are high in cholesterol. There is, however, a controversy regarding eggs. Personally, I am in favor of eggs, as long as they are not cooked in fat.

When you stop using the salt shaker, you will learn the true flavor of food, and find you are craving less salt and enjoying the foods more.

Decrease consumption of salt, and those foods high in salt (see chart). Remember, if it tastes salty, it contains too much. When you stop using the salt shaker, you will learn the true flavor of food, and find you are craving less salt and enjoying the foods more.

Don't worry about getting fat because you increased your complex carbohydrates. The fear we have eating a potato or piece of bread is unfounded. After all, fat has twice the number of calories; so if you eat the hot dog, and not the roll, you are only kidding yourself. The recommendations call for us to eat less fat, sugar and salt along with increasing carbohydrates; so we would be better off eating the roll, especially if we were lucky enough to find one made with whole grains.

Fat, sugar and salt are hidden in foods, such as hot dogs, bakery products, mayonnaise, ice cream, hamburgers, cheese, highly processed foods, and potato chips, which contain large amounts of fat as well as salt. Adding vitamins, or otherwise fortifying junk food does not change the fact that it is junk, and not worth eating. The pink color of processed meats is not from iron, as it is in "real" meat. Rather, it is from food coloring, food dyes, or sodium nitrate.

Some food colorings, such as those found in margarines are derived from carotene, and safe. Many food dyes, however, are not adequately tested, and several have been banned as they are found to be carcinogenic. New dyes are being added all the time, and the word "natural" on a label does not necessarily mean it is **all** natural. I suffered a severe allergic reaction from a juice that had "natural" in big letters on the label. On later inspection, I found the words "artificial coloring" in fine print. The FDA currently is working on legislation that would affect labeling, especially the use of the words, "natural ingredients."

Sodium nitrate, and its derivative, nitrite, will finally be banned in 1982, as they are carcinogenic. These are found in 7% of the foods we eat: smoked fish, bacon, ham, sausage, corned beef, lunch meats and hot dogs. In addition to their high sodium and fat content, this is one more reason to avoid them. If you do eat them, at least take some vitamin C at the same time, as this reduces the carcinogens.

Low carbohydrate fat diets have caused people to kid themselves into thinking that protein and fat calories don't count. One of my obese male friends thinks that if he takes off half the roll of a Big Mac, the rest won't make him fat. The same thinking carries over to all beef, which is one reason it is suggested that we eat less meat. You will notice variances in the caloric values listed for foods. Size and fat content effect these, but let's look at some general figures for meat, poultry and fish:

Lower	Middle	Higher
2 oz. broiled chicken (95 C)	2 Drumsticks, (160-180 C)	8 oz. pot pie (505 C)
3 oz. lean hamburger (no bun) (135 C)	3 oz. regular hamburger, no bun. (235 C)	3 1/2 oz cheeseburger (no bun) (320 C)
3 oz. lean roast beef (205 C)	3 oz. Swiss steak (315 C)	2/3 cup beef stroganoff, over noodles (525 C)

Lower	Middle	Higher
2 1/2 oz. broiled cod, with butter or margarine (120 C)	2 1/2 oz. fried ocean perch (breaded) (160 C)	2 1/2 oz. baked, stuffed fish (1/2 Cup bread stuffing (325 C)
3 oz. boiled shrimp (100 C)	3 oz. fried, breaded shrimp (190 C)	1/2 Cup shrimp Newburg (285 C)

Because Americans eat millions of milkshakes, hamburgers and French fries daily, the Department of Agriculture analyzed the calories in some of the commonly eaten fast foods. (To get a complete list of the foods surveyed, write: Information Office, Beltsville Agricultural Research Center, Beltsville, Maryland 20705.) Some of the findings are:

Food	Calories
Burger King onion rings	140
McDonald's French fries	238
Burger Chef vanilla shake	259
Burger King chocolate shake	298
Burger Chef apple turnover	269
McDonald's Egg McMuffin	332
Burger Chef hamburger	235
Burger King cheeseburger	327
McDonald's Big Mac	425
McDonald's fillet-of-fish	447
Burger Chef Super Chef	529
Burger King double beef Whopper	662

Even if you are not watching your weight, this isn't the most nutritious way of eating these foods. First, they are all high in fat and sodium. Second, as in the case of French fries, you are not getting the nutrients you would get from eating a baked potato with the skin. Finally, if you are counting your calories, you can see that these foods take a big hunk out of your daily budget, and you usually walk out still hungry.

Please don't think I am advocating walking out of McDonald's and back into the neighborhood deli. Two 4-1/2 inch slices of salami (without bread) costs you 175 calories. Two ounces of ham are only 135 C, but that is only two very thin 6-1/4 by 4 inch slices, and you probably would be unhappy if that's all you got.

SUPPLEMENTS

Most likely you'll be laughed at if you ask your doctor for vitamin or mineral supplements. If you persist, you may be told condescendingly that perhaps some extra vitamin C in the winter or a multi-vitamin won't hurt, the implication being it won't hurt, but it probably won't help anything, either. If you are having heavy menstrual periods, perhaps you will have your blood hemoglobin checked, and iron prescribed. No doubt you will be advised that all the nutrients you need are found in your foods, and if you "eat a balanced diet" (whatever that is) nothing supplemental is necessary.

This may be true for some or even most individuals. Many even thrive on less than the Recommended Dietary Allowances. I have a friend who has been in professional athletics all his life, is about 15 pounds underweight, and has always subsisted on small amounts of the worst junk food. His doctor advised him to take a multivitamin capsule as his diet was inadequate, and he does so sporadically; yet he is, at the age of 56, never sick and has energy to spare. My guess is there are enviable genes, since the whole family has at one time or another been in athletics, one member even having been at the top of world class swimming.

Most of us do not fall into this category: we need to carefully watch our diets and whatever supplements we take. An estimated 20 million Americans are now taking vitamins, including celebrities like: Senator Strom Thurmond, tennis pro Bobby Riggs, Wonder Woman Lynda Carter, actor George Hamilton and singer Rod McKuen. Many of them had their supplements prescribed by their doctors because their high-stress lives left them exhausted. They feel the extra vitamins and minerals give them the boost they need to carry them through fatiguing travel and long hours in front of the cameras.

One of the best known proponents of mega-vitamin therapy is Dr. Richard Passwater, a Maryland biochemist and author of five best-selling books on mega-vitamin therapy. Although he often suggests taking many times more than the RDA of SOME of the essential vitamins and minerals, he cautions that we can overdose on some of the vitamins, especially the oil soluble ones, such as vitamin A, and not everyone's stomach or system can tolerate a sudden concentration of vitamins.

Dr. Passwater advises people to begin their health regimen by adopting the common-sense practices we have been hearing about all of our lives: 8 hours of sleep, no smoking, plenty of exercise, limited alcohol, a balanced diet, and vitamin supplements that do not exceed the FDA. He feels that if you are interested in optimal health, you can then think about taking super-vitamins.

Regarding sleep, my own experiences and many studies have shown that the amount of sleep we need may average 8 hours, but there are wide individual variations. Usually men, and often older people, need less than women. Some do quite well on 6 hours a night; however, if you are regularly getting that little sleep and feel tired all the time, you may try getting more and see how you feel. Some may need 9 hours of sleep, especially if they are very physically active and light sleepers.

Taking supplements can be dangerous if you think that since a little bit is good, a lot is better. Also, if you take high doses of SELECTED vitamins and minerals, (such as just one of the B vitamins), you can create an imbalance that causes a deficiency in others. As I stated before, individual needs vary from person-to-person and time-to-time. There are times, such as when you are under stress, smoking (or around others who are), or drinking, that you may need more of the B vitamins and vitamin C. At other times, other supplements may be indicated. This is why I am reluctant to tell others what I take, other than a specific few which we will look at.

Nutritionist Jean Mayer of Harvard University doesn't prescribe mega-vitamins to the large numbers of people who read his column. Instead, he describes the functions of and needs we have for nutrients, and **highly recommends eating whole, natural foods, with as little processing as possible.** He states that when we eat whole foods to obtain specific nutrients, we are also getting related vitamins and minerals, often absent in processed (but enriched) foods. He does, however, say that a daily multivitamin-mineral supplement won't hurt. The thinking is that many people today do not have the time to eat properly, and often omit highly nutritious foods such as fresh vegetables and fruits. Also, foods that are picked green and stored for long periods of time have lost much of their nutritional value, as have vegetables that are overcooked or processed. Other than a multivitamin-mineral, the following supplements are most often needed by women our age:

IRON

Iron. We need ample amounts if we want to feel and look well, and avoid anemia. Iron makes it possible for the red blood cells to transport oxygen, so it is especially important for a women who is exercising. Some need more of this essential element than others. Premenopausal and pregnant women need more than men, as do young children and teenagers because they are

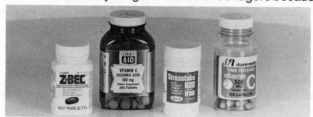

Taking supplements can be dangerous if you think that since a little bit is good a lot is better.

growing. Older people, especially if they eat poorly or have trouble with absorption, may need iron supplementation. The recommended daily requirements are:

GROUP	AGE	RDA
Infants	0-6 months	10 mg.
Children	6 months-3 years	15 mg.
Children	4-10 years	10 mg.
Teenage boys	11-18 years	18 mg.
Girls and Women	11-50 years	18 mg.
Adult Women	18-51 years*	10 mg.
Older Women	51-75 years*	10 mg.

Pregnant women are unlikely to get enough from their diets, and should be on supplemental iron. In fact, it is difficult for most of us to get enough iron, especially female athletes and vegetarians.

If you have been diagnosed as having anemia, it is important you know the type and cause. For instance, if you have pernicious anemia, you will need additional folic acid (found in leafy greens), and vitamin B-12, perhaps by injection. Anemia can be caused by chronic bleeding, cancer, various bone marrow disorders, or, as is common with older people, poor absorption. In these cases, iron or folic acid supplements may mask and confuse the issue; therefore, it is important that you follow your doctor's advice regarding testing and treatment.

The requirements for pre-menopausal women are higher because of blood lost during menstruation. If your periods are very heavy, as often happens just before menopause, your pale face, fatigue, irritability, poor appetite and short attention span tell you that you need more iron. Often iron supplements help you feel better almost immediately.

It is possible to get enough iron through diet alone, although difficult if you are on a limited or calorie restricted diet. Some medications can interfere with iron absorption, as can tea (because of the tannic acid) and egg and milk products (eaten with iron-rich meals). On the other hand, vitamin C, found in citrus, tomatoes, green peppers, melons and broccoli, enhances iron absorption. Plant sources, such as beans, peas and lentils make their iron more available to the body when they are eaten with small amounts of fish, poultry or meat. When cooking acid foods like tomatoes, use a cast-iron pot to increase the iron content.

Not all iron supplements are the same and individuals may react differently to the various kinds. For instance, some get diarrhea or constipation. Ferrous gluconate and chelated iron are usually more readily absorbed, as is iron taken with acid juice such as orange, grapefruit or tomato. A good idea would be to take your iron first thing in the morning with vitamin C and juice.

What foods supply iron? Beef liver provides the most; so it would be wise to eat a 2 ounce portion once a week. Pruce juice, oysters, and clams are also high, as is blackstrap molasses (also high in calories). Cooked lima and baked beans provide iron, but should be eaten with a little animal protein for better utilization.

Foods of medium value are beef, chicken (more in the dark meat), sardines, sunflower, pumpkin, or squash seeds, peas, tomato juice, watermelon, dried apricots and dates, and peanuts.

Sources of iron in the lower range are apple juice, bean sprouts, broccoli, leafy greens, tuna, cabbage (raw), peanut butter, raisins, sweet or white potatoes, winter squash and mushrooms.

If you eat a wide variety of the above foods you will not only be increasing your iron intake, but B vitamins, protein, magnesium, vitamin C, calcium and other vitamins and minerals as well.

Anemia, as detected by the standard CBC bloodtest, is not a sensitive criterion for iron depletion. Iron can be depleted from storage sites, and these need to be tested directly. If you feel and look tired and "run down" although your doctor affirms that you are in good health, and you are not under undue stress, you may still be low on iron.

Evaluating dietary iron is not easy because of the differences in absorption. It has been estimated that only about 10% of dietary iron is available in the body. Heme iron, which consists of 40% of the total iron of animal tissues, is absorbed more readily, and increases the availability of other iron in the meal, as does vitamin C. Intestinal mucosa will regulate iron absorption and keep the body's iron content constant when there is sufficient iron in the diet. In the event of deficiency, absorption increases, but usually not enough in cases of anemia.

If you are anemic, or are having trouble getting enough iron in your diet, avoid eating dietary and medicinal substances that decrease iron absorption such as tea, EDTA, phytates (found in whole grains and beans), antacids and calcium and phosphate salts. This is not to say you can never eat these things, just eat them separately from your iron-rich foods. Although phytates may decrease iron absorption if you are new to eating whole grain or bran products, your body does adapt, and absorption normalizes.

CALCIUM

The Department of Agriculture conducted a survey of 3,500 households in the 48 contiguous states in April-June, 1977, to determine the nutrient content of food used at home. Similar surveys have been done since 1965, pointing up changes in our dietary habits. For instance, we are now eating more protein, cheese, and yogurt, but fewer eggs. Most households, in all income brackets, consumed more than the RDA for protein. The nutrients most often found to be below allowances were vitamin B-6 and calcium. These findings are published in a number of reports by the Agriculture Department, and on the surface, they seem to be conflicting, as B-6 is found in chicken, beef and fish, and calcium is found in cheese and yogurt.

The statistics showed that only 3% of the households used food that failed to provide the RDA for protein, while 1/3 did not provide enough calcium and B-6.

These two statistics taken together should be of special concern to the woman over forty, especially if she is also dieting. The concern becomes even greater if she is on a high protein diet and also drinks diet sodas, which are extremely high in phosphates.

This statement leads into the controversial and not yet fully understood problems of calcium-phosphorous ratio, calcium absorption, protein intake, and osteoporosis.

Bone loss, especially among caucasian women, was up until recently thought to be a general phenomenon that occurred around the age of fifty. Today, however, there is a growing concensus that osteoporosis does not come on suddenly in middle age, but has been developing in older people during adult life. Some feel that the amount of bone found in older people is related to the amount present in younger adults, others that calcium supplements will not prevent osteoporosis, but relieve symptoms by inducing calcium absorption. Now there are some studies indicating that 1400 mgs. of calcium per day (the RDA is 800) may not only treat, but prevent osteoporosis. We have mentioned calcium regarding osteoporosis; however, calcium is involved in many of the body's functions. The contractibility of muscles is just one. Calcium deficiency is one of the first things we think about in treating common recurring muscle spasms, or cramps. Calcium is also being used to treat Herpes Simplex and allergies.

As with iron, we have to consider the question of absorption, which apparently diminishes in some older people. Vitamin D, which we get from sunlight (in the summer) and is found in fortified dairy products and fish liver oil, is needed for calcium absorption. There is evidence the amino acid lysine found in dairy products may increase absorption, as well as acid juice. Many older adults cannot tolerate milk, but must eat yogurt, cheese, and cottage cheese, all sources of calcium. Leafy green vegetables are also good sources of calcium and magnesium, a mineral that should be balanced with calcium (with approximately a little more than 2 parts calcium to one part magnesium). The many forms of supplements include dolomite, a source of calcium and magnesium, and calcium lactate. Dolomite should be taken with a glass of water in between meals (I take vitamin C with it). The same used to be directed for calcium lactate, although now it is suggested that you take it with meals.

In any case, perhaps 70% to 90% of the calcium in the diet is excreted in the feces. It was thought that oxalic acid, found in certain foods, such as spinach, and the phytic acid found in cereals, bound with calcium to form insoluble salts that impaired absorption. This would mean that you would have to discount the milk in your cereal and cheese in your spinach quiche as a source of calcium. It is now considered less important, if there are liberal amounts of calcium.

Urinary excretion of calcium varies widely, although it seems to be fairly constant for a given individual. The average loss of calcium in sweat is about 15 mg., but may increase during the strenuous activity. The amount of calcium absorbed through the gut is related to the amount in the diet; if you eat less, more is absorbed. This brings us again to the problems our "civilized" diet has caused.

Although the figures for humans are not fully understood, there is a desirable ratio between calcium and phosphorus. There is growing evidence that high phosphate diets (phosphorus is found in most foods, is used as an additive, and is extremely high in soft drinks and meat) and high protein diets cause bone resorption (loss) of calcium through the feces. It is for this reason that 800 mgs. are the RDA for this country, while the World Health Organization has found the people in "less developed countries" can do well on far less.

Dr. Michael Lesser, in **Nutrition and Vitamin Therapy** says that a calcium shortage can result in anxiety attacks, as well as depression, a tense and irritable disposition, impairment of memory, insomnia, and cramping in the calves. He also says that calcium helps allergy sufferers because it lowers histamine levels, but must be taken properly to insure maximum absorption.

Dr. Lutz claims if there is pain when you press hard on your shin bone, you may have a calcium deficiency.

Magnesium, which is found with calcium, is also affected by our tampering with nature. Most of it is processed and refined out of wheat, sugar and oil. Soaking, canning, cooking and boiling also causes loss, unless you drink the liquid. According to Dr. Lewis Barnett, the calciferol (synthetic vitamin D) that has been added to milk, binds with magnesium, making it unavailable. Fluoride, added to water that may be high in magnesium, does the same thing by bonding with the magnesium in the blood and forming insoluble magnesium fluoride.

The Food Consumption Survey of 1977 felt that most Americans were not magnesium deficient because of the small amounts found in coffee. Green vegetables, nuts, whole grains and seafood would be preferable sources.

Most of us have reason to be concerned about our calcium intake, absorption and loss. One factor that is usually not disputed is exercise and activity. As with all of our faculties, what you don't use you lose, including bones.

VITAMIN C

No other vitamin has received more publicity, or been the center of more controversy than vitamin C. On one end of the spectrum is Dr. Linus Pauling, who advocates taking several grams daily, while at the other end is the RDA of 60, which is 40 mgs. more than is necessary to prevent scurvy, and is considered to be sufficient for most men and women to maintain a satisfactory ascorbate body pool.

Since vitamin C is usually not toxic unless taken in very large doses (GI symptoms such as diarrhea will appear first), an excess is excreted in the urine, and there is evidence that supplements may be helpful in a wide variety of situations, it is the one vitamin that is often recommended by doctors, even if they feel the effect is that of a placebo.

The function of vitamin C is not fully understood, and there is no "set" amount that is correct for everyone at all times. Certain factors increase our requirements, such as emotional and environmental stress (high temperature), cigarette smoking, birth control pills and other hormones, alcohol, age and drugs. Exposure to air pollution as well as other people's cigarettes also increases our needs.

Vitamin C is found naturally in citrus fruits, tomatoes, strawberries, green peppers and other fruits and vegetables, but is easily destroyed when exposed to air and light, and prolonged cooking. Adding baking soda to food also destroys its vitamin C content, as does pickling, curing, salting, fermenting, and contact with copper.

It is possible to get enough vitamin C from a carefully selected and prepared diet under "normal" conditions, but who among us is lucky enough to drink pure water, eat pure food, breathe pure air and be relatively stress-free?

What are some of the benefits of vitamin C under "normal" living conditions? It enhances the absorption of iron when taken at the same meal, an important factor for women. It suppresses the tendency of the nitrates in food preservatives to form cancer-causing nitrosamines. It acts as a detoxifier on such heavy metals as lead, mercury and arsenic, and the carbon monoxide and sulpher dioxide of air pollution. It increases the therapeutic effect of some drugs such as aspirin and insulin, while at the same time reduces their toxic side effects. (Vitamin C does interfere with the action of certain drugs, and may effect the results of some blood tests, so your doctor should be informed if you are taking supplements.) It synthesizes and maintains collagen, the protein "cement" that supports and holds the body's tissues and organs together. For this reason it is considered by some to be a "youth" vitamin, as the gradual deterioration of collagen is involved with the entire aging process. It promotes healing of wounds and burns, although it may cause scarring, in which case it should be taken with vitamin E. It helps maintain spinal discs, of use to runners and sufferers of "back trouble." It is said to prevent colds, viruses and infections, a statement that is disputed by some researchers. The most common agreement is that if you do get sick, vitamin C will shorten the length of time and relieve some of the symptoms.

This brings us to the subject of the therapeutic value of vitamin C. When using vitamin C as a therapy, technically, one should be under the care of a doctor, as adverse side effects, or masking of symptoms is possible. Also, there is something called "rebound scurvy," which is caused by the sudden withdrawal of large amounts of vitamin C. To prevent this, taper off gradually over a few weeks. As far as preventing colds is concerned, I have often had success by taking more than the usual dose of vitamin C at the first symptom of a scratchy throat, etc., and going to bed, even if just for a short nap. I then maintain the higher dose for the next few days to prevent a recurrence of symptoms.

Dr. Michael Lesser (**Nutrition and Vitamin Therapy**, Grove Press), has used vitamin C to cure mental symptoms such as confusion, depression, and fatigue. He has treated the confused state sometimes seen in the elderly, used it as a tranquilizer, and as part of the treatment for schizophrenia and drug addiction.

There is evidence that vitamin C may prevent atherosclerosis and lower serum cholesterol. Many other claims are made for vitamin C, even that it increases intelligence. If benefits **are** that of "the placebo effect," they are still valid.

What is the best form of vitamin C to take, and when? If you take vitamin C with a meal, it will reduce your chances of getting diarrhea. (If you still have this problem, lower the amount of vitamin C.) Although ascorbic acid is the official designation for vitamin C, and is the component in natural vitamin C that is considered to be "active," on general principles I like to take my vitamins in their natural state, or as close to natural as possible. In this way I am getting related components, such as ascorbogen, and bioflavinoids. Don't be fooled into thinking that because a vitamin label says "natural ingredients" that it comes the way nature prepared it. Usually vitamin C is mostly ascorbic acid with a small amount of added rose hips. Most people think bioflavinoids are useless, but let's see what they can do for women.

BIOFLAVINOIDS

Vitamin P, or bioflavinoids, is found in the pulp and rind of citrus fruit, green peppers, broccoli, cherries, grapes and cantaloupe. Citrus bioflavinoids are the most biologically active, and you will see them listed as such. You may also see hesperiden or rutin, from buckwheat or green peppers. They are found naturally with vitamin C and should be taken that way, but, unlike vitamin C, they have not been determined to be necessary for humans; so no daily requirement has been set.

There is some consensus that bioflavinoids help correct problems with capillary fragility, and they are used therapeutically for this purpose. Since they are water-soluble, considered non-toxic and without side effects, I feel safe in recommending them to women who are suffering from heavy menstrual bleeding. They, along with vitamin C, correct the problem in one to three months. Naturally, you would need to know the cause of the bleeding, but if no disease is present, then bioflavinoids would certainly be preferable to a hysterectomy. The usual dose is 1,000 mgs. daily. After a while you can reduce the amount you take between periods, and take a gram a day on the days it is needed.

Many women I know have been helped by this regimen, several avoiding D and C's. Even if your menstrual cycle has become normal, do not forego your yearly pelvic exam and Pap test. Bioflavinoids may reduce bleeding, but they do not cure cancer.

We have seen that it is possible, although difficult, to obtain all the nutrients we need from a low calorie diet. Although some people need far fewer calories to meet their energy needs, the calories they do take in should be of high nutritive value and well "balanced". Fats, sugars, salt and depleted foods should be avoided, as well as fads such as "high protein, low carbohydrate" diets. The supplements most often recommended and needed are a multi-vitamin/mineral capsule, iron, calcium, vitamin C, and bioflavinoids (therapeutically).

Becoming aware of the caloric and nutritive values of common foods is a big first step. A natural second step would be to eliminate those foods that are high in calories, but have little nutritional value—what we call "junk" foods. Foods, such as raw nuts and raisins, that are high in calories **and** nutrients may be eaten with discretion, depending on the amount of weight you want to lose and the amount of energy you expend. It is just as important to increase your activity as it is to reduce your food intake, and exercise provides us with many benefits other than weight control.

Start from right where you are with small changes. Take the skin off your chicken, and cook without fat, oil or butter. Don't give up because you think you must run a marathon. Go for a brisk walk instead. Drink water between meals, and snack on celery, green peppers, cucumbers and radishes (with a yogurt dip for variety). Walk up the stairs whenever you can; in fact, look for excuses to do so.

The following is the approximately 1,200 calorie Diet Workshop plan we use. This diet may be amended to include more or fewer calories depending on your needs and the amount of weight you want to lose. I am against rapid weight loss plans that extend over long periods of time, as too much muscle tissue is lost.

BREAKFAST: 4 oz. orange or grapefruit juice, or any fruit
1 egg **or** 2 oz. cottage cheese
or 1 oz. cheese, **or** 2 oz. fish +
1 oz. bread (that is one slice, or half a
    bagel or half an English muffin)
or 2/3 oz. cold, non-sugared cereal **or**
1/2 cup hot cereal

LUNCH: 3 oz. fish, chicken (without skin), or tuna
    (in water)
or 2 eggs, **or** 6 oz. cottage cheese, **or** 2 oz.
    hard cheese, **or** once a week only, 3 oz.
    lean beef, hamburger, ham, tongue +
1 oz. any bread +
all you want of low carbohydrate green vegetables such
as romaine lettuce, kale, spinach, summer squash,
cabbage, cauliflower, broccoli, collard greens, asparagus,
cucumber, endive, lettuce + beverage and fruit

DINNER: 6 oz. cooked meat, fish or poultry
1/2 cup limited vegetables, such as carrots, beets,
tomatoes, peas, winter squash, tomato sauce, eggplant,
cooked onions, okra or leeks, brussels sprouts,
parsnips, water chestnuts. All you want of unlimited
vegetables.
Beverage and fruit

You may sprinkle on grated Parmesan or Romano cheese, and have a glass of tomato, Clamato, V-8, diet cranberry or diet Cranapple juice daily. You should include 2 ounces of skim milk daily, or if you cannot tolerate milk, two 6 ounce servings of plain yogurt.

You can make your diet lower in calories, but do so proportionately, rather than eliminating all of just one kind of food, such as bread or fruit. Free vegetables can be used as snacks; so can bouillon, although it is high in salt. If it is more convenient, you may divide your intake into 5 meals rather than three, but don't increase your total amount of food. If you feel like eating less on some days, then do so!

There are almost as many diets as there are overweight people. The most important things to remember when choosing one is that it must not be detrimental to your health, and that it must suit you and your lifestyle. If you can't live with, or make a commitment to, your diet, you will go off it and become another yo-yo.

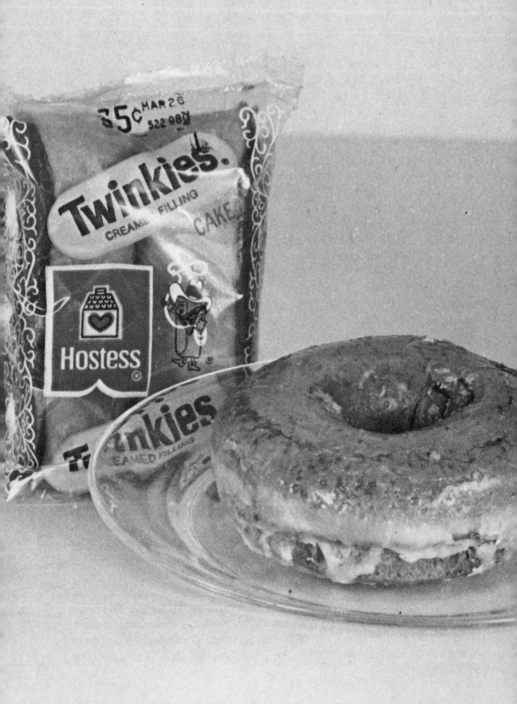

7
MUST WE BE JUNKIES?

Who are the addicts making today's news stories? Women! Women of all ages, and all social, economic and educational levels. These women are not heroin junkies, but addicted to doctor-prescribed drugs. In addition to addiction are side effects caused by the drugs or the mixing of drugs with one another or with alcohol. In fact, approximately 60% of all drug-related visits to hospital emergency rooms are made by women, and the most commonly overdosed on is Valium. Valium is a story in itself which we will tell later.

Who's to blame? Doctors and women themselves. There is a feeling by patients that if they walk out of a doctor's office without a prescription, their visit was wasted. Knowing this, doctors will often prescribe unnecessary and potentially dangerous medication. Doctors are not always aware of potential side effects and rely too heavily on information provided by pharmaceutical companies, which often spend more on advertising than they do on research. Unnecessary drugging is not only expensive, but it is dangerous in subtle ways. There is often a reaction between a prescription drug and simple over-the-counter drugs such as Tylenol or aspirin.

An example of this is a popular diet pill which the FDA has asked to have removed from the market. The pills contain a drug, phenylpropanolamine, which can cause sudden attacks of high blood pressure, and is dangerous for anyone with heart disease or diabetes. One patient died of an irregular heart rhythm while taking the drug with the tranquilizer, Mellaril, and another suffered kidney failure while taking it with aspirin and Tylenol.

Some of the products being withdrawn are: Ayds AM/PM, Control Drops, Extra Strength Appedrine Tablets, Vita-Slim Capsules, Super Odrinex Tablets, Power-Slim Packets, Bio-Slim Time Release Capsules, Diatec Diet Aid Drops and Diatec Tablets. As of this writing, 4 other companies had not responded to the FDA request.

Research on this drug, which is also found in cold and allergy medication, shows there is an alarming rise in blood pressure in young, healthy, slender people. Diet pills alone brings in an estimated 110 to 380 million dollars a year. Perhaps they have an effect in weight loss, but one could get similar results from taking a harmless placebo. In any case, drugs are a worthless means of weight control because they cannot be taken forever, and the patient learns nothing useful from taking them. If you live through it and manage to lose some weight, it will all be regained as old eating and exercise patterns are not changed.

We need to check with both doctors and pharmacists about the risk vs. benefit before we take any drug. In addition to the Physicians Desk Reference, much new literature is delineating drug side effects. Because of widespread drug abuse problems, Congress has moved to require that prescription drug labels describe potential side effects. It is our responsibility to read that information and to inform our doctor of any other drugs (or vitamins) we are taking, including over-the-counter remedies. We also need to ask if drinking, even in moderation, is safe while taking the drug.

Keep this in mind also: even though new drugs are rigorously tested, none can be simply called "safe." In an article entitled "Post-Marketing Followup" (A.M.A. Journal, Nov. 23, 1979, p 2310), there is an admission by doctors of knowledge that information concerning adverse drug side effects is obtained only after the drugs have been prescribed and tested on humans. Many adverse effects take years to manifest. Moreover, drugs (such as aspirin) which were used prior to 1927 were not subjected to the testing procedures now required for new drugs. An example is methapyrilene, an antihistamine recently banned by the FDA because it was found to be carcinogenic in test animals. This drug was a component in non-prescription cold medicines and sleep-aids such as Compoz, Cope, Allerest, Nytol, Sominex, and Excedrin P.M.

We need to look at effectiveness as well as dangers from drugs. In some, less may be better. A recent experiment showed that women with urinary tract infections did as well or better on 3 days of trimethoprysulfanathaoxole as they did on the standard, longer course.

Other evidence shows that many drugs lose their effectiveness or may even become addictive after prolonged use. Antibiotics are an example. They should not be taken unless necessary, certainly not carelessly for the common cold. In addition to the risk of side effects or allergic reactions, antibiotics destroy healthy (and necessary) bacteria, and a tolerance is built up, so that if you do need it, it may be ineffective. Some people take aspirin as a sleep aid, but it too will work for that purpose for a week only, then is useless.

Due to pressure on Congress, another drug, Saccharin, will stay on the market for another 2 years. This is despite much evidence that although it may be only slightly carcinogenic, it has a synergistic reaction with other carcinogens. The consumers are looking for miracles, and they are willing to pay any price.

This need for a miraculous surcease from the problems, large and small of living (and dying), is inducing women to seek help that is, in itself, causing greater problems. Let's consider a related situation that is starting to come out from under the rug: the alcoholic woman. Exactly what the relationship is is unclear, but twice as many women alcoholics as men are also addicted to Valium and Librium. This may be due in part to the woman who denies her alcoholism and relates other symptoms to the doctor, including her vague anxieties. Largely at fault are doctors who tend to think of women as more emotionally unstable than men and have little time to treat them properly. It's easier to dash off a prescription for a tranquilizer.

Alcoholism is a growing problem. Among women, it's not only the drinking but others' reactions to it that makes it worse. People look differently on female drunks, placing a moral judgment upon them as failed mothers, wives and people. We tend to be more tolerant of their male counterparts. In the case of a marriage, nine out of ten wives will stay with their husbands, but when the roles are reversed, so are the ratio numbers.

According to Marian Sandnaier, author of "The Invisible Alcoholics: Women and Alcohol Abuse in America," although there are close to four million American women classified as problem drinkers, the problem and the drinkers for the most part remain in the closet. This, despite the candor of such prominent women as Betty Ford and Joan Kennedy. Families as well as alcoholics deny the disease, leaving the woman protected and untreated.

What can we do for an alcoholic friend or relative? One can go to a mental health center and talk over the problem with a counselor. Often a member of the family will need help with his own emotional needs in trying to live with the alcoholic. If you don't want a personal approach, there is literature available. Many chapters of Alcoholics Anonymous now have women's chapters, and most cities have local councils on alcoholism and drug abuse. There is a new national network of support groups for alcoholic women called Women for Sobriety. It can be reached by mail only in care of Box 618, Quakertown, Pa. 18951.

No prescription is required to obtain alcohol, and unfortunately, this is often true for the number one prescription drug in the world, Valium. Because it is thought of as being innocuous and "harmless," it is often passed out among friends and family members as readily as aspirin. An estimated one in eight Americans will take or has taken this drug, with 45 million prescriptions written in 1978 alone. It was claimed to be "safe and

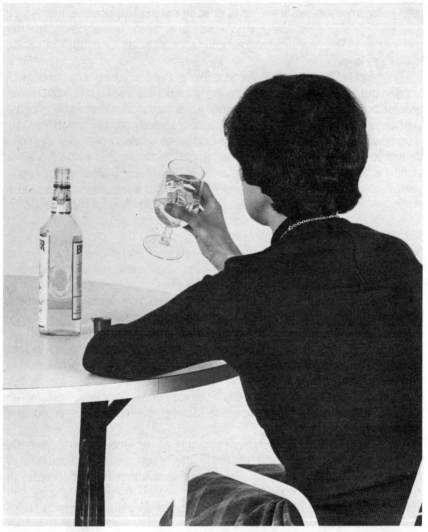

Authorities claim that there are close to 4,000,000 American women who can be classified as problem drinkers.

effective" by its manufacturer, Roche Laboratories. This propaganda was accepted by the general public as well as their physicians, and today no one knows how many are taking this drug or are addicted to it, because it is often purchased illegally and its use (and misuse) unreported.

This is not to say there is no valid use for Valium. It can be used legitimately as a muscle relaxant, sleeping aid and to help control anxiety.

But even for these uses, in most cases, natural means such as exercise, herbs, relaxation techniques and diet would be preferable. Psychotherapy may also be the preferred treatment for many situations treated lightly with Valium. In fact, Valium often masks symptoms, leaving the deep underlying problem unresolved.

Valium overdose can be fatal, especially when it is mixed with alcohol and other drugs. But just as appalling as the numbers seen in emergency rooms is the number of addicts, both known and unrecognized. Prescription data suggests that 20 million Americans take Valium, and some estimate as high as 30% misuse it. The recent formation of "Valium Anonymous" points up the fact that Valium addiction is a very real problem. In addition to its newly recognized addictive quality in fairly moderate doses, Valium can blunt symptoms that can be useful. For instance, a certain amount of anxiety is normal in daily living. It is what impells us to study for exams, obey the law, and take care of ourselves in other ways.

Although we have singled out Valium, the reference here is to all drugs that act on the mind, whether they are called psychotropics, sedatives, hypnotics, depressants or just plain tranquilizers, ordered by prescription, or weaker over-the-counter versions.

For some women, short term therapy may be in order, usually 10 days with no refills. Who should NEVER take them? Of course, those with a known sensitivity should avoid them, as should those with an addictive personality, whether to alcohol or other drugs.

At a congressional hearing, Senator Edward Kennedy, Chairman of the Senate Subcommittee on Health and Scientific Medicine, said that Valium and Librium have produced a "nightmare of dependence" for millions of Americans. As a result of this, Hoffman LaRoche is developing a program to educate the public on the proper use of Valium. Kennedy is also planning a campaign warning of the dangers of mixing alcohol and tranquilizers. Knowledge is the first step in avoiding abuse and addiction!

Addendum: Due to Congressional pressure (much of it from Senator Kennedy) as of the summer of 1980, tranquilizer makers must warn doctors and the public against unnecessary use of anxiolytic (antianxiety) drugs. Five producers of the drugs Valium, Librium, Serax, Ativan, Centrax, Traxene, Azene, and Verstran gave their word to the FDA that their advertising and labeling will contain the statement: "Anxiety and tension associated with the stress of everyday life usually does not require treatment with an anxiolytic drug." The FDA is expecting warnings for similar products, both branded and generic.[1]

[1]U.S. News and World Report, July 28, 1980.

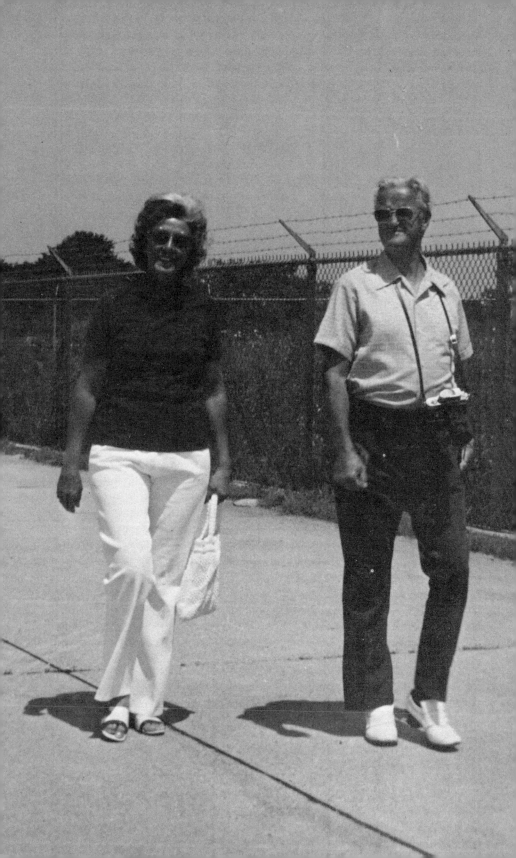

8
ALTERNATIVES: HOLISTIC MEDICINE AND THE *WELL*NESS REVOLUTION

A friend of mine went to his doctor recently with the same complaint he'd had for years: muscle spasms, especially at night, and pain in his legs after walking short distances. Other than these inconveniences, he felt fine. Surely, he wasn't acutely ill. Within the hearing of other patients the doctor yelled: "Nurse, get this hypochondriac out of here." He won't return to that doctor but does not know where to look for help, since he is not "sick"—but not well, either.

Let's define terms. When speaking of "wellness," one does not mean absence of disease. There are many gradations from vibrant health and energy to life-threatening illness. If you suffer from chronic fatigue, headache, lack of energy, obesity, pain, irritability, sleeplessness, or if you smoke or drink excessively, you may not be sick, but you are not well, either. Since most doctors are trained to diagnose and treat disease, they aren't the best judges of whether or not you are well. ONLY YOU ARE! No one knows your physical and mental state better than you do.

A growing number of "traditional" doctors are utilizing this philosophy, accepting alternative treatments that were once assigned to the "fringe," and helping patients in self-diagnosis and treatment, such as blood pressure measurements.

One of these doctors in the Washington (D.C.) area is Dr. Elliot Dacher, chief of the Georgetown University Community Health Plan in Reston, Virginia. He says: "The greatest healer is inside, and I don't think our doctors know our bodies better than we know them ourselves." Not the words one would expect to hear from a doctor with a traditional medical background!

Dr. Dacher asks his patients to accept responsibility for participating in their own illness or health, and when they do, if they choose "wellness," he will guide them. He says, "But if you choose to participate in being an ILL person, I will take care of your symptoms if you have them . . . ."

One of the tools Dr. Dacher uses to achieve deep relaxation is self-hypnosis, which he thinks is quicker and better than T.M. He feels that this, and other self-help techniques can solve many of the major health problems of our civilization today: anxiety, depression, stress, obesity, alcoholism, heart disease and cancer. He says that many of the infectious diseases of the past did not go away because of antibiotics alone, but as a result of better sanitary and living conditions, food supplies and water—in other words, not only medicine, but the whole context of people's lives. Many of his patients now meet in "wellness" groups. (To get on the mailing list and receive the newsletter, write: The Wellness Network, P.O. Box 2531, Reston, Va.)

Dr. Dacher also conducts training seminars for professionals and interested lay-people which are step-by-step learning experiences, where the participant explores the concept of wellness, develops a personal wellness program, and learns a variety of relaxation techniques, including self-hypnosis. Hidden talents are used towards changing and improving the daily experience.

Holistic Medicine is synonymous with wellness. Doctors who practice it in Holistic Medicine Centers around the country are interested, as Dr. Dacher is, in the patient's getting well, and staying well, with emphasis on the latter. Holistic doctors consider the whole person, instead of treating a diseased part. They see a patient as an individual, and consider the total environment: stresses, goals, fears, living, and inter-relating patterns. Holistic doctors often use unconventional diagnostic tools, and "natural" as well as "standard" therapies.

Often those who seek holistic medical help are already concerned about nutrition and a healthy lifestyle. Many are exercising, and taking vitamin and mineral or food supplements. Often they are confused about what, how much, and when to take them, and the holistic doctor can offer guidance in the form of individual analysis. Many of the analytic techniques are not used by traditional medical doctors, but that does not mean they are invalid—just slow to be accepted by the medical establishment.

One diagnostic tool is the Muscle Response Test (MRT), another is hair analysis. For hair analysis, a small amount of new growth is taken from the nape of the neck, and by one of several methods it is analyzed for mineral content, as well as toxic metals, such as lead, mercury and cadmium. Using this method, the specific needs of the patient are assessed and treated accordingly. Another diagnostic tool used in Russia and other European countries, but rarely accepted here, is Kirlian photography, also known as corona discharge photography and electrophotography. It is the application of electricity to an object on an unexposed sheet of film resting on an electrode. The resulting luminous discharge is recorded in color and detail on the film.

Leonard Koniliewicz, director of medical photography at Polyclinic Medical Center in Harrisburg, Pennsylvania, (the only U.S. hospital where Kirlian photographs are routinely ordered for diagnosis), says he has found correlations between finger-pad corona discharge auras and disorders such as cancer and cystic fibrosis. He claims he can accurately time the ovulation cycle, and by these minute variations in skin conductance, find a correlation between physiologic changes associated with illness, often undetectable by other means. Kirlian photography is related to Chinese acupuncture, another tool often used by holistic medical practitioners. Unfortunately, it has been linked to mysticism and occult phenomena in this country, which has hurt its reputation.

Along with acupuncture, a holistic doctor may use traditional Chinese herbal medicines as well as our own drugs. An orthomolecular physician will treat nutritionally, plus advise stress reducing techniques, such as deep relaxation and exercise. One of the things one would learn from these doctors is not only the prescription for exercise, but the correct method (often neglected by many doctors). I have seen many people with back problems incorrectly doing exercises that were on a sheet of paper handed out by their doctors. Often they were doing more harm than good.

An important aspect of holistic medicine is the new and burgeoning interest many doctors, especially orthopedists, podiatrists, and cardiologists, have in sportsmedicine. Only a few years ago, Dr. Jokyl, who was the sportsmedicine consultant to UNESCO told me "there is no sportsmedicine in the United States." It is not true today, as there are sportsmedicine centers associated with universities, hospitals, and clinics all over the country. The magazine **The Physician And Sportsmedicine** reaches every doctor, and conferences and seminars are available to doctors to update their training.

A conference entitled "Sportsmedicine For Rural Physicians and High School Athletic Directors" was held in Boston, in April, 1980. The director, Jerry Ingalls, M.D., an Illinois surgeon with a special interest in this field, believes an important aspect of sportsmedicine is that "You are not dealing with a sick person, but a well person. You don't put 90% of him or her out of commission because 10% is injured."[1] Hopefully, the day is gone when a

[1]**AMA Release: 33rd National Conference on Rural Health.**

doctor thinks that a person with a low resting heart rate is necessarily sick, or that if you injure yourself while running you are restricted to a slow stroll forever. It is important for those of us who are active and want to stay that way to find a sympathetic and knowledgeable doctor.

We often go overboard in our enthusiasm to make changes. Arm yourself with knowledge before you throw away your medicine and run to the herbalist. Herbs, vitamins and minerals can be as toxic as drugs (in fact, in large doses, they ARE drugs) if taken indiscriminately. Examples pro and con were in two recent AMA news releases: Pro: Studies confirm marijuana ingredient is helpful for some cancer patients. The acive ingredient (THC) was given to patients who were suffering nausea and vomiting from drug therapy. According to John Laszlo, M.D., and Virgil Lucas, three-fourths of the patients in the study (who were not benefited by standard drugs for nausea) reported relief; of these, 19% had no further nausea. (If they had used "natural" methods, they would have had them smoke, rather than give them pills.) Con: On the other hand, according to a March 31, 1980 release, the movement towards self-help medicine, and an awareness individuals have in changing their lifestyles to improve health risks, has its hazards. Mentioned were the illness and death of three women using an herb to induce abortion. That article concluded, however, "We should assume that, on the whole, informed consumers will make health choices in their own best interests."

INFORMED is the most important word. Companies that pay medical care costs are making efforts to cut costs by improving the health of their patients. One way they are doing so is by disseminating information in the form of lectures, newsletters, and free publications. A program has been initiated in Missoula, Montana by Blue Cross. This is a three-year self-care education program offered to 200 volunteers. The courses emphasize personal responsibility for health, lifestyle, and medical self-help skills.

Hospitals, clinics, health maintenance organizations and health fairs are providing free lectures, testing, and information regarding subjects such as hypertension, obesity, arthritis, heart attack and cancer risk. Many industries provide noon and after-work exercise, stress-reduction, smoke-ending, and obesity classes.

Some health insurance companies are requiring patients to seek a second or third opinion before undergoing surgery. This is wise, even though a 1974 study published by Dr. Eugene McCarthy of Cornell Medical School showing that 17% of recommended surgery was not confirmed by a second opinion, was recently disputed by another study (1,600 Medicaid patients in Massachusetts). They found that only 11% were told they didn't need the operation, a meaningful statistic if you are one of that 11%!

There are several ways to get a second opinion. One is to ask the doctor making the original recommendation to refer you to another specialist. Another is to see if your health insurance carrier has a "second opinion" procedure set up. In addition, there is a nationwide hotline set up by HEW in 1978. You can call toll free 800-658-6833 (800-492-6603 in Maryland) to find the name of a second opinion referral center near your home.

What changes can we make to stay healthy? Changes in our bodies and environment begin in our minds. According to Dr. Dacher, for many, being ill illicits unconscious reactions. Out of fear of disability, pain and death, we are motivated to become patients. The "patient" gives the responsibility of healing to medical professionals, relinquishing the right to make decisions

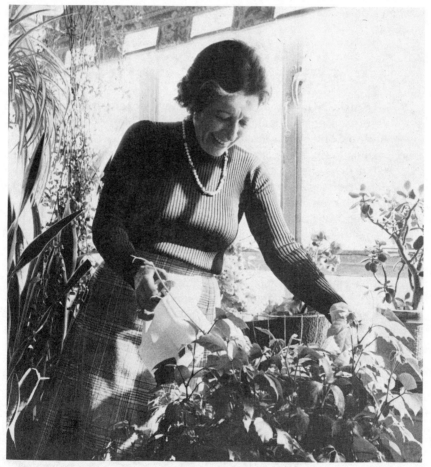

What changes can you make to stay healthy? Changes in your body and environment begin in your mind.

and judgments regarding therapy and lifestyle and denying the inherent capacity for healing and well-being. There is a feeling of having no control over being ill or well.

Just as being a patient is a choice, so is being a well person. You can learn the value of being well and "wellness behavior" even if you are not ill. No matter what therapy you may be currently undergoing, remember: the real healer is within.

Group Health, a Washington, D.C. Health Maintenance Organization, informs its members via lectures and newsletters on ways to stay healthy. Of primary importance are: STOP SMOKING, MAINTAIN NORMAL WEIGHT, AND EXERCISE. Under that they place environmental factors, occupational factors and auto driving habits. Let's start with:

WAYS TO PREVENT
SERIOUS LUNG DISEASE

STOP SMOKING. You can do it! Dr. Donald Vickery, president, Center for Consumer Health Education makes the following statements in the booklet **Who Controls My Health?**

- Smokers have 2 to 3 times the chance of dying from heart attack and 25 times the chance of developing lung cancer than non-smokers.
- Emphysema is a probability, and if a woman is pregnant, the chances of producing a dead or sick baby are increased.
- Smokers, their clothes, cars and homes smell offensive.
- Women who smoke develop earlier and more facial wrinkles than those who don't.
- If you use an oral contraceptive, you have a death rate as much as 6 times higher than those on the pill who don't smoke.
- Menopause occurs earlier in smokers.
- Kissing a smoker is repulsive. (Many people will not date smokers.)
- Smoking is expensive. Two packs a day cost over $500 a year! Think of the fun vacation and wardrobe you could have instead!
- Smoking is a major cause of residential fires.

All of these points apply—plus the simple truth that you will have much more energy if you stop smoking, and you, and everyone around you, will be generally healthier.

If you need help to stop smoking, the booklet "Clearing The Air" offers many hints. Send for it to:

"Clearning The Air," Box A, National Cancer Institute, Bethesda, Md. 20205.

AVOID polluted, smoke-filled rooms, burning of trash, dust, and smog. Finally, there is scientific documentation of what those of us with common sense, allergies, and many doctors have already known: The "passive" smoker is suffering lung damage as well as the "voluntary" smoker (New England Journal of Medicine, March 27, 1980). In the March 13, 1980, issue of the same magazine there is a discussion on allergic reactions to cigarettes from which many unknowingly and unwittingly suffer. There are other harmful chemicals in cigarette smoke, including carbon monoxide, and they reach all of the organs of the body—not just the lungs. These chemicals increase the total susceptibility to cancer, affecting the passive smoker as well. Courts, federal and local governments are finally acting in favor of the victims of others' smoke. Low tar cigarettes are **not** the answer. Scientists are questioning the validity of the assertion that they are less harmful, and other toxins, in addition to tar and nicotine, remain the same.

- See your physician if you have any of the following symptoms: persistent or recurring cough, tightness or pain in the chest, shortness of breath, or coughing up blood.
- Avoid being overweight, as this causes the lungs to work harder and makes breathing more difficult.
- Keep the environment clean: (free of dust, animal hair and dander, and other pollutants that may be inhaled).

Group Health stresses occupational factors as presenting hazards to health. In addition to respiratory tract pollutants, they are exposure to carcinogens, and stress-producing factors such as noise, crowding and boredom. These problems are being addressed by the Environmental Protection Agency and the Department of Labor in conjunction with labor unions and other groups. For your own protection, Group Health offers the following suggestions:

- Wear face masks, and use proper ventilation where air pollutants (dust or chemicals) may be a problem.
- Be aware of, and follow, on-the-job safety regulations.
- Use personal protective equipment.
- Be sure engineering controls are followed.

Many "on the job" safety requirements can be wisely put to use in the home, where most accidents occur. Often it takes a little effort and a lot of common sense to avoid injury.

Finally, Group Health notes that a large number of deaths and disabilities due to car accidents can be avoided, and the following suggestions are made:

- Encourage people to use other, safer means of transportation.
- Drive the speed limit, making allowances for weather and road conditions.
- NEVER DRIVE IF DRINKING.
- Use seat belts for adults, and special harnesses for children. I recently attended a health symposium sponsored by the local AMA. One doctor

put using seat belts as the most important thing you can do for your health!

Common sense practices are just a beginning towards promoting "wellness." Other factors are:

DIET

Overeating and underexercising does more than make you unattractively fat. Overweight people have a greater risk of heart attack, pulmonary and gall bladder diseases, diabetes, and vascular diseases. Even if you are not overweight, your diet affects your health in many ways other than the so-called classical deficiency diseases such as scurvy and beri-beri. For instance, the National Cancer Institute says there are five "prudent principles" of diet one can observe to reduce the risk of cancer:

- Avoid excessive body weight by balancing caloric intake with exercise.
- Avoid a high intake of fat.
- Include generous amounts of fiber in the diet.
- Maintain a well balanced diet through proper intake of vitamins, minerals, fatty acids and protein, plus fresh fruits and vegetables.
- Consume alcoholic beverages in moderation, as there is a high correlation between heavy alcohol consumption and an increased risk of certain types of cancer.

According to findings by the American Health Foundation and scientists from fifteen nations, junk diets and the contemporary lifestyle are the seeds of killer diseases. They feel that cancer, heart disease, and stroke will be even more prevalent when today's children reach maturity.

The conclusions were based on a report of the first cross-national evaluation of risk factors for heart disease, cancer and stroke among 15,000 boys and girls examined during a "know your body" health evaluation in schools. The program was conducted under the auspices of the Foundation, and health experts in Finland, France, Greece, Italy, Yugoslavia, The Netherlands, Norway, Kuwait, The Federal Republic of Germany, Kenya, Nigeria, Japan, Taiwan and Thailand. In the U.S., it took place in New York City, Westchester County, New York, Evanstown, Illinois, and Kansas City, Missouri.

The children showed abnormal findings in measurements of cholesterol, smoking, hypertension, obesity, cardiovascular health and dental hygiene. These findings mirrored the incidence of disease in the adult population, leading the scientists to the conclusion that diet and lifestyle from childhood are implicated.

So, what's new? We've been admonished all of our lives to eat properly, exercise, get enough sleep, and relax. Biofeedback, for one thing! We now

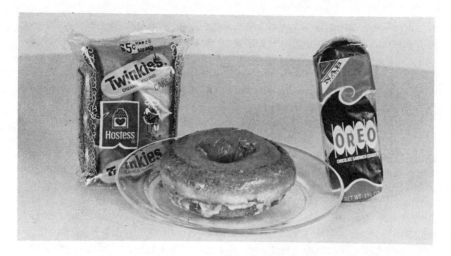

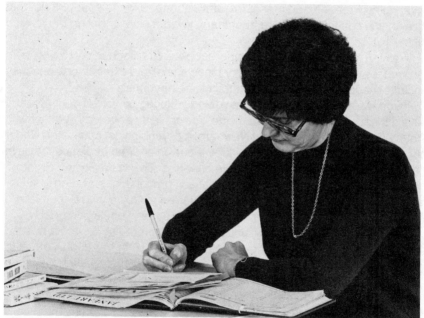

Junk diets and the contemporary lifestyle are the seeds of killer diseases.

know we can use our mind to control our autonomic nervous system, and affect body functions of which we never dreamed we could gain control.

Biofeedback is not learned easily and safely from a book, for its misuse can have negative consequences. Biofeedback has been used success-fully in the treatment of many stress-related illnesses; it is in widespread use in pain clinics, used by orthopedists where other treatments have failed, and in the successful management of circulatory diseases such as Raynaud's Syndrome and migraine headaches. Research is even being conducted involving cancer treatment with biofeedback. If interested, find someone who is legitimate and experienced in its use. Often biofeedback works where nothing else has.

Most of the self-awareness movements today are holistic. Because some of the practices are quite esoteric and "way out," much of the medical profession has been turned off. However, if you are newly motivated, and want to explore the subject further, here is a sampling of information you may learn at conferences or read.

Starting with the familiar and going towards the exotic: The Health Activation Network (P.O. Box 923, Vienna, Virginia, 22180) sells books, training materials and tools, beginning with a family "black bag" health kit which includes many of the things you saw in your doctor's bag years ago: everything from a blood pressure cuff to a tongue blade spoon. If not that brave, you can take a course from them, join the club, or get on the mailing list.

Training seminars led by people such as Dr. Dacher are being held around the country. They are highly motivational and explanatory, and may include meditation and an introduction to self-hypnosis.

If you want to become further involved in taking control of your life, at a little distance from "western" medicine, you could try a five-day seminar with John Adams, Ph.D., and Janet Newberg, a psychological counselor. Under the auspices of the NTL Institute, they focus on a target audience that is in the process of undergoing major life changes. Their Life Styling Program takes the holistic approach towards disease prevention, including relationship building, nutrition, non-competitive games, relaxation and meditation. The emphasis is on integrating all of the sub-parts of one's personality.

You can help yourself even if you are seeing a therapist. Janet Rainwater, a Los Angeles psychologist, explains how to do so in her book **You're In Charge: A Guide to Becoming Your Own Therapist**. (Guild of Tutors, 221 pages, $8.50 paperback.) To become more aware of yourself, she advises keeping a journal of thoughts and activities, and writing an autobiography. She suggests asking yourself two major questions:

"What am I thinking right now?"

"Do I want to continue?"

If the answer is "no", switch to thoughts that bring pleasure, indulge in some creative or relaxing daydreaming, or even something practical like "What am I going to make for dinner?"

The healing experience can be carried even further (out) by "Wellness Consultants" such as Sharon Bush and Tom Goode, in Fairfax, Virginia, who use techniques like progressive relaxation, energy balancing, and auric cleansing. They may not be for the uninitiated!

You've made a good start by reading this book. For additional holistic reading, I suggest:

- **High Level Wellness: An Alternative To Doctors And Disease**, Donald Ardell, Rodale Press.
- **The Mirage Of Health**, Rene Dubos, Anchor Press.
- **The Stress Of Life**, Hans Selye, McGraw Hill.
- **Aerobics For Women**, Kenneth Cooper, Balantine.
- **Maximum Performance**, Lawrence Morehouse, Ph.D., and Leonard Gross, Pocket.

There are an infinite number of holistic approaches and mind-body relationships. With the discovery of endorphins, western science is indentifying on a chemical level what eastern mystics and doctors have known for thousands of years. And for the romantics—yes, you can be "lovesick". It's not only in your mind!

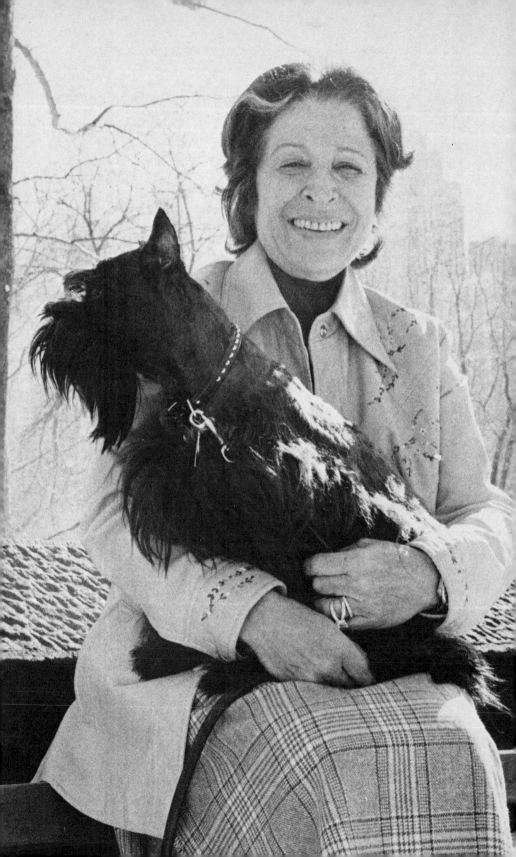

9
ENDORPHINS: DRUG WITHIN

"You are as young as your faith, as old as your doubt; as young as your confidence, as old as your fear; as young as your hope, as old as your despair. In the central place of every heart there is a recording chamber; as long as it receives messages of beauty, hope, cheer and courage, so long are we young. When the wires are all down and your heart is covered with the snows of pessimism and the ice of cynicism, then and then only are you grown old."
Douglas MacArthur

Until recently, most scientists would have placed little or no scientific credence on the above quotation. Nor would they be overly interested in researching "positive thinking" or take seriously the prophet Edgar Caycey's statement regarding the emotions effecting the pituitary gland, and conversely, chemicals produced by the gland effecting emotions. They laughed at Norman Cousins laughing away his fatal illness, and would be reluctant to prescribe Hans Selye's (and my Aunt Anne's) emotionally induced remission of a fatal type of skin cancer. When people recovered after taking a placebo instead of a drug, doctors thought they would have recovered spontaneously, anyway.

They recognized psychosomatic illness (often mistakenly), and came to realize that more and more "real" illness, such as heart attack, back pain, ulcers, and even a lowering of the body's own immunological responses were stress-induced. They saw older people who felt abandoned and depressed, give up and die, and those who remained active and interested both mentally and physically stay healthier and live longer. Dr. Butler, head of the National Institutes of Health's Institute of Aging, places prime importance on these factors regarding the health and well being of older adults. Could these health responses be caused by chemicals within the body itself; and if so, what induces their production and reception?

The answers to this and a host of related subjects are actively being sought by scientists in a wide range of fields. They are just beginning to scratch the surface, but the findings are truly exciting!

What are these chemicals and where do they come from? The average human brain is comprised of ten billion nerve cells called "neurons," no two of which are exactly alike. Each neuron sends thousands of bio-electric messages to other neurons passing at the synapse, a millionth of an inch gap between neurons. It is here that key chemicals that aid in the transmission of messages are activated. These chemicals, called neuro-transmitters, reach the next call with an excitatory or inhibitory reaction. There are receptors within the neuron that act like "keyholes" to specific chemicals or peptides.

Research is progressing on many fronts. In 1973, Candace Pert, who is now a pharmacologist in the Biological Psychiatry Branch of the National Institute of Mental Health, along with Solomon Snyder, a Johns Hopkins psychiatrist who was her dissertation adviser, discovered the first verified system of opiate receptors within the brain, that is, receptors for morphine and other opiates. Shortly afterwards, two British scientists, Hans Kosterlitz and John Hughes, discovered the brain manufactures its own opiates, a natural chemical they called "enkephalin" meaning "in the head."

Their discovery held a special meaning for Dr. Choh Hao Li, Director of the Hormone Research Laboratory of the University of California in San Francisco. He had discovered and synthesized a hormone, Beta-lipotropin, which is active in moving fat away from the tissues to the liver, where it is burned up. However, working with camel brains, he found that he had only some of the peptides in the chain. Drs. Hughes and Kosterlitz's peptide, metaenkephalin, corresponded to numbers 61 to 65 in the camel hormone fragment. These were opiates within the camel's brain. The 31 acid sequence they later called beta-endorphin was 18 to 33 times stronger than morphine.

Scientists are searching for more "endorphins" (morphine within) and receptors. They are finding that it is produced in the pituitary, hypothalamus, and perhaps to a lesser degree, in the spinal cord and elsewhere. Pharmacological firms are racing to produce it, and some is already being used in the treatment of pain. Doctors at the Tulane University School of Medicine in New Orleans, and at the University of California in San Francisco have achieved significant pain relief by inserting electrodes into patients' brains to stimulate their own secretion of endorphin. They think this may be one of the ways acupuncture works.

Dr. Li is excited with the results of endorphins on drug addicts and methadone abusers. After one or two injections, the addict wanted no more narcotics. The known effect has lasted for two to three months, but whether it will last forever is uncertain. Neither is it known for sure why it works, or if it will work on all drug addicts. Other questions arise: Will it work for alcoholism, or mental illness, such as schizophrenia?

What is even more exciting, researchers are looking at peptides with relation to all kinds of brain functions. Some feel it may be the key to eliminating mental illness altogether. They are looking at receptor and neurotransmitter systems that may control all emotions; that is, pleasure, depression, memory, perception, and even intelligence. They have even found a peptide that is an effective aphrodisiac, LFR. Dr. Ruben may be right when he says the most important sex organ is the brain!

There is evidence that we can affect our own endorphins. Long distance runners and other heavy exercisers become addicted. Dr. William Morgan, Professor of Physical Education at the University of Wisconsin, Madison, writes on "The Negative Addiction in Runners." (**The Physician and Sportsmedicine**, Feb. 1979). He feels there is a definite chemical addiction in long distance running. The "high" is real, and may occur (according to different sources) anywhere from thirty minutes to an hour out. Dr. Morgan considers this condition negative when the runner runs despite injury, and at the expense of job, social life and family. He mentions the mental depression, restlessness and other symptoms exercise addicts experience when deprived of their activity. He states that running should be the means to an end, and not the end itself.

Not all experts are in total agreement. Certainly, one should have a little sense and moderation. The "Negative Addiction in Runners" was mentioned at the First Annual Conference for Physical Fitness and Sports for All, sponsored by the President's Council on Physical Fitness, in Washington, D.C., February, 1979. Karl Stoedefalke, Ph.D., of Pennsylvania State University talked of his colleagues who now take a two and one-half hour lunch break to run, whereas an hour was once sufficient. The problem is: the better you get, the longer it takes you to feel as if you have really exercised. This is a typical response to a drug, but one of the reasons you enjoy running in the first place is because it is a mood elevator. George Sheehan, one of the best known running doctors, refuted Dr. Morgan's article. However, one must consider Dr. Sheehan at the other end of the spectrum. He considers running a valid and valuable end, and should not be relegated to the role of "means."

Arnold Mandell, M.D. is a controversial brain chemist and founding

Chairman of the Department of Psychiatry of the University of California, San Diego. He has researched in the field of drug abuse and became apparently overinvolved in the use of amphetamines by professional football players. He is now especially interested in the neurotransmitters morepinephrine, seratonin, and dopamine. There is a remarkable similarity between dopamine and d-amphetamine, a drug which stimulates the central nervous system. In the lab, high levels of dopamine injected into rats' brains mimic the symptoms of amphetamine psychosis: they get restless, agitated, attack and even kill each other. Mandell feels that it is high dopamine levels that lead to character traits of competitiveness, aggressiveness, and violent territorial impulses.

Seratonin, on the other hand, has the opposite effect. A lack of seratonin can cause insomnia. Mandell feels that you can induce your own brain to produce seratonin instead of dopamine by making certain life decisions. By selecting activities such as religion, philosophy, running, and listening to classical music, as opposed to (an extreme example) getting up the hate necessary to play football, one can encourage the action of one chemical and discourage another.

Norepinephrine[1] is another neurotransmitter that is produced in response to the stress of exercise. The nervous system apparently adapts quickly and begins to produce less as early as the second bout of exercise.[1] Are these chemicals produced within our own bodies addictive? The evidence is in the affirmative. Is the addiction good or bad? The question is debatable; however, to make a value judgment, I would say "good." If you are exercising to relieve depression—and it does, albeit, in some cases, temporarily—then one needs to exercise long enough to produce the necessary chemical effect. If the chemical then becomes addictive, it is preferable to valium addiction, alcohol, or a nervous breakdown.

The term "brain over matter" could be put to use regarding endorphine, since there is some evidence that "brain" and "mind" are not one and the same.

Dr. Li isolated chemicals, then later realized their purposes. His "chemical approach" began with isolating molecules, then maintaining the faith that their biological function would be discovered. Other researchers work from the biological approach, that is, looking for a chemical only after its biological activity is known.

Anthropologist Lionel Tiger feels that the discovery of endorphine substantiates his theory that there is a biological basis for human optimism. He views the history of humans as a hunting species: one that would not have survived without hope. Although he feels that hope is genetic, he also

[1]**The Physician & Sports Medicine, Vol #9, Sept. '79 p. 57.**

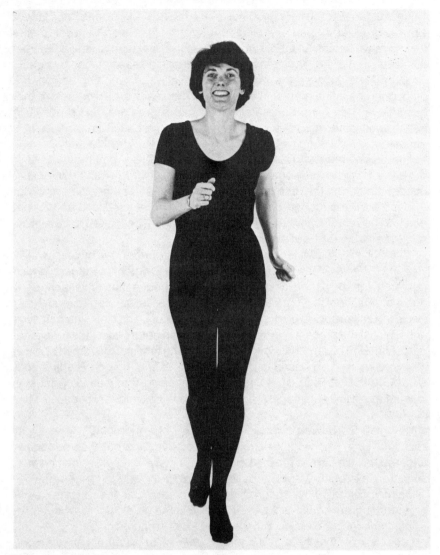

There is evidence that you can affect your own endorphins.

places great emphasis on environmental factors, especially the early experiences of life. Young people who get a feeling that they're worthwhile and competent seem to have a kind of health that may have a physical basis, an "exercising of the optimistic muscles." This type of early "strengthening" tends to carry through a lifetime, making these people better able to withstand hostility, duress, and loss.

In substantiation, a longitudinal study of 204 men done by Harvard University (over 40 years) indicates a strong correlation between mental and physical health. Of the 59 who showed the best mental health between the ages of 21 to 46, only 2 developed a chronic disease or died by age 53. Of the 48 who showed the worst mental health (anxiety, depression, and emotional maladjustments), 18 became chronically ill or died before their mid-fifties. They felt that mental health had a greater effect on physical health than other risk factors such as alcohol, tobacco and longevity of ancestors.

The biochemical implications of mental health are enormous. Loss of hope is damaging and sometimes even fatal. A disproportionate number of people die during the first year after retirement, and others die from grief. Abused and abandoned children often become abused and abandoned adults. The reasons for these phenomena have been looked at from many angles, and Lionel Tiger's is only one.

Although his credentials are impressive, he is surrounded by controversy. He is the Director of the Graduate Anthropology Program at Rutgers, directs research for the Harry Frank Guggenheim Foundation and lectures at dozens of schools each year. He is a pioneer in the controversial new discipline called sociobiology, one that blends social and biological sciences, and looks at the present nature of humans as an outgrowth of the prehistoric past. Although he strongly sympathizes with the feminist movement, he was criticized by women because of his male "bonding" theory. His fifth book **OPTIMISM: THE BIOLOGY OF HOPE** is causing a sensation. Tiger says that optimism is a survival strategy that still holds true today, because it is in our genes.

How can we benefit from our awareness of endorphins? After all, an injection, if you can get it, is extremely expensive. How can we use our own endorphins in the areas most crucial to us, the relief of depression and pain, an increase in energy levels, obesity control?

Gaining control of our endorphins is one of the most basic things we can do regarding our "wellness" or self care. It is the glue holding together the whole package of exercise, nutrition and stress reduction.

Let's look at obesity from a chemical viewpoint. We mentioned Dr. Li's hormone, Beta-lipotropin, which is involved in the "burning up" of depot fat. Another chemical, cholecystokinin, seems to be a "course regulator" of weight, that is, a deficiency was found in people who were more than 20 pounds overweight. At Temple University, a research team led by David Margules, Ph.D., found that genetically obese rats (those bred to overeat) had up to 4 times as much of an endorphin in their pituitary glands as lean mice on the same diet. They also found that certain endorphins and receptors exist in the gastrointestinal tract. What can we do about these chemicals, many of which are still undiscovered?

I was a believer long before researchers found real evidence of cures with placebos (the placebo effect). I did a study with 20 of my students, and a comparable group of "controls." For two weeks they kept a record of their weight, caloric intake, and activity, to establish a baseline. For the next five weeks they kept a similar record but were given a placebo which they were told would automatically burn up extra calories without any conscious effort on their part. Although this study needs to be done again under carefully controlled conditions, what I did find was very interesting. At least a third complained of "stomach rumblings, gas pains" and other minor G.I. disturbances. The ones that accused me of giving them a placebo lost no weight. Those who had been my students for the longest period of time and had the most faith in me lost the most weight, averaging two and a half pounds a week, with no recorded change in diet or activity.

In another instance, I spoke to a man who at that time held the "Guiness Book" record for walking barefoot on coals for the longest time. I asked him if he was able to use this control in weight reduction. He had in fact done an experiment. For one week he increased his caloric intake by at least a thousand calories a day, eating large amounts of cake, gravy and ice cream. Each night before he fell asleep, he went into deep meditation and visualized himself the way he was in college, a much thinner man. By the end of the week he had lost a large amount of fat. (I think it was at least 8 pounds.) You don't have to walk on hot coals to prove to yourself that you can do it too.

Regarding weight control, the missing link between success and failure lies within your own mind! I recently made this statement at a talk I gave at my spa. One of my guests was the head of a large corporation, and part of his function was to train executives. He confirmed my belief by stating that if a person did not think like an executive, he or she could not become one. "As you think, so you are," he said. This principle is stated in the Bible. I added, the key word is not "think" but **BELIEVE.**

Let's move away from endorphins and the esoteric for a minute and see what happens when you think like a fat person. Obviously, you're going to act like a fat person. You're going to head for the nearest chair, and the closest parking place. You'll ask the kids to fetch whatever you need that's up or down stairs. You'll watch the tube every night instead of walking, dancing or bowling. You'll eat everybody's leftovers, and have that ice cream sundae. After all, you're fat anyway, so what's the difference? You will find your most pleasure in eating, but you eat so fast, and in so many places, that most of the time you're not even aware you are doing it. You pop candy each time you sit (which is most of the time), but you tell yourself it's O.K. because you bought it in the health food store. Have you ever noticed that thin people walk up the escalators while fat ones ride? When you think fat, you act fat and you become fat.

Some of these statements are obvious. After all, it is harder for a heavy person to go up and down stairs, and easier to sit than stand. How can "endorphins" change that?

Keep in mind that not all endorphins are beneficial. One, for instance, plays a role in causing "shock" which may be helpful at times, but in extreme, leads to death. Apparently, we have the means within ourselves to activate endorphins, both to our benefit and detriment.

Hans Selye, the world's leading expert on stress, makes an important distinction between "distress" which is harmful, and "eustress" (from euphoria) which has a beneficial, tonic effect on the mind and body. He emphasizes that **what is distressful for one person is not necessarily bad for someone else.** He is the archetypical, racehorse "A" personality type. He finds boredom extremely stressful, and thrives on what may cause a heart attack in someone else. He links all illness (including cancer) to the body's inability any longer to handle the stress placed on it, whether it be mental, physical or environmental (food, chemicals, drugs, smoke, etc). We shall discuss stress further in the chapter "More about stress." It is important to mention it here to reinforce the emphasis on the inseparable correlation between mind and body.

Selye used his mind to cause a remission (if not cure) of a fatal type of skin cancer. My Aunt Anne did the same thing with the same type of cancer. True, she may succumb eventually, but in the meantime, she has had more than ten years of life as a gift, during which she traveled all over the world, painted, sculpted, and enjoyed.

Norman Cousins took large amounts of vitamin C and laughed himself out of a fatal collagen disease. Doctors are no longer laughing at him, and he is invited to speak at medical school graduations all over the country. Studies are being conducted investigating the link between mental attitude and breast cancer. Preliminary evidence shows that women who accept the diagnosis without further question, and those who think they will die, have the highest mortality rate within five years. Those who either deny they have cancer, or fight it in every way they can, including diet, and the investigation of research, have shown to have the highest "cure" rate.[1] The correlation between mind and body, although mentioned many times in the Bible, and practiced by yogis and primitive peoples around the world for centuries, is now being documented by Western scientific evidence. How can we use it creatively, and to our advantage?

Although we do not have full understanding of what happens in our bodies when we practice mind control, we are learning all the time, and seeing results. Endorphins are being discovered and identified. Changes in brain

[1]Prevention, April 1980.

194

wave types are being measured and recorded. Research is ongoing in biofeedback; that is, instruments are recording and returning information to us regarding bodily changes induced by the mind. Changes that are taking place in the autonomic nervous system that were once thought to be out of our control are now shown to be influenced by the conscious mind. These include respiration, heart rate, blood pressure and temperature, muscular tension and relaxation, and more.

How do you begin? The keywords are:

- VISUALIZE

- BELIEVE (FAITH IN THE RESULTS)

- RELAX

Let's start from where we are, here and now. Find a full length mirror, stand nude in front of it and look into it honestly and unemotionally . . . writing down the things you see that you like on one piece of paper and those that you would like to change on another. Sometimes something as simple and honest as an open, free evaluation such as this can induce an "AHA!" experience, as Fritz Perles called it. We can see the obvious, and often easily changeable, when our minds are not cluttered with other thoughts and emotions. We may discover things we can easily improve upon such as hair style or color, make-up, facial hair, and facial **expression.** I had my first experience with this technique when I was about thirteen. I was beginning to discover the opposite sex, and was experiencing the usual self-doubts, insecurities and unhappiness over the way I looked. One day I decided to see what I really looked like. I stood nude in front of my mother's mirror and took a hard look. I saw a lot of split ends on my shaggy hair. I saw round shoulders and a slouch that was intended to hide my newly forming small breasts. I saw a disproportionately large derierre, that was the trade-mark of all of the females on my father's side of the family. I also saw a person that was not fat, and had good legs from many miles of walking and bicycling. In fact, I noted that my legs were my best feature, and the first thing I did was vow to keep them that way. What else did I do?

First and easiest, I had a good haircut. I bought a padded bra, a turtleneck tee shirt, and stood tall. At the same time, I went to the library and took out every book I could find on physical fitness, and sent away for exercise devices advertised in magazines. Of course in those days they were for men, and I couldn't budge them. I learned that sitting would increase the span of my butt, and I haven't sat down since—well, hardly ever! (I am sitting now.) In addition, I did the exercises in the books, and with the improvement in posture, soon saw my waist and buttocks get smaller and firmer, and my abdomen flatten. I began a lifetime habit of exercise—one that you can begin NOW, TODAY, no matter what your age.

Note that which you want to improve upon, but don't dwell on your imperfections, as they will then become even further entrenched in your mind. Instead, TAKE SPECIAL NOTICE OF YOUR GOOD FEATURES, AND VISUALIZE AS ALREADY CHANGED THOSE YOU WANT CHANGED.

How can you picture something in your mind that is not apparent in your mirror? Make use of "creative fantasy;" that is, mentally picture yourself as being, looking and acting the way you would like to. NEVER PICTURE YOURSELF AS DOING SOMETHING YOU FIND UNDESIRABLE, such as stuttering, or stumbling. If that's the picture you hold, that's what you will create.

To carry this even further, if you wish to appear beautiful to someone, when you are with that person imagine they are thinking of you as beautiful. Thoughts, impelled by belief and emotional desire, are alive; and they affect not only us ourselves, but reach out to those around us.

If it's a more attractive figure you want, visualize yourself as already having it, and reward yourself mentally by fantasizing as reality the pleasure you will obtain from achieving your goal. These pleasures could be wearing more attractive, stylish clothes, compliments from women or men friends, male admiration, whistles or whatever.

Suppose you cannot dredge up a picture of yourself with an attractive body. If at one time you were thinner, find an old picture of yourself and put it on your bathroom mirror where you can see it often. Put another one on your bedroom mirror, and one on the refrigerator door as a reminder. Keep this image in your mind. An alternative to this is to select some attractive "bodies" from magazines, and put the picture of your head on top. Be realistic, though. If you are five feet tall, don't try to become a New York stick model.

You have completed the first step, that is, VISUALIZATION. But as I said before, thinking is not enough. You have to BELIEVE, AND HAVE FAITH IN YOUR BELIEF. You may have difficulty with this, especially if your logical mind tells you it just is not so. This is one reason why **realistic goals are important**, so you do not become discouraged before you begin. How can we increase our ability to BELIEVE? Looking at those pictures frequently is one way. RELAXING AND MEDITATING IS ANOTHER.

The thoughts and images we hold before we go to sleep at night will be working towards becoming reality through our subconscious. Going back to endorphins, the chemicals we stimulate will be activated, either for our good or detriment. The body is the computer, BUT WE ARE THE PROGRAMMERS!

We shall discuss further the various techniques of deep relaxation and meditation in the chapter on Stress; however, some brief hints here will get you started. The purpose is to relax your physical body and your conscious mind, and replace undesirable thoughts and emotions with a picture of yourself that represents your goal. If you go into this with the idea that it won't work, it won't. REMEMBER, BELIEF IS THE KEY INGREDIENT. Let me give you an example. I have a friend who was a subject in experiments using biofeedback at the National Institutes of Health. The study was having some success helping people with Raynaud's Syndrome, a circulatory disease. Betty knew it wouldn't help her, and of course it didn't. She wasted her time. This person not only failed to receive help from this study, she is an example of what I am speaking of—but on the negative side. She does not have a clear image of herself and has gone from very thin to fit, always thinking of herself as "fat." She expects to fall and become injured and always does. She anticipates and receives all kinds of problems and calamaties. She honestly believes they will befall her and they do! Some of these problems are a result of our early childhood training. If you see yourself in this same cycle, you may need help. Often psychological counseling can help one see oneself and relationships in a more beneficial light.

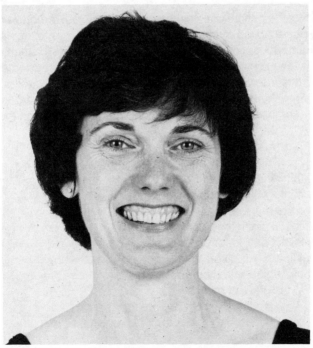

You have to believe that you can achieve your goals and HAVE FAITH IN YOUR BELIEF.

If we have a healthy outlook, we can visualize good for ourselves. The best time to begin is before sleep, RELAXING, AND VISUALIZING.

- Take a deep breath in, and hold it 4 seconds.
- Exhale completely and very slowly, and hold the air OUT 4 seconds.
- Do this 4 times, lengthening and slowing each inhalation and exhalation.
- Relax your body, beginning with your feet and working up to your head, telling each part to relax 5 times.
- Let your body feel limp and heavy, and sink into the bed. Visualize nothing, or black velvet.
- Be aware of your entire body. If any part still feels tense, tell it to relax.
- Breathe in slowly, and as you do so, **visualize yourself the way you want to be.** Repeat 3 times.

It is absolutely crucial that the statements (or affirmations) you make, and the pictures you visualize are positive, rather than negative. In autosuggestion, or self-hypnosis (and this is a mild form of it) we create what we affirm: "I am thin" rather than "I am not fat."

If health is your goal, say "I am in perfect health in every way" and visualize yourself that way. If you want to relax, say "I am relaxed." Never say "I am not tense."

This technique can be used several times a day, but remember to get into a relaxed physical and mental state first. The best times for implanting your goals in your subconscious mind are the last thing before sleep, and when you are just awakening in the morning. These are the times when the conscious mind relinquishes control. Don't negate your active mind, however, because your thoughts and the emotions they impell affect us in many ways, they are just beginning to be understood. Reflect upon the following poem:

STATE OF MIND

If you think you are beaten, you are.
If you think you dare not, you don't.
If you'd like the win, but think you can't,
It's almost a cinch that you won't.
If you think you'll lose, you've lost.
For out in the world you'll find
Success begins with a person's will—
It's all in the state of mind.

—Author Unknown

Another way our mind affects our weight is obvious; yet many are still unaware the significance of the mind—that is, the effects of our moods on our eating patterns. Often, a negative mood signals hunger. Many people eat when they are angry, depressed, hurt, tired or bored. Awareness of this fact is the first step in substituting alternatives for eating. How about lying down and visualizing yourself doing something that gives you great pleasure, looking and feeling great while you're going about it. Next time you are bored or irritated, if possible, do it! Or, run around the block.

Let's return to that person you saw in the mirror. How was the picture? Was your chest down near your navel, were your shoulders and upper back round (kyphosis), was there a sway in your lower back (lordosis), or perhaps a lateral misalignment (scoliosis)?* If any or all of that fits you, read on.

Good posture, or body alignment, is more than just correct structural and muscular balance. It begins in the mind! Even a person with the most exemplary posture will slump or slouch when depressed. The reverse is also true: A "down" body position has that effect on the mind and emotions. Furthermore, your body will expend more energy to maintain an imbalance, and your breathing will be shallow so that you will be lacking in vital, energy-giving oxygen.

There is a customary stoop in people with depressing, purposeless, degrading lifestyles. The word "downtrodden" literally reflects on the body.

On the other hand, a "regal bearing" means just that. You see few queens or those with a high self-esteem slumping and slouching along. Your self image is crucial: IF IT IS NEGATIVE, CHANGE IT DURING YOUR PERIODS OF AUTO-SUGGESTION!

In addition to the mechanical, there is a biochemical relationship between the mind and posture. Your state of arousal is controlled by the central nervous system, which is governed by the "Reticular Activating Mechanism" or RAM. The RAM receives impulses from the sensory nervous system and discharges motor impulses that affect muscles. When the RAM is activated, there is an increase in tension. When you are depressed, your muscular tension decreases. If it decreases enough, you slouch, and move slowly and half-heartedly. The reverse occurs when you are happy and confident: your posture and alertness reflect your mood.

We can deliberately excite our "RAM." Cheer yourself on! Actually shout some encouragement, or some happy thought. Imagine vividly that you won the lottery or accomplished some exciting feat. Imagine the way you would feel at that time, and then if it is at all possible, go out and do something that brings you pleasure. Don't go out and eat something fattening or spend an excessive amount of money, because these acts will make you feel guilty, and you will be right back where you started.

What other connection is there between posture and the mind? Dr. Lowell

*Deviations may be muscular rather than structural, and correctible by awareness and exercises.

199

Ward is a chiropractor who has had much success with his principles of "spinal stressology." He believes misalignment of the spine can affect the mind and emotions and conversely, strong psychological traits can cause spinal abnormalities, such as scoliosis. For many patients, he recommends counseling along with other therapies.

The evidence confirms the idea that we can consciously strengthen our own abilities to create that which we desire. We can take control of our own reins!

10
STRESS
AND RELAXATION

Stress: Every day we read something new about it. We all know, too, when we suffer from it acutely—loss of a job, or applying for a new one, divorce, death, sickness, all potential sources of acute or chronic stress. However, many of us are still not aware of the fact that the body and mind are inseparable, a point I cannot emphasize enough. Stressors (causes of the stress reaction) can be in the mind and affect the body, or, like weather, affect the body first. In any case, there is a body-mind reaction.

What is STRESS? Webster's defines it as "a physical, chemical or emotional factor that causes bodily or mental tension, and may be a factor in disease causation." Taber's Medical Dictionary says it is believed that a certain amount of stress is needed to maintain well-being. Excess can cause pathology.

Hans Selye, the grand vizier of stress, originated his concepts thirty-five years ago when he documented the body's physiological responses to physical or emotional pressures. He termed the biochemical reaction to stress the three-stage "general adaptation syndrome."

• First stage, the alarm reaction, or "fight or flight." During this stage the adrenal-cortical system produces hormones essential to fighting or running away. The heart rate increases, blood sugar elevates, pupils dilate, and digestion slows. This reaction can have a negative effect on the body, because in today's society, most of the time we are unable to fight or run from stressors. One of the results of this unused energy is tense, shortened and painful muscles. Another may be an excess of adrenalin stored in the heart muscle itself. This syndrome can have positive benefits, also. Sometimes running is the right thing to do to relieve chronic stress. For instance, a change of job or marital status may be in order.

• The second stage is the resistance, or adaptive stage. The body begins to repair the effect of arousal, and the acute symptoms disappear. If, however, stress continues, adaptation fails in its attempt to maintain defense. This stage may continue for years, or until:

• The third stage, exhaustion, (commonly called burn-out), occurs when the body can no longer respond to the stress. Diseases or a nervous breakdown may then occur.

Today, Hans Selye points out that these diseases are not just the ones we commonly think of as stress related, but include all diseases, even cancer. An interesting study was done along this line by Dr. Richard Topman, of Linacre College, Oxford. His results, reported in **New Scientist**, showed that antibody level was not as accurate a predictor of cold severity as was psychological well-being. He found that introverts who handled stress badly and had trouble adapting well to change were more likely to contract severe colds than extroverts.

Of interest to all of us is simply the wear and tear caused by stress, and the body's reaction to it.

"Fight for your highest
attainable aim
But do not put
resistance in vain."

Hans Selye

It is important for us to realize that **what is dis-tress (harmful) to some, is eu-stress (from euphoria, beneficial) to others.** Dr. Selye's first rule is: "RUN IN YOUR OWN DIRECTION, AT YOUR OWN PACE."

Stress may be broken down into three general types: *emotional stress,* which may cause gastrointestinal symptoms, headache, heart attack, hypertension; *physiological stress,* such as infection, pregnancy, malfunctioning thyroid or low blood sugar; and *physical stress,* caused by injury, extremes of climate, hunger, noise, thirst, pollution, radiation, alcohol, coffee, drugs, strenuous exercise and lack of sleep. Almost all stress, from whatever the source, affects both body and mind, as they are not separate entities.

Long term stress from hunger and inadequate housing is an example. There is evidence that if physical needs of the body are frustrated, whether they be the need to rest, to move and exericse, or even sexual in nature, the whole organism is thwarted, and an anxiety or stress response results, to a greater or lesser degree.

In order to find out what stresses caused illness, Dr. Thomas Holmes of Seattle, Washington, worked out a LIFE CHANGE UNITS SCALE, OR THE SOCIAL READJUSTMENT RATING SCALE. He and his staff put down all the events, both happy and unhappy, that are likely to have impact on most people. In his study, he allowed the public to rate the importance of the

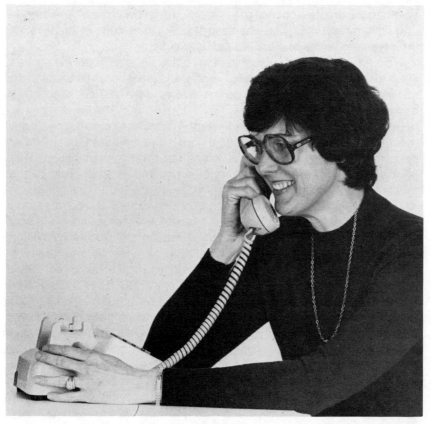

It is important to realize that what is dis-tress (harmful) to some is en-stress (beneficial) to others.

various events. On a point value starting at 100, death of a spouse was considered to be the most stressful. The life events included such things as jail terms, changes in residence, wife beginning or stopping work, and business readjustment. Even major purchases and changes in the lives of children and grandchildren were included.

Using 3,000 men stationed on three U.S. cruisers in San Diego, Dr. Holmes found that those who scored the highest on his scale during one year had the greatest chance of being sick the following year. The body has only limited resources, and when used up, the third stage of stress results. When our resources are totally used up, we die.

We learn to resolve or adjust to many of the large stressful events in our lives. It's the everyday unresolved hassles and pressures that keep us in the second stage of stress, and cause low-level anxiety that needs recognizing and dealing with.

Remember, some stress is necessary. We adapt to a changing environment, changes that may stimulate and increase the quality of our life and performance. Many people thrive on higher levels of stimulation. These people are enthusiastic, interesting, creative, and have an ability to solve problems.

The concept of the human function curve indicates that a certain amount of arousal stimulates us to work at our best. For instance, how long would you listen to a speaker who stood there yawning and slouching? With just the right amount of stress he or she is dynamic, with too much, nervous, stumbling and faltering. The important thing is to reach the correct amount of stress necessary for the event. The RETICULAR ACTIVATING MECHANISM in the brain helps regulate this by sending impulses to the muscles. We can stimulate our own RAM by shouting encouragement to ourselves, even if inaudibly. Unfortunately, as we grow older our stress reserves diminish, and we go into the areas of excess stress more easily.

"Recognizing" harmful stressors is the key. Most of us are not in touch with our bodies. Although we take vacations, lead a more or less relaxing lifestyle, and have no trouble sleeping, we still may not know the feeling of complete relaxation. Usually our minds and muscles are at some point or another between the relaxed state and painful tension. If your muscles are shortened and tight, or going into acute spasm, there may be acute stress involved, or long-term chronic tension. Until you experience self-hypnosis, or auto-suggestion, or one of the progressive relaxation techniques, true deep relaxation may be an unknown. Before we learn how to relax, let's look at some of the common and not-so-common causes of acute or chronic tension.

It is worth repeating that what is harmful to one may be beneficial to another. Divorce, for instance, although high on the stress chart, may bring relief from stress. Stressors, in themselves, are neutral. It is our perception of them that makes things, events, or situations "good" or "bad." Time pressures are an example. Some people work better when under a deadline. They may also need to have their lives organized around the clock. Others, like myself, are happiest when there are no set times to do anything, and no clocks around. Clocks are inanimate. When it's 8:30 on Sunday morning, your reaction is "it's early, I'm going back to sleep." On Monday morning, however, you jump out of bed, adrenalin coursing, and you curse because you are late for work. It's relative and personal, highly individual, the result of environment, heredity, and chemistry.

Let's look further at some stressors, both common and not-so-common. Then we will look at our response, and finally, what we can do about it.

One stressor we all know: traffic delays. Add rude drivers, heat, and our own tight time schedule, and we're looking at real stress. What can we do about it, other than fume? First of all, look for an alternate route, if possible. If you are truly trapped, and there is no action available, then escape! How? Put on some relaxing music, lean back and enjoy it. If there is scenery, or interesting people and buildings are around, enjoy them. If it is hot, think cool thoughts — the color blue, snow, the ocean with a cool breeze. Sometimes anger at other drivers can be relieved by yelling your favorite derogatory term. Just close the window so they don't hear. After you've done that, forget it! If you continue to dwell on it, you will become angrier. Instead, talk to yourself. Slowing your breathing and saying the word "relax" will help. Imagine you are in a place or situation that brings you pleasure and calm. Put yourself there until you are out of the traffic jam. Do not fight in vain! Retreat and escape instead. Your body will respond to the relaxing thoughts, instead of the stressful situation.

Our clothing can be a source of stress. If it is too tight, our body responds by contractiong in an attempt to move away. Foot abnormalities caused by wearing tight shoes is an example. Wearing high heels causes another type of stress. The pelvis is thrown out of position, contributing to backache, tension, and muscular imbalance. (See the chapter "Aching Back.")

All of these are sources of physical stress. Clothing can cause emotional stress, as well. If you are a blue-jean type of person and are forced to wear a dress every day, you may feel stressed. The same is true if your clothing is dirty, torn, or unsuitable for the occasion or environment.

Change is stressful. So are boredom and loneliness, or many unfinished jobs. You may be stressed if you are being stifled or inhibited, or if you are expected to work beyond your capabilities. If you think a person is causing your stress reaction, take positive action by talking to him or her. Explain your feelings. Communication can resolve many problems.

Other physical causes are poor body alignment, exposure to harmful chemicals and weather. Food allergies and coffee cause a stress response, as does noise. Sound over 70 decibels closes peripheral blood vessels.

Let's look at weather, as we are all forced to live with it. We know the body works to adjust to extremes of temperature, either hot or cold. You may think it is unimportant today, as our cars, homes and workplaces are usually artificially cooled and heated; but we are not indoors all the time, nor should we be. If you are not outdoors at least an hour a day during warm weather, your body won't adapt to the season by lowering the sodium content of the perspiration and producing more salt cells. When you go out on the weekend for a game of tennis, you are much more likely to suffer heat stroke or exhaustion.

Weather does more than that. Those "witches' winds" known in several areas of world are truly devastating. They come loaded with positive charged ions, which have a negative effect on health and emotions.

Police have always seen an increase in assaultive behavior during hot, sticky weather, and psychiatrists have known that a stretch of bad weather can tip an unstable person over the edge.

According to Dr. Stephen Rosen[1], an expert of weather and human behavior, day to day atmospheric changes can have a great impact on the way you feel and behave. The weather yesterday or the day before can affect the way you feel today. It can also affect the potency and side effects of many common drugs, and aggravate medical conditions. Industrial accidents are more likely to occur during periods of warm air and heat thunder storms (also charged with positive ions) and to decrease during long periods of cold air movement.

Some people are more sensitive to weather conditions than others. Dr. Rosen finds that the most weather susceptible person tends to be the woman who is either slender or very heavy, either in her teens or over 60, and is shy, inhibited, anxious and depressive.

Some weather-sensitivity symptoms are: fatigue, irritability, head pressure and/or pain, forgetfulness, insomnia, disinclination to work and others. You may be more sensitive to pain, have less endurance and muscle tone, and if susceptible, suffer from such things as migraine, arthritis, asthma, chest and nerve pain. Common drugs, such as aspirin, can cause weather sensitivity. It dilates the blood vessels, and quickens the loss of body heat, so should be used carefully in cold weather. On the other hand, some experts feel it is dangerous for athletes to take aspirin in hot weather. Marijuana and alcohol reduce body temperature, and can be extremely dangerous in cold weather.

What can we do to offset some of the effects of weather? When it's hot,

1. U.S. News & World Report - July 2, 1979 pp 37-40.

our appetite is normally diminished; so we eat less. Replace fluids hourly, whether thirsty or not. Eat more vegetables, salads, and carbohydrates. I highly recommend eating celery and drinking V8 as electrolyte replacement, especially if you are exercising. In cold weather, protein and fat foods produce body heat; five small meals a day are more efficient than three. During heat waves, avoid other stressors; exercise and work less strenuously, especially in the beginning of summer. Be aware that your food allergies may be aggravated. Moisten the air in winter. Vary vacation spots, trying seashore, mountains, various climates. Keep in mind that blood pressure will fall in a warm climate and rise in a cold climate. When traveling, allow two days for your body to adjust to the change in climate. If you want to know more about how weather affects us, read **"Weathering: How The Atmosphere Conditions Your Body, Your Mind, Your Moods—and Your Health,"** by Dr. Stephen Rosen.

It's our perception of the stress that causes emotional stress. A career woman may envy the housewife who sleeps late, but unemployed women between the ages of 25 and 60 are the biggest users of Valium. Often women work out of necessity rather than desire. The jobs may be unfulfilling, and the woman may have guilt feelings regarding her family. Sometimes the woman has all of the responsibility of home and child care, as well as holding down a full time job. If she tends to be a perfectionist, she will be frustrated in her attempts to maintain a spotless home, bake and cook, and do well on the job. If the husband refuses to help at home, often resentment will be added to guilt and frustration. The woman may be "enlightened" and contemporary, but if the man is not, there will be trouble. The solution to the problem has to be reached by both people involved.

One of the causes of physical and emotional stress is working without rest. Our bodies were intended to have a rhythm of work and rest; it is apparent in all of nature. Because our society and needs dictate otherwise, we have ignored this law and pay for it in destroyed health. You cannot go on forever working night and day. Eventually the weakest link in your chain will give way to the stress, and break.

"Perfectionist" personalities create stress for themselves (often abdominal) and others. If you work in the home as well as outside, you will have to lower your standards of home-making and elicit the help of all other members of the family. Ironing and waxing are unimportant when you are dead on your feet and risking illness. Help and concern from your partner is all-important. If this is not forthcoming and causing friction, the next step is counseling for both. Often the man will be locked into his role ideas of "man's work" and "woman's work" and refuse to change. If the situation is intolerable for the woman, then divorce may be the only answer, when all other avenues have been investigated. Bear in mind that there will be new

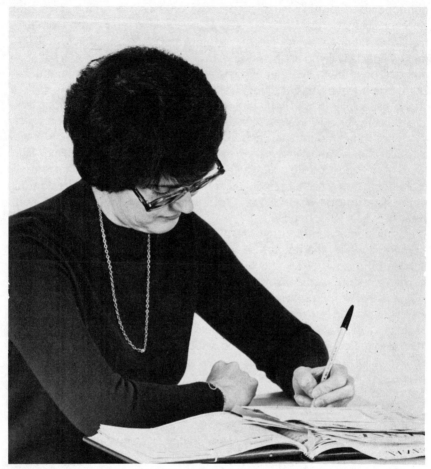

Occupational stresses are very real and very personal.

problems — those of a single parent. They may or may not be easier to handle.

Just as the perfectionist personality creates stress, so does the anxious person. This type of person relives all of the problems of the past, and creates new ones for the future. The body responds to this type of imagining as though the stress were real. Be aware that we suffer real physical and mental stress from our imaginings, and that we create that which we hold in our mind. Always ask yourself: **"What am I thinking? Is this what I want to think, and to happen?"** If the answer is "no" **then replace the thought with another.** The more you practice this, the easier it becomes.

Occupational stresses are very real and very personal. Some individuals feel stifled and thwarted when working for someone else. If they are self-starters and have the means and motivation, then they should be self-employed. Others feel more secure with less responsibility. They are happier if someone tells them what to do, and they can go home and forget the job. Examples are friends of mine, both lawyers. The husband works for a high pressure firm and brings work home at night, weekends, and when on vacation. The wife works for the government, and never thinks about the job when away from it. Neither would trade places with the other. He may be a typical "A" type personality, the "driven" kind that often has heart attacks. On the other hand, he may be like Hans Selye, who describes himself a super, race horse "A," and thrives on work and achievement.

Factory workers suffer frequent stress related illness. It is felt the reason for this is that people are forced to work at the pace of a machine, which is out of tune with their own rhythm.

Truly fortunate is the person who is able to work successfully at a job for which she is suited and which she likes. This person is rare. The person who loves solitude should be a forest ranger; those who thrive on crowds should work in the city. Pity the claustrophobic who works in a tunnel! Do not be afraid to change!

Someone who likes to be alone may find it impractical to live in the woods, but she should avoid living in crowded apartment complexes and keep away unnecessary long-staying house guests. She would probably be happiest having a small family, or no children at all. In fact, she may prefer living alone altogether. Today, there is no stigma attached to a woman being unmarried — it is our choice. It is a good feeling to be independent, and not obligated to anyone. It is not necessary to be half of someone else; we are complete in ourselves.

We are finally being accepted in traditionally male occupations but are still earning less. Believe me — money, in the form of compensation for work done, reduces stress! In addition to the material things it allows us to get (plus vacations), it provides psychological rewards. Many woman have to work harder than their male counterparts in the same position. Unfortunately, in their attempts to succeed, women are driving themselves into the stress-type illnesses that have typically plagued men, such as heart attack. It is now felt that after the age of 44, women are at the same risk of heart attack as men. Men are giving up cigarettes, while more women are smoking and at an earlier age. Women in the workplace are desperately in need of stress reduction techniques, and many industries and government offices are now providing them.

Lack of sleep is a form of stress that causes individual symptoms. Eventually we adjust to inadequate sleep, but if we listen to our bodies, we will know that we are not functioning at optimum capacity. My own response to two nights without enough sleep is a sore throat by the end of the second day. There is not enough reserve for the body to maintain homeostasis, and the weakest link breaks. My friend boasts she needs only four hours of sleep, but she is always "exhausted" and never associates this with improper rest. Our need for sleep varies. Men, and sound sleepers, need less. Athletes in training need more. Sometimes people sleep too much: a symptom of a psychological problem, perhaps boredom. If you are always sick, see if you aren't being stressed by inadequate or improper sleep.

Environment is a source of stress. I can't tolerate clutter, but others feel right at home with it. Some find pleasure doing group activities with many people; others prefer walking alone. Know yourself, and do what feels best. If a rigid, structured job with many restrictions has you feeling as if you are going to scream by the end of the day, you may find a glass of wine relaxing. Keep in mind that the relaxing benefits from alcohol tend to be reversed if you have more than one or two drinks. Probably the most enjoyable way to drink is with a close friend. Drinking alone can be depressing and lead to a habit you may not want to acquire. Don't feel you have to do the "bar scene" because everyone else does. If you are not comfortable there, you will be creating further stress for yourself.

We have only so much ability to adapt to stress. There are many factors affecting this, including genetics and age. If we are stressed, then allowed to rest and recover, (as is done with exercise), we grow stronger and can then withstand more stress (to a point). However, if stress is unrelenting, we use up our stress reserves produced by the adrenal glands and elsewhere in the body. If this continues, the end result may be premature aging, or death.

A plastic surgeon who spoke at my spa told of his youngest facelift patient, a woman in her thirties who aged quickly after her husband was killed in Viet Nam. Stress took its toll not only on her face, but on her whole organism as well.

Stress can cause a vitamin deficiency, particularly B complex and C, and can be created if the deficiency already exists. The stress response suppresses the immune response, which is why people under stress get sick more often. One of the reasons may be that the body's immune system becomes weaker from the overproduction of cortisone (one of the hormones secreted when under stress).

Sickness is only one sign of stress. Another stress sign is the appetite, and gastro-intestinal reactions. Some people eat when they are under stress, and often are totally unaware that they are putting anything in their mouths. A way to identify this behavior is to keep an accurate record of EVERYTHING you eat, and **how you feel at the time.** True, eating should be a pleasure. But often people derive no satisfaction from their habit, only

was one of the reasons he was — hardly an ideal way to maintain weight.

We need to know what events, emotions, and foods cause symptoms, and then, as much as possible, take control over them to make positive changes. Many foods we can eat safely when we are relaxed become enemies when we are under stress. Some women find the symptoms worsen the week before menstruation, and during menopause. Stressful foods, like events, are individual but the ones that cause the most trouble for everyone with a sensitive stomach are cigarettes, alcohol, and coffee, all substances you can easily live without.

The best technique for knowing ourselves: keeping a diary. You are working at a behavior modification, whether or not you want to lose weight. Over a period of several weeks, record what you eat (including snacks), where you ate it, time, what else is going on in your life (including menstrual cycle) and how you feel. You may find you can eat small amounts of foods safely, but suffer with cramps if you eat a huge serving. You need to be more cautious when you travel, are angry or hurried. A relaxed and pleasant setting is important, as is serene and pleasant conversation. Things you can safely eat in the afternoon may make you sick in the morning. If you have a hiatal hernia, eating a large meal before going to bed can cause you to be uncomfortable all night. Instead, eat earlier, and go for a walk afterwards. As with all symptoms of stress, once you have done all you can to change the situation or environment, change yourself. You may have to alter your perception of the stressor. Our "stress" instructor told of the time a large man pushed in front of him in a movie ticket line. He politely asked the man if he would go to the back of the line. The reply was a dirty look. He again asked him to move, and was answered with an angry, threatening look. At this point he decided it wasn't worth fighting about, and he ignored the issue, because it really wasn't that important. The instructor was assertive, but stopped short of being aggressive. He coped by changing his perception.

Change wherever possible, alter your perception if it is **realistic,** and try stress reduction techniques such as exercise, deep relaxation, yoga, and biofeedback.

For further information, contact the American Digestive Disease Society (ADDS), Dept. S, 420 Lexington Ave., New York, N.Y. 10017. Free brochures are available.

What other signals does our body send us to let us know it is being stressed? I mentioned frequent illness, including allergies and colds. Other physical signs are falling hair, white spots on the fingernails, skin eruptions, fatigue and irritability. During acute stress, there will be a change in body temperature, heart rate, breathing, and perhaps blood pressure. The following is a list of some bodily tension responses, and how you may relieve them:

- Tightness or pain in the forehead, or arching brows.
  To relieve: Tighten even further, once or twice, then relax. Massage your temples gently.
- Eyes squinting or staring.
  To relieve: Look at an object slightly above your line of vision until your eyes get tired. Then let them close gently.
- Clenched jaw, or biting the inside of your mouth.
  To relieve: Clench your jaw as hard as you can, once or twice, then let your jaw go slack.
- Tight neck, swallowing, or clearing your throat.
  To relieve: Tense your throat, pushing your tongue against the roof of your mouth. Then let your throat relax. Take a deep breath; hold it in, then exhale, and hold it out for a few seconds.
- Hunched, tense shoulders.
  To relieve: Pull them towards your ears. Hold four seconds, then let them drop. Repeat twice more, then let your shoulders and arms hang loosely at your side.
- Tight and painful upper back.
  To relieve: Reach around your body as though you are hugging yourself. Try to reach your scapulae if you can. The feeling is a stretch in the back. Hold that position tightly and rock your arms back and forth so there is movement in the back.
- Clenched hands.
  To relieve: Make your hands into tight fists, holding that feeling for a few seconds. Repeat and let your hands go limp.
- Tight, painful lower back.
  To relieve: Slowly bring one knee, then the other, towards your chest. You may do this standing, sitting, or lying. If lying, follow by slowly bringing both knees towards your chest.
- Tightened thighs, legs or toes.
  To relieve: Tighten as hard as you can, two times, holding a few seconds each time. Then let your legs feel heavy and limp.
- Sitting rigid in your chair.
  To relieve: Starting with the head, then progressing one vertebra at a time down your back, do a toe touch between your legs while sitting in your chair. Do this slowly, exhaling through your mouth as you lower your body. Hang there loosely for a few seconds, then tighten your abdominal muscles, and roll back slowly to a sitting position, one vertebra at a time, beginning with the lower back first. Now, relax, and feel the weight of your body against the chair.

When relaxing any part of your body, direct the word "relax" to that part. When slowing your breathing, be aware of the abdomen going out when you inhale, and coming in when you exhale. Hold at the end of each phase, and repeat as often as you want.

The following are more signs to look for in determining if you are under stress, some worth repeating:

· STRESS WARNING SIGNS

- Feeling of tension in forehead, back of neck, chest, shoulders, face, stomach, or other parts of the body
- Sweating
- Rapid heartbeat
- Feeling or hearing the heart pounding
- Warm or flushed face
- Cool and damp skin
- Shaking or trembling in hands, legs, or other parts of the body
- Nausea, or the stomach feels like you are stopping in an elevator
- You are gripping something tightly
- You are scratching part of your body
- You are moving a certain part of your body
- Biting nails or grinding teeth or clenching jaw
- You have trouble speaking, or feel as if you are going to choke
- You feel faint or dizzy
- You are breathing fast or heavily

Those are some physical signs of stress. Others are personality types of symptoms which may be harder to recognize as either causes or results of stress. Remember, SOME STRESS IS NECESSARY. WHAT IS STRESS-FUL AND HARMFUL TO ONE PERSON, MAY BE HELPFUL TO AN-OTHER. You have to judge by physical symptoms, and other things going on in your life (such as your health) whether your stress is distress, or eu-stress.

In addition to illness, stress in the workplace leads to absenteeism, alco-holism, and accidents. In Japan, some industries give their employees time each day to spend punching a stuffed effigy of their foreman. This not only expends the physical energy, but helps relieve some of the hostility and frustration. What do we do, other than drink or jog?

One organization, Tenneco, a Houston-based oil company, has hired a psychologist to work with the 2,500 people in the home office staff.[1] Michael Haro conducts noon-hour seminars with the focus on creating awareness; that is, awareness of their own levels of stress, and what they may do about it. He emphasizes that although people may fall into the moderate-to-high

1. **Washington Post - July 2, 1980**

risk category in his tests, they don't necessarily have a problem. The problem comes, he says, "If you feel at any level it's getting in the way. Then you ought to address it."

The first part of his test determines whether you are a "type A" personality. This person is "supposed" to be in the high risk category for heart attack, women even more so than men. (Before you panic, remember, Hans Selye thrives on being this type of person.)

The Type A personality **may** be hostile, impatient, or irrational. They are restless during leisure hours and feel guilty about relaxing. They are usually competitive, aggressive, and feel they have to win. Sometimes they grind their teeth, pound their fists, and they are always in a hurry, even when eating. Some develop extreme anxiety symptoms, such as nervousness, sleep disturbances, and depression. Coronary disease most frequently occurs before the age of 70 in type A personalities. High blood pressure, heavy cigarette smoking, and high cholesterol levels increase the risk factors.

You may have some characteristics of the "Type A" personality, and not others. Haro places **Aggression** in a separate category, and has his participants evaluate themselves for their level of aggressiveness. Notice, **I am not saying assertiveness.** Often people didn't know there is a difference. Some of the qualities of an aggressive person are: hostility, enjoys combat and argument, easily annoyed, seeks revenge, and sometimes willing to hurt people to get his or her own way.

Anxiety is another indicator of stress. These people experience uneasiness of a diffuse sort. Often they relive unpleasant experiences from the past, as well as dwell on those that may or may not happen in the future. Frequently the anxious person has severe physiological reactions such as trembling, sweating, and irregularities in breathing and heart beat. (Often these symptoms disappear when coffee is eliminated.)

Haro considers **Autonomy** as a possible indication that the person may be under stress. This person tries to break away from any restraints, confinement or restrictions of any kind. He may be rebellious, independent, and nonconforming. In this category, as in the others, the individual must determine whether the "stress" is hindering or helping.

COPING BEHAVIORS

Relieving the physical symptoms of stress is only part of the answer. In some cases, it may be all you need to do, but usually there are additional ways of coping.

If you see your doctor, you may receive a prescription for Valium or Librium. THIS IS NOT RECOMMENDED! We can adopt any number of psychological defenses, such as denial or rationalization, which are valid,

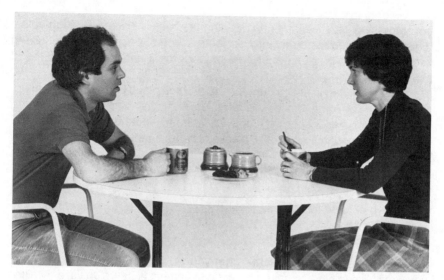

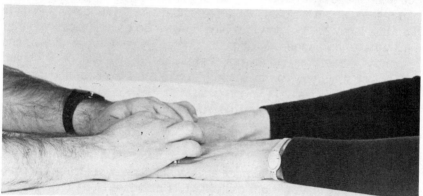

Expressing your feelings and opening the lines of communication are constructive ways of coping with stress.

but beware of overuse. The fight or flight response may be used positively or negatively. Fighting or attacking may take the form of blaming someone else. Flight or escape can be physical or psychological. If your office or home is filled with a build-up of pressures, go into another room or place, even for a few minutes, then think about something else, someone else, somewhere else! You will return refreshed and better able to cope. You can mentally escape by fantasizing that you are at a special place that brings you peace and relaxation. This is especially helpful if you have **no control** over the outcome of your problem. If there is nothing you can do about it, fretting and worrying won't help.

Expressing your feelings and opening the lines of communication helps. This can be used constructively or destructively. Specific problem-solving techniques may involve better time management and the setting of short term and long range goals.

Problem solving is difficult unless the problem itself is clear in your mind. Donald A. Tubesing, an educational psychologist and president of the Whole Person Associates in Duluth, Minnesota conducts stress skills workshops throughout the country. He asks his participants to fill in the blanks in the following statements:

- Maybe I don't need to...................................... anymore.
- Maybe I do need to......................................some more.
- Maybe I need to.................................... sometime soon.
- Maybe I need to......................................once again.
- Maybe I need to..................................... sometimes.

These statements help clarify what you would like to change, and what you would like to have remain. There is a statement of future goals, a recalling of a resource from the past, and an area that allows you to move in more than one direction. We see in writing that we **do** have choices; we may simply have to change our attitudes, unreal personal expectations, and responses to certain circumstances. We may find we are not trapped after all.

Tubesing feels you can take charge of your reactions to stressors by using four techniques:

REORGANIZATION: Control the way you spend your time. Isolate your goals, then draw up a short term and long range plan to achieve those goals. The goals may be broken into daily, monthly and yearly. I find it imperative to write things down. Make a list of things you need to do including making phone calls, then scratch them out as they get done. You may not accomplish everything; that's all right, as flexibility is important. Don't forget to save time for relaxation and pleasure. Your time is precious. Place value on it! We all have obligations and duties; however, many people waste time on things that have no pleasure, meaning or value simply because they think they "must do" what others do, or expect them to do. If you really hate something that is supposed to be recreational, don't do it! You may lose some "friends", but it's worth it. Evaluate the way you spend your time, decide what is important, then separate the wheat from the chaff. You may decide against polishing your silver so often, or spending every Sunday in front of the tube.

Planning is essential, both at home and on the job. Studies have shown that managers agree that the major time wasters are interruptions, inefficient or unnecessary meetings, crisis, ambiguities, poor delegation and poor communication.

CHANGING THE SCENE: This may be in the form of a vacation (note the word vacate inherent in vacation), or a relocation of home or work. It may mean marriage or divorce, depending on your particular stressors. When you take that vacation, go someplace that has the attributes you need. It may be stimulation or relaxation, but it should be different. Leave your work and if possible, your children at home. You may want to go without your husband. Women who come to my spa often tell me that by the middle of the week they miss their husbands, and develop a renewed appreciation of them.

CHANGING YOUR MIND: This means re-labeling or changing your attitude about what is bothering you. Look for the good that is inherent in most situations. If you have a lemon, make "lemonade." When you have internal dialogues with yourself, say complimentary, positive things, instead of derogatory or self-defeating statements. Remember, whatever you hold in your mind tends to become true in the external. Visualize things the way you would like them to be; then imagine they are that way now. A sense of humor goes a long way. Laugh at yourself, and place yourself apart from your problems, see them from a new perspective and you may be able to laugh at them too. Many people find religion is very helpful, as long as it is not punitive. Look for passages about faith and love. I particularly like "metaphysical" books and groups. You might find helpful the writings of Emmett Fox, Jack and Cornelia Addington ("**Your Needs Met; The Time for Miracles is Now**"), Norman Vincent Peale, or Lao or Walter Russel. Poetry and classcal music are relaxing. Enjoy them at home, or for a change, go to a concert. Most areas have free ones, especially in the summer. It really helps to totally immerse yourself in something or someone else. This can be a friend, lover, child, or someone in need of your help, but don't let yourself become a sounding board for everyone else's petty problems. Added to your own, they can drag you down.

BUILDING YOUR STRENGTH: This includes physical, mental, psychological, spiritual, skills.

The key to selecting an effective energizer is your reaction to it. If what you are doing is no longer working, look for new strengths and develop new skills. Don't be a perfectionist. You don't need to be able to run a marathon to derive pleasure and benefit from running.

I'll never forget a weekend in my life that was a particular turning point for me. I was depressed following the breakup of my marriage, and walking in a nearby natural area near the river. Walking in nature was something I'd always done when faced with large problems, as it helped me to relax and look at things from a new perspective. This time it wasn't working. On that particular walk, I met a man who was teaching rock climbing on the nearby cliffs. I watched, thinking "I'll never do that!" However, by the end of the day, I had made two climbs. What a "high" that much-needed accomplishment gave me at that particular time! The next day I attended a workshop sponsored by a metaphysical group featuring this particular aspect of art.

Painting and drawing happen to be two of my minor skills, so again, there was pleasure and satisfaction. I never returned to my previous "low." That weekend was special. Ordinary activities would not have supplied the resources I needed. Each of us needs to look within (and without) to find and develop her own special sources of strength.

For the most part, nature is my psychiatrist. I don't mean a crowded ballpark on Sunday afternoon, but a "wild" area where there are neither sights nor sounds of other humans. It is best to go alone so that through nature, you can relax and get in tune with your own rhythm. It takes a while to learn to do this, and if you're very tense, you may not relax as quickly as you would like. I have done this all my life, and it works for me.

Frank Capra, the director of the American film classics, **Mr. Smith Goes to Washington**, and **Meet John Doe** uses the same technique to relax. He describes the feeling of knowing nature with all the senses in his article "See My Psychiatrist" in **Spectator** magazine, (summer, 1980). He says:

> "This is Nature, the psychiatrist, talking to you; cleaning your mind and body, replacing the cankers of fear, meanness, envy and doubt with the purity, courage and joy of natural life; and saying to you; 'Be glad you're alive. Think clean and live with God.' "

A friend of mine, a psychologist (and one of the wisest women I know) does just the reverse. She lives on a farm and is close to nature all the time. When she is going through a particular stressful time, she plunges herself into a course at the local university, an excellent resource and a stimulating change. I suggest you take something that is especially appealing to you, perhaps a subject you have always wanted to learn more about.

Having fun is a therapeutic skill that many adults don't have. Often people feel guilty when they enjoy themselves, thinking that fun is for children only. It is especially nice to have fun with a close friend, or your husband. Fun can mean doing simple things that are more pleasant than the daily routine. How many people do you know who spend every evening in front of the tube? I think the best marriages are those where there is a sharing of many things that bring enjoyment and pleasure. Problems arise when one partner wants to enjoy life, and the other doesn't know how or doesn't share the same interests. Sometimes counseling helps; however, as change is involved, the situation is often unresolved other than in divorce.

If your fun includes physical activity, you are ahead of the game. Stress causes excess adrenalin to be stored in the heart muscle itself, and exercise squeezes it out. But stress affects our coordination, often causing us to make mistakes; so if you are under acute stress, look for activities that require less skill and are non-competitive. Walking and slow jogging are excellent, but don't push past the pleasure!

A few more words about running for relaxation: There seems to be no question that running relieves depression, especially the temporary kind.[1] According to Dr. A. H. Ismail, Ph.D., Professor at Purdue University, the physiological and biochemical changes that take place when a person begins an exercise program can affect the whole personality!

Definite changes were seen in men over a four-month period when they exercised three times a week, one and a half hours each session. They reported feeling more secure and relaxed, and most said they did not care as much about what others thought of them. Dr. Ismail further commented that there are fewer insurance claims among active people.

In addition to taking a vacation when one is needed, take time off each day. Preferably do something that brings pleasure, but escape may be in the form of light "escape" reading or even "soaps" on T.V. I don't care for television and usually watch only the news or an occasional movie. However, the news is hardly relaxing, nor are most movies today.

Support in the form of a group, a counselor or friend is needed for those undergoing chronic life stresses. It helps to know that your experiences are not unique, and you are not alone. There are support groups for families of alcoholics, child-and wife-abusers, and crisis centers when immediate help is needed. These services are available in rural areas as well as large cities. Don't be ashamed to utilize them if needed.

Support is crucial even if you are not undergoing major stressful situations. Most often the support of a friend, co-worker or family member is what is needed rather than a group or professional. Unfortunately in our changing social environment, most people have too few relationships they can count on as sources of support. Some of the traditional functions of family and religion are no longer available or even valid.

According to several studies performed by the Institute for Social Research (University of Michigan) at NASA, poor interpersonal relationships can lead to ill health.[2] Dr. Cassell found that women who received little warmth and support during their pregnancies were much more likely to experience complications in childbirth. He found (in other studies) changed hormonal levels in people deprived of warmth and support, and determined that the death rate is three to five times higher among divorced men than among married men of the same age.

I mention support of co-workers, because today most women do work outside the home, and the workplace can be a major source of **unnecessary** stress. In a study of hospital managers, (John Adams, 1978), it was found that the following "change events" were felt to be the most stressful by the respondents: 1) requirement to work more hours than usual; 2) major

[1]**Family Weekly, March 30, 1980.**
[2]**Social Change, Ideas and Applications, Vol. 8, No. 4, 1978.**

changes in policies and procedures; 3) increase in pace of work; 4) new supervisor; 5) new subordinates; 6) major reorganization of department; 7) change in nature of job; 8) new co-worker.

It was concluded that the stress induced by these events was variable, depending on the amount of communication and preparation that took place. Of prime importance was reducing the surprise element of necessary change. In the same study, the following DAILY CONDITIONS were found to be the most stressful: 1) work overload; 2) feedback only on unsatisfactory performance; 3) lack of confidence in management; 4) role ambiguity; 5) role conflict; 6) unresolved interpersonal conflict; 7) "fire-fighting" rather than working from a plan; 8) interunit conflict.

It was felt that these daily stresses usually could not be resolved by bureaucratic change, but through intensive modification by individuals on every level.

Managers could also learn to become sensitive to signs of stress in the behavior of their subordinates. One or more of the following forms of **NEW** behavior in an employee indicates a high level of stress, possibly calling for counseling: 1) disregard for low (or high) priority tasks; 2) reduced amount of time given to each task; 3) change of boundaries or shift to avoid responsibility; 4) blocking out new information; 5) superficial involvement or appearance of giving up; 6) negative attitude or cynicism about customers/clients; 7) depersonalized or detached behavior; 8) going by the book; 9) inappropriate humor; 10) being overly precise (intellectualizing); 11) absenteeism.

The NTL Institute (P.O. Box 9155, Rosslyn Station, Arlington, VA 22209) offers one day (and longer) training sessions on "Understanding and Managing Stress."

In addition to conducting seminars, Dr. Adams recommends follow-up activities such as additional or continuing stress management training for individuals or groups; stress assessments; revision or development of job description or standards; creation of exercise programs and facilities; required annual physical exam, with counseling provided to those exhibiting symptoms of stress-related illnesses; serving fresh fruits and juices as an alternative to coffee and cake at meetings and seminars; quarterly interchange between senior management and first line supervisors to discuss issues, policies and decisions.

Dr. Adams states that "The stress provoking norms in most organizations . . . tend to be both pervasive and consistent."[3] It is important that a follow-up program be explicitly managed and consistent and that the amount of time required to make changes not be underestimated. He sums up the following:

[3]**Social Change, Ideas and Applications, Vol. 8, No. 4, 1978.**

Suggestions For Effective Stress Management

- Self management
- Vigorous regular exercise
- Nutrition: good eating habits, vitamin and mineral supplements
- Letting-go techniques: centering and focusing, relaxation/meditation/ prayer, finishing unfinished business
- Self awareness: needs, desires, idiosyncrasies, congruences, assertiveness
- Personal planning: time management, positive life choices
- Creation and use of support systems
- Altering stressful organization norms, policies and procedures

CHARACTERISTICS OF EFFECTIVE STRESS MANAGERS

- Self-knowledge: Strengths/skills/liabilities
- Varied interests-many sources of satisfaction
- Variety of reactions to stress-repertoire of responses
- Acknowledgements and acceptance of individual differences
- Being active and productive

The more self aware one is, the better she is equipped to make positive life choices and avoid stressful situations. We keep returning to the fact that each of us has different stressors and different responses. If the country bores you, then tackle the challenge and excitement of the city. Conversely, if the noise, rush and stress of the city "get to you" in any or all of the myriad of ways it can, then search for more peaceful surroundings. If it is impossible to move, then perhaps a weekend retreat in the woods will help relieve the stress and renew you for Monday mornings. Our knowledge of ourselves is never complete and is ever-changing, although many characteristics remain the same throughout a lifetime.

My basic nature is to "act." Once I have made a decision to do or buy something, I do it as soon as possible. Having things "pending" makes me nervous. For instance, buying an old house and taking forever to fix it up would drive me crazy; so I would not do it. Along this same line, I take action when something is bothering me, rather than keeping things churning inside. The technique is to look at all of the possible consequences of your action and if you can live with the worst possible one, then act! Perhaps you have seen the advice: "If someone or something is bothering you, get it out of your system by writing a letter, then tear it up." That's good advice if nothing you can say or do can change the situation, and your letter will only fuel the stressful situation. However, if you can make positive changes by airing your feelings and opinions in a letter, then do it! If the consequences are drastic, be prepared to live with them. You may be surprised to find that by taking the initiative you have gained respect and the changes you are seeking actually occur. The point is: if something can be done, do it!

Although unfinished business (in both relationships and jobs) are common stressors, don't increase either the mental or physical stress by setting impossible deadlines for yourself in order to get everything done at once. Dr. Selye refers to the moving of a woodpile. If it is too large, don't overstress yourself by doing it all at once. Instead, take two days.

Exercise and correct diet does not prevent stress, or even protect us from specific stressors, but it does enable us to better withstand the effects of stress. Exercises such as TaiChi, Yoga, and stretching can produce the relaxation response, while vigorous (aerobic) exercise can take the mind off the problem immediately, have a tranquilizing effect, relieve depression and help throw off excess adrenalin stored in the muscles and heart. Aerobic exercise also develops greater cardiovascular efficiency; the heart muscle itself is strengthened; the blood pressure and heart rate are lowered, thereby making us more fit to withstand the strain of stress. This will be explained further in the chapter on **exercise**.

NUTRITIONAL ASPECTS OF STRESS

Nutritional deficiencies and imbalances can **cause stress** as well as be an **effect of stress**. Fad diets, or even well balanced low calorie diets can create a deficiency in vitamins, minerals and fiber. Processed depleted foods not only are missing many of their natural nutrients, but rob the body of vitamins when they are metabolized. Examples are coffee, sugar and alcohol, which rob us of vitamin B-1. Diets deficient in calcium, magnesium and fiber are not uncommon, and calcium and magnesium in particular are needed to "calm the nerves."

The adrenal glands normally contain a high amount of vitamin C, which is used up when under stress. If their supply is inadequate, vitamin C will be taken from other tissues. Vitamin C is found not only in the adrenal glands, but in all organs of high metabolic activity, such as the pituitary gland, brain, eyes, ovaries, and other vital tissues. When under stress, from whatever the source, whether it be physical, emotional or weather, there is a sudden precipitous drop in vitamin C.

When extra nutrients are needed because of stress, the body works to preserve the brain and other essential organs, robbing other parts of the body. That is why people under stress will often exhibit such symptoms as lifeless, thinning hair, skin problems, brittle or white-flecked fingernails. Often there are symptoms of hypoglycemia (low blood sugar). Fatigue and depression are common, as well as decreased libido.

Along with vitamin C, the B complex and zinc are needed in times of stress. Zinc intensifies the action and absorption of other vitamins, and vitamin B6 aids in the absorption of zinc. Zinc may be a brain sedative, influences hormones, and is involved in regulating blood sugar. Zinc is helpful in skin problems, possibly because it aids in the transport of vitamin A to the skin. Women on the pill who are bloated and depressed are often helped by the addition of B6 and zinc.

A specific type of nutritionally induced stress is food allergy. Symptoms can vary from fatigue, brain fag, depression, mania, hallucinations, confusion and migraines. Food allergies also cause hives and nasal congestion, and in extreme cases, anaphylactic shock, which can be fatal. Food allergy changes the histamine level so that we are more susceptible to other allergens, such as pollen and dust. When food allergy symptoms are chronic, they are often mild and not easily recognized. One long distance runner added speed and mileage to his running when he stopped eating chocolate.

Usually food allergies cause us to become addicted to or crave those foods to which we are allergic. The cravings often occur by the clock, at the same time every day. There will be a "high" after the food is eaten, then a compensatory letdown.

The foods to which people are most commonly allergic are wheat, milk, chocolate and eggs. However, one can be allergic to any kind of food, even specific water. One doctor I know routinely takes his hay fever patients off milk. They usually respond immediately by having no more symptoms of hay fever.

How can you tell if you are allergic to food without rushing immediately to an allergist? Addiction is a clue, but the best way is to go on a total fast, then introduce one food at a time. When you re-introduce a food to which you are allergic, chronic symptoms may then become acute and easily recognizable. The pulse is another indication. If, after eating a specific food, there is an increase from the normal resting pulse by about sixteen beats or more, the chances are that you are allergic to that food. Alcohol increases our sensitivity to the foods to which we are allergic, as does exercise immediately after eating. Some years ago I had a severe allergic reaction to shellfish when I drank at the same meal and then danced. I had a similar reaction again under the same circumstances, although at other times I can eat shellfish with no difficulty. At the time this occurred, my doctor denied that there was a connection, although today it is well documented, as more people are exercising and having similar reactions.

The logical thing to do is identify the foods to which you are allergic and eliminate them from your diet. Often people with allergies and who are under stress are helped by supplementing vitamin C, pantothenic acid and niacin (B vitamins), as these nourish the adrenal glands. Remember, vitamins are not just simply foods, and it is possible to overdose and cause toxic reactions, or create an imbalance. Unless prescribed by a physician, it would be preferable to take a balanced B supplement or brewers yeast or desiccated liver. (This should come from South American sources, usually Argentina, as there is less danger of chemical or hormone pollution in the liver.)

A good general rule, whether you are under stress or not, is to cut way back on, or eliminate sugar, coffee, alcohol (beyond one glass of wine), and highly salted or processed foods. In this way, your diet will not be adding to your stress.

THE RELAXATION RESPONSE

Just as we have a "stress response" which elicits the "fight or flight" reaction, we have a relaxation response. We can learn to relax to the point where we can go to sleep, lower our blood pressure and heart rate, and achieve an altered state of consciousness.

There are several ways of doing this which include meditation and deep relaxation. First let's review a few "letting go" techniques that can be utilized easily and quickly, depending on your needs and what is available. They help us let go, if even for just a few minutes, of our immediate problems and tensions. Often, because of this release, we find the solution which has been hidden from our conscious mind by our own restrictions.

Short walks, in nature, if possible. Walk briskly, letting your arms and legs move freely, think about and enjoy your surroundings, rather than your problems.

Deep breathing, inhaling and exhaling slowly. Don't overdo this in the beginning, as you may become dizzy or hyperventilate. Some techniques to try are:

- Inhale deeply. As you slowly exhale, say a calming word such as RELAX, CALM, PEACE, ONE, or any word that is particularly soothing to you.
- Inhale slowly, holding your breath at the point of maximum inhalation for a few seconds. Exhale slowly, holding the air OUT for a few seconds. Repeat a few times, concentrating only on your breathing.
- Belly breathing. Let your belly expand as you slowly inhale, tighten as you exhale.
- Take a deep breath, hold it, then let it out as S*L*O*W*L*Y as you can. Repeat a few times.

When you focus on breathing, you take the attention away from your problems. Breathing deeply and slowly increases the negative pressure in the chest, which helps draw blood toward the heart through the large veins. An increased supply of blood to the heart helps maintain the pressure of blood to the brain, and away from muscles that are seeking blood for "fight or flight."

Pause: Even for a moment. Look out the window, talk and think about something pleasurable.

Diary Writing: Put down your thoughts, feelings, actions, what is bothering you, or who, what you want to do, or anything that you feel must be put down.

Take a break: Juice and fruit are superior to coffee and cake, but a break doesn't necessarily mean food. It may mean just going into another room and removing yourself from the source of your tension.

Action: This can be running, walking, pacing the floor, going through your tennis serve (without the racket), running the vacuum, or stretching. Action is especially important if you have been sitting for long periods of time, which is a source of tension and restriction in itself. Two types of action:

- Stretch, standing. Reach the palm of one hand towards the ceiling. Without standing on your toes, try to lengthen that side of the body. Hold the stretch for up to thirty seconds, then do the same on the other side. Do a forward bend in your chair. Let your head hang down between your legs, and reach through your legs towards the back of the chair. Tighten your belly muscles as you roll slowly up to a sitting position, one vertebra at a time.
- Range of motion movements. Our joints as well as our muscles tighten when we sit for long periods of time, or are under tension.
- Turn your head SLOWLY from side to side as far as it will go without pain. Let your chin **slowly** drop towards your chest, then make a circle in front of you with your head. Don't tilt your head back so that you are looking at the ceiling, as this may cause pain in the neck.
- Stand with your knees slightly bent. Slowly reach down the side of one leg, then the other.
- Do a forward toe touch with the knees flexed, letting your head hang towards the floor, and your arms flop loosely. Gently almost straighten alternately one leg and then the other so there is some movement in the hip area.
- Reach behind your back with one hand. Take the other hand and gently push back on your elbow to increase the stretch in the shoulder. Do the same with the other arm.
- Bring one knee and then the other towards your chest. This can be done standing, sitting or lying. Simply move any part of your body that feels tight, tense or stiff.
- Invent your own movements. Your body will tell you what feels good.

- Meditation and prayer: This can be anything from the Bible to poetry or some of the metaphysical books I mentioned. Find writings that say and mean something to you. Read them several times, meditating on the meaning until you respond. Try the works of other cultures and be open to similarities and differences. Listening to classical music or watching a beautiful ballet can be spiritual experiences. They are excellent ways to relax and forget the "stresses of life." Again, appeal is an individual consideration. Try the classics, but be open to the newest and most contemporary.

DEEP RELAXATION

There are many different ways to achieve deep, wholebody relaxation. Here are two:

FIND A QUIET PLACE, TAKE THE PHONE OFF THE HOOK, REMOVE YOUR SHOES AND CONSTRICTIVE CLOTHES. Sit comfortably in a reclining chair with your entire spine supported, or lie flat on your back with a pillow beneath your knees and your arms lying relaxed at your sides. LET YOUR ENTIRE BODY FEEL HEAVY: FEEL THE WEIGHT OF IT AGAINST THE FLOOR. Consciously SLOW YOUR BREATHING DOWN, BEING AWARE THAT YOUR BELLY IS RISING AS YOU INHALE, AND LOWERING AS YOU EXHALE. Slow your breathing down even more, and **pause at that point where you can no longer exhale any more.** VISUALIZE YOURSELF BEING ALONE AT A PLACE THAT IS ESPECIALLY RELAXING TO YOU. IT MAY BE THE SEASHORE, OR THE MOUNTAINS, OR A PEACEFUL VALLEY. TRY TO RELIVE THE SOUNDS, SMELLS AND VISION OF IT. You may imagine yourself drifting with the current on a gentle stream, or lying on a raft in the ocean, timing your breathing with the rise and fall of the soft waves. Next, go on to either method 1 **or** method 2 of the following deep relaxation techniques:

METHOD ONE

After you have done the preliminary relaxing, say the following to yourself **SLOWLY:**

My face is relaxing; my face is relaxed; my face is COMPLETELY RELAXED.

My neck and throat are relaxing, my neck and throat are relaxed, MY NECK AND THROAT ARE COMPLETELY RELAXED.

My shoulders are relaxing; my shoulders are relaxed; MY SHOULDERS ARE COMPLETELY RELAXED.

Let your arms feel heavy, and be aware of the floor beneath them; if there is carpet, feel the texture. Say:

My arms are heavy; my arms are relaxing; my arms are relaxed; my arms are completely relaxed.

My upper back and chest are relaxing; my upper back and chest are relaxed; my upper back and chest are completely relaxed.

My back is relaxing; my back is relaxed; my back is completely relaxed.

My belly is relaxing; my belly is relaxed; my belly is completely relaxed.

My legs are relaxing; my legs are relaxed; my legs are completely relaxed.

My feet are relaxing; my feet are relaxed; my feet are completely relaxed.

If you are not asleep, be aware of your entire body. If you feel tension in any part of it, direct that part to relax. You may use this and the following techniques to aid in sleeping or as a twenty minute break during the day.

METHOD TWO

First do the preliminary relaxing as in method one, then perform the following sequence **SLOWLY:**

Tighten your feet as tightly as you can, then let them relax. Tighten them halfway; relax. Tighten them just a little, then feel them completely relax.

Tighten your lower legs as hard as you can, then relax. Tighten halfway; relax. Tighten just a little; relax completely.

Tighten your thighs and kneecaps. Relax. Tighten halfway; relax. Tighten just a little; relax completely.

Tighten your buttocks and abdominal muscles. Relax. Tighten halfway; relax. Tighten just a little; relax completely.

Tighten your upper back and chest. Relax. Tighten halfway; relax. Tighten just a little; relax completely.

Pull your shoulders towards your ears. Let them drop. Pull towards your ears again; let them drop. Lift them just a little, let them relax completely.

Tighten your arms as hard as you can; relax your arms. Tighten halfway; relax. Tighten just a little; relax completely.

Make your hands into tight fists. Let your hands relax. Repeat twice more, then let your hands feel relaxed and limp.

Tighten your throat and clench your jaw. Repeat once more, then let your jaw feel relaxed and slack.

Tighten your face muscles as tightly as you can. Screw up your nose, purse your lips, draw your brows together. Relax. Now do just the opposite; lift your brows, open your mouth as wide as you can; hold for a few seconds, now let your face relax completely.

Be aware of your entire body. If there is tension in any part, increase the tension to its maximum, then relax completely.

There are some shortcuts if you don't have the time to go through whole body progressive relaxation. The following techniques can be done quickly.

THE SECRET IS BODY AWARENESS.
- If the tension and/or pain is in your back, stretch it and move it slowly and gently.
- Tension in your shoulers: Lift and drop, roll them forward and backward, and shake your arms.
- Tension in your hands: Make tight fists two or three times, then let your arms and hands hang limply.
- Tension in your jaw: Clench it tightly once or twice, then let it relax, and hang slack.
- Tension in your thighs: Bend your knees slightly, then relax your thighs.
- Tension in your temples: Massage your temples, then with your hands, stretch the frontalis muscle, (the one across your forehead).
- Tension in the trapezius muscles across the top of your shoulders and up your neck: Massage and knead them gently. Better yet, get someone else to do it for you.

You can relax your whole body quickly, using the mental and visual method by "playing dead," the way you may have done when you were a child. Let your body be loose, limp, relaxed and out of your physical control, or you can pretend you are a rag doll, boneless, loose and limp. The easier it is for you to visualize and "get into" your role, the more you will relax.

You can use the muscle contraction method of relaxation, doing the whole body at once:

Tighten every muscle in your body as tightly as you can, squeezing your eyes shut tightly, clenching your fists and jaw and curling up your toes. HOLD THE CONTRACTION FOR FIVE SECONDS ONLY. DON'T HOLD YOUR BREATH; INSTEAD, EXHALE THROUGHOUT. LET GO SLOWLY AND RELAX.

NEXT

Repeat the muscle contraction, but this time instead of tightening everything, you will lengthen the muscles as you contract. Open your mouth wide, lengthen your arms, legs, fingers and toes, and lift your brows. AGAIN, HOLD FOR FIVE SECONDS ONLY, WITHOUT HOLDING YOUR BREATH. **NOW LET YOUR WHOLE BODY BECOME LIMP, LOOSE, HEAVY AND RELAXED, SINKING INTO THE FLOOR.**

A shower massage is a good way to relax tight muscles in the morning or during the day. Stay in for twenty minutes, if you can. In the evening, a bath is more relaxing. It should be neither hot nor cool, but comfortably warm. Bath salts or oil enhance the experience. I use "Batherapy," which can be purchased at health food stores, when my muscles are very sore. Avoid high-detergent bubble baths as they can cause urinary tract infections. Don't stay in longer than twenty minutes, as you may feel weak when you get out, or have stiff joints from remaining in a restrictive position.

A glass of wine or two, sipped slowly and shared with your husband or a good friend, can be very relaxing at the end of the day. The setting should be serene and attractive, and the topic of conversation pleasant and light. Of course, we are aware that alcohol is addictive and that too much will have the reverse effect of what you are trying to achieve.

Never take your work or studies to be with you. Finish your work day an hour or two before you go to bed and make your bed time reading light, religious (or spiritual) or even boring. The bedroom should be pleasant and quiet, and not a work place. Proper ventilation is important if you want to awaken refreshed. I firmly believe in opening a window at night, summer and winter, unless your house is sealed to remove allergens. My allergist, who was a maverick (and ahead of his time in many ways) advised me to sleep with two windows open for cross ventilation. Again, know yourself and do what feels best for you. But if you awaken feeling as though you never slept, look for the cause. Tension and stale air are two possibilities.

One point I cannot over-emphasize is the mind-body relationship. Either the mind or the body can initiate the stress, but they are inseparable. More is being learned about this through the work being done with the body chemicals endorphins and enkephalin. Many women in our age group have been taught to deny our bodies and I'm amazed at some of the brilliant, successful women who have no knowledge of their bodies, or what they can do. The women themselves are amazed when they find that with "awareness" and gentle persuasion, they can do things they never thought possible. Hopefully, at some point in this book you will have a "Gestalt;" that is, you'll say "Aha, now I know what she means!" You'll know you've got it, because it's a body-mind experience.

I'll conclude with these comments on the Stress Responses: Fight or Flight, sexual arousal, and crying.

Recently I foolishly got myself into the situation of being trapped between high, unknown cliffs and the rapid approach of night and a severe thunderstorm. If I had been unable to get out, there was no way down at that point, and the night would have been spent in the rain, vertically, among rocks, rattlers and copperheads. I started to panic. The story that a drowning person will grasp at a straw is true. To get to the top of the cliff, I climbed a crumbling ledge that I normally would not have attempted. To my shock, at the top of THAT cliff was a deep sheer chasm, with another sheer cliff beyond. At this point, panic became real. In times like this I have a special prayer I say; whatever else it does, it tends to bring me a certain amount of calm. I looked for a way out. To my right was a small, half dead tree which bridged the chasm and led to what looked like a clearing above. I recall little of the climb and scramble, only the immense relief at finding myself on firm ground again. Even the dense, flesh-tearing brambles were a joke. The fight or flight reaction got me out of there, because rational thought never would have let me do what I did. On the other hand, had the tree broken, I may have been seriously injured. Who knows, perhaps the prayer is what made the difference. I know I don't want to experience that feeling again!

Arthur Schlesinger, the historian, commented on a related theory at the time of the Democratic National Convention, August, 1980. There was widespread complaint about the passivity of President Carter when he was renominated. He says:

"There is a cyclical rhythm in politics., Action, passion, then (they get) worn out. The American people are tired now. They need a rest . . . Emerson said that politics are largely physiological, it's vitality vs. exhaustion. The country gets tired, it needs repose." He went on to comment:

"Depending on whether it's an activist or an exhausted stage, you get a president who responds."[4]

It was interesting to note that Ted Kennedy, who did not get the nomination, gave the most impassioned speech, one that brought tears to the eyes of both his and Carter's supporters.

Crying is a stress response that occurs both during "dis-tress" and "eu-stress." Although scientists know the cause of continuous tears, the kind that keep our eyes moist, and irritant tears, like those when chopping onions, they do not know the reason for emotional tears.

We cry at the best and worst of times. At weddings and at births, in pain and at death. Some women cry during orgasm, others at the sight of a beautiful painting or scenery, or when listening to music (either happy or sad). Men do not cry as often because our culture frowns on it. There is speculation that because of this inhibition, they suffer more from such stress-related illnesses as ulcers and have a shorter life expectancy.

According to Dr. Selye: "Crying can reduce stress. Crying is sort of an external realization of internal emotion, a cutting loose. If someone wants to cry, suppressing it may call forth a stress reaction."[5]

Biochemist William H. Frey, II theorizes that tears are nature's way of excreting bodily chemicals that build up in response to stress. He is basing his hypothesis on the fact that people usually feel better after crying, and that the other exocrine functions, such as sweating, exhaling, and urinating, involve the removal of toxic materials.

[4]The Washington Post, Aug. 15, 1980.
[5]The Washington Post, Aug. 13, 1980.

He is testing his theory at Minnesota's St. Paul-Ramsey Medical Center where he is collecting and analyzing tears from subjects who cry when peeling onions, and when watching tear-jerker movies such as "Brian's Song." He is also getting laughter tears. So far, they did find statistically significant amounts of protein differences in the different types of tears, but there is no definitive conclusion as of yet. If it is determined that his theory is correct, and there is a difference in the chemistry of tears, we will have new and valuable insight into "stress."

What does stress have to do with sex? Usually when under acute stress, or suffering some of the symptoms of chronic stress, there is an inhibition of sexual desire. However, many of the physiological responses to sexual arousal are identical to those of stress. Often stress reduction is part of the treatment for men who are suffering from secondary impotence; that is, they are unable to have or maintain an erection for which there is no pathological reason. Now, some studies have shown that inducing a mild stress response may be just the impetus that is needed. Exciting movies (not porno) were used to help initiate and enhance the arousal stage. Here again, what was achieved was "eu-stress."

We can't stay at high levels of eu-stress forever either, although we may want to, but this is what adds the spice and joy to life.

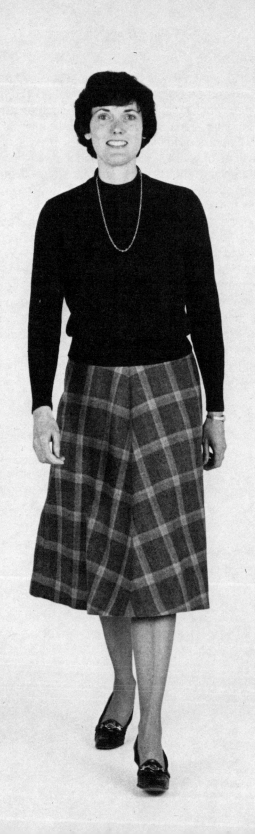

11
LIBIDO AND LIFE
AFTER FORTY

This chapter is not intended to be a "sex manual," however, in my counseling of obese women—and women in general— I find that sex, (or the lack of it) is a major problem.

Nowhere is the mind-body synchronization more apparent than in sex or sexual attraction. In fact, the mind is the most important organ.

When we are excited mentally, chemicals (endorphins) are produced that are powerful aphrodisiacs. Also, many people in love produce strong, addictive chemicals, and when love is withdrawn or thwarted for one reason or another, they suffer withdrawal symptoms, such as depression, similar to that of amphetamine withdrawal. Like all things related to our psychology and physiology, there are vast differences between individuals. Some are inherent, others ingrained due to parental, societal, and religious restrictions.

I do not believe that frustrated sexual energy is released in more creative ways, nor do I believe if sex is prohibited it becomes more enjoyable. In fact, it appears that in societies that are less sexually inhibited, there are fewer sex related difficulties. Some even hold the theory that sexual repression also diminishes the capacity to love, making people more likely to be hostile and aggressive.

Behaving as though sex is dirty or non-existent can lead to impotence, frigidity, or vaginismus (painful intercourse due to spasm of the sphincter muscles).

Forget the notion that your sex life ends when you can no longer reproduce. Many experts feel that women have stronger sexual drives than men, although the amount of intercourse varies greatly among individuals. A woman's sex drive peaks when she is in her thirties and remains constant until she is in her sixties or even older, with a slow decline thereafter. The male decline may be slow or non-existent, depending on testosterone levels.

Many of our ideas of sexless middle and older years reflect society's attitudes. We should not expect deafness, blindness or senility to be a normal part of aging, nor should we anticipate diminished sexual desire or ability.

In fact, sex should improve, because women no longer have the fear of pregnancy, children are out of the house, and many inhibitions have been discarded. At this age, women have more time and energy to spend on their husbands, and men are more sensitive, less preoccupied with personal gratification, and have greater control over orgasm.

Love, affection, touching, and sex is meaningful to people of all ages, and intercourse is a valid form of pleasurable exercise. (Don't consider it your aerobic exercise, however, because the increase in blood pressure and heart rate is due to stimulation by the adrenal glands.)

One of my students, a recently widowed older woman, confided that one of the things she missed most was her good sexual relationship. When she mentioned this to other widows her age, she was treated like a sexual pervert. Most said they were glad to be free of the bother. I convinced her SHE was normal, although unfortunately unique.

What causes this abnormal, but all too typical situation? First, many women our age received no sex education, other than the idea we were pure, sexless and passive. Sex was to be endured within the marriage for the man's pleasure. Men, on the other hand, were sexual, (which was bad), and were to be held at bay until the wedding night, at which time all was bliss for the man and we were ready to bear children.

Men often knew nothing about touching, affection, caring, or even technique. These things were not considered important to young men, who were most often preoccupied with their own personal self-gratification. Fortunately, these concepts have changed for many young men today, as "roles" are not as clearly defined, and tenderness is no longer considered a woman's quality.

There was high value placed on virginity, but men all tried "to make out." However, when the girls acquiesced, they were considered "bad" or "dirty." This makes for an unfortunate situation, because there is evidence that intercourse comes naturally to women, whereas men have to learn.

These inhibitions, brought on by parents and society, often cause the person's sexuality to be in contrast with the rest of the personality. A person who is outgoing and active otherwise may be reticent and inhibited regarding sex. More naturally (and usually) the sex activities reflect the general personality. But beyond intercourse, women and men need touching, affection, caring and sharing. This is not only during foreplay but following orgasm as well. Touching should be part of the life of a couple, not necessarily leading to intercourse. Many women tell me their husbands never touch them except when they want sex, and then it is over within a few minutes. This reduces intercourse to copulation, and women to receptacles.

It is no wonder they become sick, frustrated, and fat, and are glad to be rid of it altogether. A man may want a more sexually aggressive partner, and if his wife is inhibited, he may look for extramarital relationships.

Many men say they are no longer attracted to their wives because they are fat, whereas the women say they are fat because their husbands have not touched them in years. Of course, this is an excuse, but women do need loving and touching. Often the men have no technique, or if they do, spontaneity may be lacking, not only during intercourse but at other times as well. Although some studies have shown that the most happily married couples have sex on a more-or-less routine basis (averaging twice a week), it seems to me that would be a bore.

Probably the most important factor is that both have similar needs and expectations, as there is more than one way of loving the opposite sex. Feelings may be romantic, strongly sexual, or those of friendship. If one partner feels one way, and the other another, problems may arise. A good relationship should have an underlying basis of friendship, no matter what else exists. That means common interests, bonds, and liking each other, although many other kinds of sensual turn-ons take place. Some people feel inhibited with a person they love, and only relax and let go with a stranger. Some have the desire to act out their fantasies, no matter how bizarre; but for most of us, they are just temporary escapes from reality. Sharing fantasies with your partner can be very exciting to both. The more we are aware of and familiar with our bodies, the more likely we are able to know and convey that which gives us satisfaction. Some women have one or two orgasms, but most are capable of many. Most men have one or two, but some men too, are multi-orgasmic. Of course, reactions vary according to the way we are feeling, and the stimulus. A multi-orgasmic person may be tired, and satisfied with one orgasm, or extremely stimulated and reach one high peak. Women no longer feel that sexual gratification is for the man only. If a woman is attracted to a man, her whole body is sensitive and responsive. He needs to know which technique excites her, and not sulk if he is rebuffed. There is certainly a need for sex counselors, because of the lack of premarital education; and couples should avail themselves of their services if necessary.

Impotence appears to be on the increase. Some blame this on dietary deficiencies, chemicals or drugs. Others blame the women's movement for making men feel obligated to perform. Frankly, from what I have observed, I think our traditional rules of etiquette concerning dating, through which we have been taught to assume that males must do the asking or inviting, are wrong. First of all, girls mature more rapidly and are more likely to be assertive rather than aggressive.

Boys, and later men, either come on too strong, inviting a reaction of defense or hostility, or are too shy to ask at all. Many take an initial refusal as a personal rebuke and never try again. Some men never mature enough to outgrow these patterns set in their teens.

I observed a typical scenario recently. I was sitting at the beach near two teen-age boys. Nearby were two girls the boys wanted to ask out. They spent all afternoon discussing how to go about it. The girls had made an initial contact by asking the time, and the boys took this as a sign they could proceed. After much deliberation, they decided they wanted to go down the water-chute with the girls, but—how to go about asking them? By the end of the afternoon the only plan they came up with was to ask the girls what time the chute closed. Eventually, they asked the question, the girls told them, and that was the end of that! The boys went home alone.

My son goes to an engineering school where the men outnumber the women ten to one. Because of this, they feel that the women will be over-booked and consequently don't ask them out. Most of the time the women have no dates at all.

I spent much time watching my son and his roommates go through maneuvers similar to the one I observed on the beach. It appears the men are very afraid of a refusal. They told me unanimously that they would much prefer to have the women do the asking. My own experiences have been the same. I love to dance, but men tell me they need several drinks before they get up the nerve to ask. If I want to dance, I do the asking, and don't take "no" as a personal rejection, certainly nothing that would affect my sexual capacities.

If you are over forty and newly widowed or divorced, you may not be aware of some of the recent acceptable changes in dating customs. Women no longer feel self-conscious about dating younger men. You may or may not have to pay your way, or perhaps go to a less expensive restaurant, but so what, if you have the money and he doesn't?

Young men often have a great deal of respect and admiration for the maturity and experience of older women, and if your sex life has been deficient, it may be just the spark you need. Again, mutual respect and liking are big "plusses."

Women today insist on being accepted for themselves as people, not toys or things. Also, women who take care of their bodies are looking for men who are trim and neat. No longer are money and power alone enough to turn on a woman. I may enjoy a stimulating conversation with an interesting man, but if he is flabby, saggy and soft, that's where it ends.

Changes take place when hormonal production slows. Hormone-

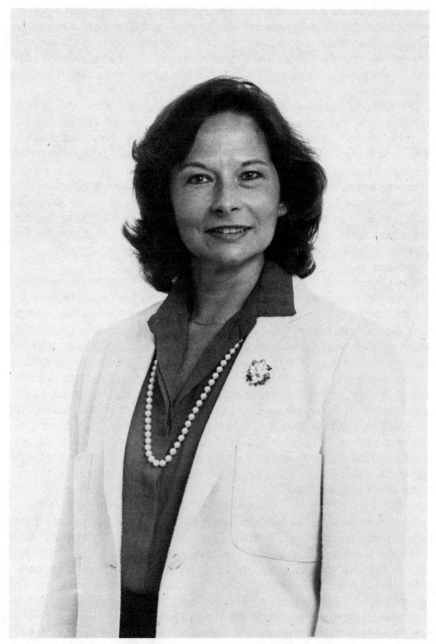

Women today insist on being accepted for themselves as people, not toys or things.

producing tissues start to atrophy, and the adrenal glands resume part of the function of producing estrogen. The uterus, genital tissues, and breasts may shrink and become less firm. Vaginal walls may become thinner and less pliable, and the cellular lining produces less lubrication upon stimulation. Even the clitoris can get smaller, although still transmitting sexual excitement.

K-Y jelly (not vaseline) helps replace diminished lubrication, and proper nutrition can offset some age-induced depletion of collagen and hormones. Keeping sexually active stimulates the glands of both men and women. **What you don't use, you lose.** This is true for all human aspects, whether they be physical, mental, emotional or sexual.

New techniques or positions with a husband or long-standing partner can add excitement to a humdrum routine. Don't try too many new things at once, or sex may become gymnastics. Technical facility is great, but not when it becomes a slick routine. Inspiration, and following the mood of the moment, evoke the greatest pleasure and the most surprising and pleasurable sensations.

Many people feel they cannot have intercourse unless they are in love. They spend years searching for the person who fits their idealized image, and if they find that person, they are often disappointed when they realize their "Gods" have feet of clay. Love makes a sexual relationship special and meaningful, even suffused with spiritual energy, but don't plan on a life of celibacy while you are waiting. You may have a long and frustrating wait.

Love, even the idealized kind, can be both erotic and pure, and should be free of anxiety and inhibitions. In a normal relationship, lovers' roles vary and change. At times, one will be the lover, and the other the receiver of love. Within minutes, roles may change, or both may simultaneously give and receive love. The more you are in tune with your partner, the more comfortable and natural your roles and responses will be. Rather than getting stale, love and sex should improve with age and familiarity: a definite possibility if both want it.

Lovers may be friends, or have an interchanging parent-child relationship. When relationships become fixed, problems arise, particularly if the roles are not mutually agreed upon.

We still see many variations of the "daddy-doll" relationship. To me, the sight of a normal, intelligent woman acting like a silly, dumb and helpless little girl to please a man, is disgusting. Unfortunately, when these women repeat this script often enough, they become the part they are playing. If roles please both, the relationship can be mutually agreeable. However, if one decides to change and the other does not, you have a whole new ball game, usually ending in extreme dissension or divorce.

There are men who like to view their wives as eternal "mothers," and women who see their husbands as all knowing, father-knows-best fathers. Some young men still feel this way, if they grew up in this type of household. If, in their view, this is normal, expected, and healthy, they had best make their future wives aware of their expectations. They can be very threatened by after-the-marriage surprises. Most older men who are set in this way of thinking will not change, and I, for one, don't even enjoy a casual date with this type of man.

Often men expect their wives to be passive, obedient, docile and non-assertive at all times except in bed. They may then expect the wife to be liberated enough to be aggressive! This is unrealistic, unless the woman really enjoys playing this game. Most women need to have a good and realistic image of themselves if they are to enjoy sex and maintain a healthy and attractive body.

Of course, the man, too, will reap the benefits.

Diet affects your sex life as it does your reproductive cycles, a fact that veterinarians have always known. Second-rate nutrition leads to second-rate reproduction: third-rate may yield none at all.

Common drugs may also have an adverse effect on sexual desire and performance. Dr. Nyla Cole of the University of Utah's College of Medicine lists the adverse effects that have been associated with certain drug classes: antihistamines can alter normal sexual functions; antidepressants lower desire; antihypertensives suppress activity; and antipsychotic drugs diminish erections and alter hormone levels. Often drugs that affect erectile functions in men create a reduction of vaginal lubrication in women.

Drugs deplete and alter nutrient levels, in addition to other side-effects. Stay off medication unless it is absolutely necessary. Ask your doctor if there are safer, natural means you can use to achieve health. You may find that drugs were unnecessary, after all.

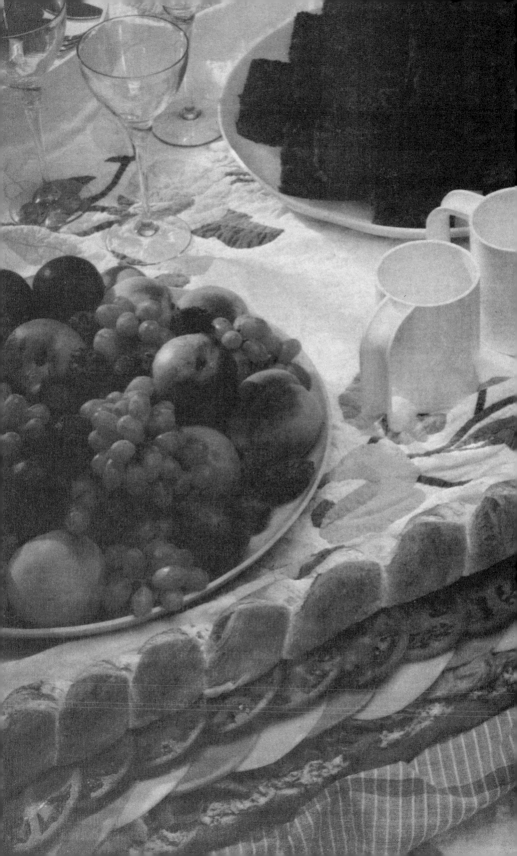

12
DIET FOR SEX

Many women claim they are too tired to enjoy sex. Unless you are truly overworked, either physically or mentally, or in the middle of a tiring and stressful situation (such as moving), this should be an occasional, not chronic complaint.

Even a small iron deficiency, or a slightly underactive thyroid can make you "too tired." It is very difficult for menstruating women to get enough iron, as much of our dietary intake is not absorbed. In addition to fatigue, one of the symptoms of iron deficiency is a disinterest in sex. Liver is the best source of iron, then red meats, almonds, beans and green vegetables. Iron is not readily absorbed from vegetable sources, and if you are a vegetarian, iron supplements should be taken to avoid anemia. The best way to take iron is first thing in the morning with some acid juice and vitamin C. Vitamin C supplements with meals help you to absorb the iron in the food, or you may prefer to add foods high in vitamin C to your meals, such as green peppers, citrus fruit, or tomatoes. Animal protein with your beans helps make iron in the beans more readily available to the body. When you are on a long term diet that is low in iron, the body learns to adjust and make do with less, but if you feel too dragged out to do much of anything, look for iron deficiency first.

If your thyroid is truly underactive, you will need to see a doctor, and perhaps medication, such as thyroxin, will be indicated. Your thyroid may be "sluggish" due to age, improper diet, or lack of exercise.

As in iron deficiency anemia, one of the main symptoms is lassitude and fatigue. Exercise may be just what you need, plus the addition of foods high in iodine, such as seafood, sea plants (dulce, kelp), and string beans. According to Dr. Michael Lesser, **Nutrition and Vitamin Therapy** (Grove Press, Inc., N.Y.), physical exercise and cold weather stimulate energy because they increase thyroid function. He treats with organic iodine, as well as thiamine (B1) and other B vitamins, if there is an indication of deficiency. Don't try to doctor your thyroid with supplements, however; diet and exercise alone may do the trick.

Cabbage, carrots, lettuce, beans, beets, spinach, strawberries and peaches contain goitrin, an antithyroid factor that depresses its function. Don't be afraid to eat these nutritious foods unless your diet is extremely unbalanced in their favor.

The pituitary gland secretes a number of hormones itself and influences the other glands, thus having both a direct and indirect influence on sexual and reproductive functions. The pituitary produces adrenocorticotrophic hormone (ACTH), which with the B vitamins pantothenic acid and niacin, stimulate adrenal hormone production. The pituitary also produces growth hormones, which control human growth.

The pituitary hormones, the gonadotrophic hormones, directly affect sexuality. In women they stimulate the production of female sex hormones and the development of the egg; in men they stimulate the production of sperm and the male sex hormone.

Vitamin E and zinc are found in high concentration in the pituitary gland. E is essential to hormone production, and because it's an antioxident, it protects the pituitary and adrenal hormones from destruction by oxygen. Zinc is involved in the function of several other glands and is abundant in the prostate and testis.

Vitamin C works with zinc and selenium in the formation of the collagen component, elastin. Collagen is the cement that keeps tissues firm and elastic.

Selenium is synergistic with vitamin E, enhancing its action. Selenium, which is found in seafood and whole grains that are grown on selenium-rich soil, has been shown to prevent breast cancer in mice—one more indication that we can help prevent cancer with diet.

Premature aging and an early menopause may be signs of an underfunctioning pituitary. Foods to nourish the pituitary are complete proteins (meat, fish, milk, cheese), whole grains, nuts and seeds. The B vitamins, which are found in these sources are important; so are green vegetables. B vitamins are also abundant in wheat germ, brewer's yeast and desiccated liver.

The adrenal glands produce adrenalin and noradrenalin in the medulla, or core. Adrenalin is produced in response to stress and inhibits sexual desire. Unlike adrenalin, noradrenalin slows the heart, promoting a relaxed feeling; but it, too, decreases the desire for sex. The cortex, or shell of the adrenal gland produces the hormones glucocorticoids (cortisone), mineralcorticoids, which control mineral balance, and some sex hormones. Some of the symptoms of chronic adrenal exhaustion are fatigue, irritability, poor appetite, periods of depression, no strength for sex, dizziness when rising quickly to a standing position, and inability to tolerate bright lights. Factors precipitating adrenal burn-out are junk food diets high in coffee, sugar, and alcohol, physical or mental overwork, exposure to toxic chemicals, infections, lack of sufficient rest or exercise. (Note that all of these conditions are mentioned in the chapter on stress.)

The first and most obvious thing to do to nourish the adrenal glands is to simply eat a more nourishing and whole-food diet. Unless over-exercise (or over training) is causing your exhaustion, exercise will aid the function of the adrenal glands. Many of the Yoga exercises are designed specifically to stimulate glands.

The B vitamins, particularly pantothenic acid, riboflavin, and niacin, vitamins A, E, and especially C, nourish the gland. Vitamin C is highly concentrated in the adrenal gland, and easily depleted.

Do not take large amounts of any vitamin, especially the fat soluble ones (A and D) without a doctor's prescription. Each of us has special requirements and individual levels at which a substance becomes toxic.

I suggest that you find a doctor or chiropractor who can test your glandular function and prescribe accordingly. The adrenal glands also require some cholesterol (soft-boiled or poached eggs to which no fat has been added), and the essential fatty acid, linoleic acid (found in cold-pressed wheat germ or vegetable oils, seeds and nuts).

We shall discuss cholesterol in the chapter on nutrition, but it must be mentioned here because the sex hormones are made from cholesterol. New evidence indicates that it is not dietary cholesterol that causes plaques to form in the arteries, but the inability of the body to metabolize the cholesterol properly, which may occur when the diet is deficient in magnesium and vitamin B6. Eating fewer calories, stress reduction and exercise help to lower cholesterol. There is no need to give up eggs, nature's most perfect food.

The ovaries produce the hormones estrogen and progesterone that determine the reproductive functions, including menopause and the menstrual cycle. Estrogen has to do with sexual activity, and the development of feminine characteristics, such as breasts. Progesterone regulates ovulation, menstruation, and maintaining a normal pregnancy. Women also produce small amounts of androgens, or male hormones, which increase sexual desire.

The B vitamins folic acid (found in leafy greens) and niacin are important in the formation and utilization of estrogen. Folic acid is especially important during pregnancy. Vitamin E is important to sexual health, and zinc aids in maintaining healthy vaginal tissues.

No woman over forty should be on the birth control pill, as the possible side effects such as blood clots, cancer and depression are greatly increased with age. The pill changes the acid-alkaline balance of the vagina, making the user more susceptible to vaginal infections and venereal disease. I have known young girls on the pill who were constantly struggling to rid themselves of chronic vaginitis. The pill also disturbs the vitamin and mineral balance, lowering some of the B vitamins, C and E, and increasing iron and A. Also, there is a raising of blood copper and lowering of zinc, which may cause depression and irritability.

Although effective as a birth control measure, it seems to me the known and possible dangers from the pill far outweigh its virtues.

Safer means of contraception are being investigated, but their use is not yet widespread. Even tubal ligation, once cited as being "safe and effective" has a common (some estimate as high as 50%) after-effect of causing menorrhagia (heavy menstrual bleeding), which may occur about two years after the surgery. More research is needed for male birth control; after all, even though they don't get pregnant, they are definitely involved!

A word about male sexuality. Most of us share our lives with men, whether they be husbands or lovers. Primary impotence in men may be caused by alcoholism, the use of drugs, (hypertensive drugs or even marijuana), diabetes, or vascular diseases. Some of these conditions are reversible and should be medically treated. Others, such as too much alcohol (if he is not alcoholic) are temporary. Alcohol plays a dual role as far as sex is concerned. A little may be relaxing and loosen inhibitions. Too much often has the reverse effect, nullifying everything.

Secondary impotence, that is, when a man is able to have an erection, but unable to have satisfactory intercourse for one reason or another, is often psychological in nature, and may be treated successfully with therapy. Do not negate the placebo effect. Placebos, as well as affecting the mind, do cause corresponding chemical changes in the body. (See the chapter on endorphins.) Of course, he must believe the pill you are giving him is some powerful Oriental aphrodisiac you were only able to purchase at great cost and personal danger! If, however, he has lost all sexual interest in you, it may be difficult or impossible to revive it unless he, as well as you, really wants this to happen.

The male sex drive may wane if he does not exercise or get enough rest, eats improperly, is under stress, and abstains. This is only common sense, but it is not always recognized. He may think he is "over the hill," when all he needs is some zinc in his diet, and a long vacation. According to Dr. E. Cheraskin in **Psycho-Dietics,** the male glands cannot perform without zinc. In addition to zinc, B vitamins, especially B6, are helpful, as well as vitamin E and manganese. Potassium and magnesium are needed for nerve and muscle cells to work properly, and they are helpful if he is also depressed. You may see improvement immediately, or he may take two or three months to respond to dietary changes. It may depend on how soon he recovers from depression and anxiety.

A natural, unrefined, whole food diet is as important to our sex life as it is to general health. Nutrients that are refined or boiled out of foods are not available to us, and the body may rob itself of existing vitamins to metabolize empty foods. Men should avoid foods such as hot dogs, bacon and sausage that are filled with sodium nitrate (salt peter).

The Orientals eat meat or fish for sexual vigor. They break foods down into Yin and Yang; yang being active, hot, and masculine; yin, cool, passive, and feminine. Meats and vegetables are predominately Yang, while starches, sweets and fruits are Yin. Ideally, there is a balance, which is achieved through diet, meditation, and specific exercise rituals such as TaiChi.

Are there such things as aphrodisiacs? It has been suggested that B15, or calcium pangamate is one. I must say that although the Russians claim it helps athletic (sexual?) performance, in this country its use is controversial.

Some studies claim it is beneficial, as it is involved in energy creation within the cell; others say it is worthless. There is the possibility that the formula is not always accurate, affecting the results. Ginseng is a tonic for the whole body, and as such, is supposed to affect sex. The Chinese consider it a masculine, or Yang, herb, although women take it also. The Chinese also give special acclaim to Bird's Nest Soup, which is made from the sea swallow nest of seaweed glued together with fish eggs. It may not sound appealing but it is a super-potent source of vitamins, minerals, and proteins!

The Chinese also consider onions, garlic, seafoods, bamboo shoots and ginger to be aphrodisiacs. Garlic and onions are sulphur foods, and claims have been made through the ages about their ability to maintain youth and health. These foods are metabolic stimulants, and garlic, especially, is being acclaimed in health circles as being beneficial in preventing heart attack and stroke.

Some of the foods mentioned in The Kama Sutra for increasing sexual vigor are milk, sesame seeds, honey, butter, and beans. The Indians suggest a glass of (whole) milk after sex, for a man to restore himself. These foods provide nutrients needed for the glands and fluids to function properly.

You can have fun making your own gland-nourishing candy. (It is not low in calories!) Get some sesame seed meal at a health food store. Add chopped almonds or walnuts and raw wheat germ and moisten with just enough honey so that you can form balls about the size of walnuts. You may add a little vanilla or almond extract for flavoring if you desire. Keep them chilled in the refrigerator, and eat as a snack or dessert. Incidently, this is a healthful candy to give to your children, as it is filled with protein and vitamins, linoleic acid, and many other nutrients.

13
SEXERCISES

Bobbie Prudden calls exercises designed to prepare your body for a full and sufficient social life "sexercises". In the course I taught for the recreation department they were called "Exotic Exercises For Women Only." I used belly dance music, some of the belly dance movements, both fast and slow, some Yoga, and lots of hip, thigh, back and abdominal strengthening and stretching exercises. The belly dancing was fun, and it specifically emphasized the areas we were working, plus it taught body awareness and control through the practice of isolating muscles. Yoga, more than any other discipline, brings the body and mind together, and as well as vastly increasing flexibility, it strengthens muscles and stimulates and nourishes glands.

Yoga teaches the unity of body, mind and spirit, and as such does not teach exercise for sexual pleasure alone. There is a form of sexual Yoga, called Tantric Yoga, and sexual pleasure books such as the Kama Sutra, and there is no question that the beginning student of Yoga almost always is aware of sexual stimulation. Some Yogis believe that sexual energies should be sublimated to higher forces, and that these energies rise up the spine in the form of the Kundalini.

Others hold that one can have a higher purpose and still use the sex force for what it was intended, that, sublimated or not, it still lies in the subconscious. Many specific exercises are given to "householder" or married Yogis, who believe that sex is best utilized when there is a mental and spiritual union as well, in other words, love. Anyone who has experienced the "Rising of the Kundalini" after sex can tell you it is a beautiful experience, filling the whole body and consciousness with high energy. This experience is not likely to be achieved as the result of casual sex.

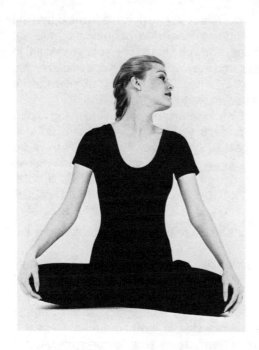

Yoga teaches the unity of body, mind and spirit, and as such does not teach exercise for sexual pleasure alone.

Sexercises are not only good for sex, but are excellent for postural and lower back problems, helpful in dancing and many sports (including tennis, jogging, and horseback riding) and are especially beneficial to women, who due to aging or giving birth, have prolapsed organs and lack of bladder control. In addition, they firm and reduce the hips, abdomen, buttocks, waist and thighs and increase energy. Men can benefit from these exercises, in other than the obvious way, for the same reasons that women can. Yogis also claim they prevent or cure impotence.

The muscles we are strengthening (and stretching where indicated) are the abdominal muscles, both in front and on the sides of the abdomen, the buttocks, again, both directly beneath us and on the sides, the hip, inner and outer thigh, plus front and back of the thigh. In addition, we shall be strengthening the sphincter muscles (all three sets) and the levator muscle at the base of the pelvis called the pubococcygeous. Strengthening the sphincter muscles will make sex more pleasurable for both of you, and the pelvic tilt exercises may make your lower back pain go away forever.

In the beginning, you may have trouble isolating the rectal sphincters from those of the vagina, but that doesn't matter. Strengthen them together, along with those involved with emptying the bladder. Many women have a weakening or tear of the muscles at the front of the vaginal wall which separates the bladder and urethral tube from the vagina. If the condition is mild and affects only the urethra, exercise may help. Keep in mind that the symptoms of urinating when coughing, sneezing or jumping may not indicate the severity of the condition, and you should see your physician. In any case, the exercises may help, and they won't hurt. (A specific exercise for this problem is: once or twice a day, when the bladder is full, interrupt the flow by stopping several times when voiding.)

To help isolate the other sphincter muscles, pretend you are trying to pick up a coin with the vagina. Or, pretend you have to go, can't get to a bathroom, so you have to hold back. Tighten all of the muscles involved whenever the directions say to tighten the sphincter muscles. Unless indicated, do all exercises on a mat on the floor. If it hurts, don't do it. EXHALE WHEN YOU HOLD CONTRACTIONS. NEVER HOLD YOUR BREATH.

This is a specific for the buttock or gluteal muscles, but it works the abdominals and thighs also.

Lie on your stomach, head resting on your arms, toes touching, heels relaxed and apart. Tighten the buttock and sphincter muscles, at the same time pulling the heels together. Hold for 5 seconds only, then relax all muscles completely, letting the heels fall to the sides again. Do this 3 times, then try contracting the abdominal muscles at the same time. Repeat 3 times, holding each for 5 seconds, and being sure to relax completely between contractions. After you finish, roll over to your back and bring both knees to your chest to stretch and relax your lower back.

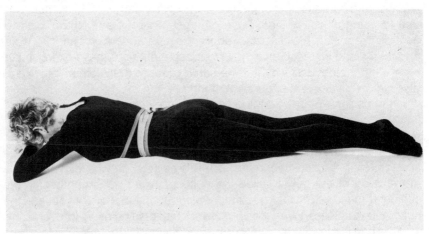

This works both the upper and lower abdominals as well as the sphincter muscles. Exercise #1 is for beginners or those with back problems. Exercise #2 is advanced, and requires strong abdominal control and the ability to visualize.

#1. Lie on your back, arms at your sides, one knee bent so the foot is flat on the floor. Exhale, slowly raising your head and upper back from the floor, at the same time lifting the outstretched leg 4 inches off the floor. Hold for a few seconds, then relax, slowly returning your head and leg to the floor. Maintain your lower back on the floor throughout. Be sure to contract the sphincter muscles each time you lift, and relax them as you lower. Build up to 5 times with each leg.

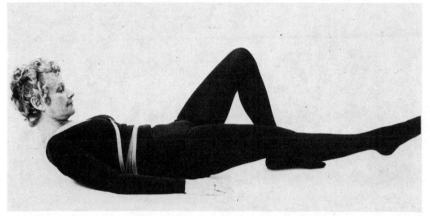

Exercise #1: abdominals and sphincter muscles (for beginners).

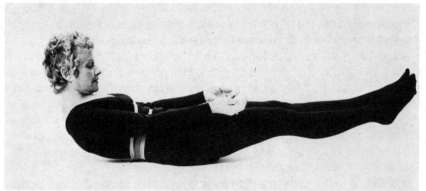

Exercise #2: abdominals and sphincter muscles (for advanced).

#2. Lie on your back, with legs outstretched, palms by your side facing up. Exhale hard through your mouth as you sharply tighten the buttock, abdominal and sphincter muscles. The force of your contraction should swoop your arms, legs, and upper back off the floor. The lower back does not arch, nor leave the floor. Hold the lifted position for a few seconds, then lie back and relax. Repeat 3 or 4 times.

This is the pelvic tilt, lying on your back. It may be done standing or sitting. Excellent for the lower back.

#1. Lie on your back with your arms at your sides. Tighten your buttock, abdominal and sphincter muscles. You should feel your lower back press into the floor. Hold for 5 seconds, then relax. (Photo below.)

#2. Contract even harder, so the lower part of the pelvis lifts off the floor. Tighten the sphincters! Repeat several times slowly.

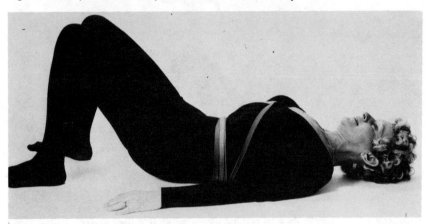

Exercise #1: pelvic tilt—lying on your back.

These exercises are designed to stretch the muscles of the inner thighs. If you find them difficult, do just the first one for a few weeks.

#1. Sit on the floor with your knees bent and the soles of your feet touching. If your joints and muscles are tight, you may have to place your feet a little distance from your body. Otherwise, bring them in towards your crotch as closely as you can. Rest your hands on your knees, or in your lap, and lift your rib cage so that your back is straight and you are stretching the upper abdominal muscles. Sit there until you feel tired or uncomfortable. Gravity will be stretching for you, and eventually your knees will get closer to the floor. Breathe in and out slowly, and relax.

#2. Sitting in the same position as above, again, bring your feet closely into your crotch, and holding on to your feet, slowly lower your head towards your feet. This may seem impossible at first, but the important thing to remember is NEVER FORCE IT. If you feel a stretch on your inner thighs and your back, you are successful. Two things will help: First, visualize your body doing what you want it to. Then, breathe in deeply, and exhale slowly, repeating several times. Each time you exhale, let your body RELAX and your head come closer to your feet. Hold the position for 30 seconds or longer, twice.

#3. Lie on your back, arms resting at your sides. Bring your legs overhead to 90 degrees, and let them spread apart as far as they can, and hold the position. If your hamstrings are very tight, your legs will not be up quite so high, and your knees will bend a little. That's fine, let them bend. Gravity is helping you stretch. After you get tired in this position, which may be from 20 seconds to 2 or more minutes, add a stretch to your hip, waist and outer thigh by **slowly** lowering your right leg to the floor beside you, then letting your left leg come across to lie directly on top of the right leg, and turn your head to the left. Hold this position for 20 seconds, then **slowly** lift your left leg, and then both, back to the center position, head centered. Next lower the leg slowly to the left; the right joins it, with the head turning to the right. Slowly return to center. Bring your legs together and relax.

This exercise stretches and strengthens the thighs as well as the whole pelvic area. If you have weak knees, do not do it. **Avoid arching your back.** Go from position A to position B, which relaxes and stretches the entire spine, as well as lengthens the abdominals. Do each position 2 times.

#1. Kneel down, then sit back on your heels. Have the toes close together, and the heels apart so there is sort of a saddle to sit in. From this position, reach your arms straight down behind you, using your hands for support. Tighten the buttocks, abdominals and sphincter muscles, and slowly raise your hips. Hold the position as long as comfortable, then sit back on your heels and go to position B. (Photo below.)

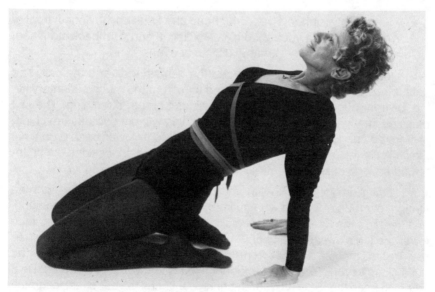

Exercise #1: stretching and strengthening the thighs and pelvic area.

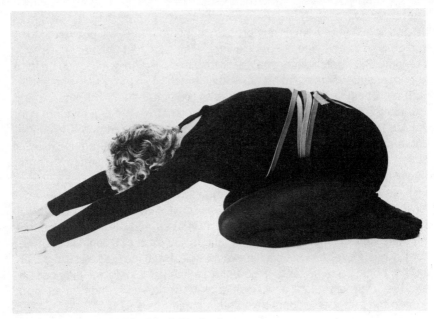

Exercise #2: stretching the abdominals.

#2. Sitting on your heels, rest your head and arms on the floor in front of you. Work on keeping your abdominals pulled in and your back stretched. Hold at least 30 seconds. Breathe! (Photo above.)

Stretches for the back of the thigh, (the hamstrings), and the calf. The hamstrings can become shortened and tight from too much sedentary living, or from engaging in active sports without proper stretching. The calf muscles often become shortened from running without enough stretching, or from wearing high heels. Both can contribute to lower back problems. Flexibility in this area helps increase your repertoire of positions during intercourse, and eases back strain. Go from exercise A to exercise B.

#1. Lying on your back, with your left knee bent, bring your right leg straight overhead. Stop at whatever point you feel your knee has to bend, and keeping the knee straight, hold that position for a few seconds, then lower the leg slowly to the floor. If your hamstrings are very tight, your leg may be less than 90 degrees from the floor, if you are very flexible, it may be quite close to your face. The important thing is that you feel a stretch. Do 3 times on each leg, SLOWLY, then bring your knees to your chest to stretch the lower back. (Photo on page 255).

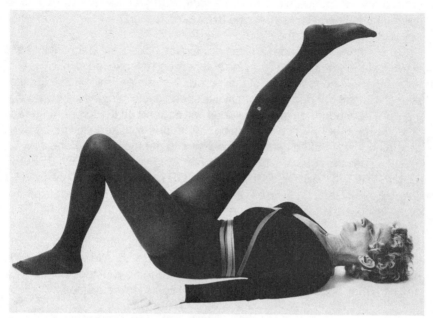

Exercise #1: stretching the hamstrings.

#2. On your back, left leg bent, feet flat on the floor. Swing your right leg up towards your face, once, twice, and on the third swing, catch it with both hands and hold it. VERY GENTLY pull your leg towards your face. **Never use undue force, or pull until there is pain.** If the leg does not move, don't force it; it means the muscles are very tight. Hold for twenty seconds or more. Do 2 times with each leg.

Taking a 20 minute warm bath or shower is very helpful before stretching exercises. Being warm, the muscles are more flexible and responsive, and there is less chance of injury. This is especially beneficial for those with tight joints and muscles, and lower (or upper) back problems.

Actually, your sexercises (and day's exercises) should begin first thing in the morning before your get out of bed, (not necessarily by the act of sex itself). You body temperature drops at night, and your movement is reduced, causing your joints, muscles and connective tissue to become stiff and less elastic. Many women, especially as they grow older, awaken with stiff and painful hip, back and neck joints. This can be caused by one or more of many reasons. There could be osteo- or rheumatoid arthritis, or osteoporosis. Your bed may be too soft or too hard or too small, not allowing you freedom of movement during the night. Your pillow could be too large, poking your neck up in an unnatural position, or too small, allowing your neck to hang down when you sleep on your side. Poor ventilation, with a lack of fresh air circulation can cause you to awaken feeling more tired than when you went to bed. (See the chapter on arthritis.)

In the winter, sleep under an electric blanket, because it is lightweight and warm. I sleep with nothing on in the summer and a loose tee shirt in the winter, so there is no restriction of movement. No matter how much exercise I plan on getting during the day, I always spend a few minutes in bed loosening up. The amount of time you spend will depend on the temperature and how you feel that particular morning. My in-bed routine followed by deep breathing in front of an open window helps to get me going for the day. Do these in correct sequence, beginning with "A." THE RULE "FLEX BEFORE YOU STRETCH" IS OF PRIMARY IMPORTANCE. YOU CAN EASILY CAUSE A STRAIN BY STRETCHING A COLD MUSCLE. Do not expect to be as flexible first thing in the morning as you are later in the day.

#1. Lie on your back with your knees bent and together. Slowly roll your knees from one side of your body to the other. Do not allow your pelvis to retract. Start by moving just a little, gradually bringing your legs closer to the bed on either side. Roll a few times, or until your back feels loose.

#2. Still on your back, knees bent, arms at your sides. Bring alternately one knee and then the other to your chest. Then bring both legs. You may gently use your hands to help bring your thighs closer to your chest, but **don't force.** Hold the position with both thighs close to your chest; then bring your head towards your knees. (Photo below).

#3. Roll your neck slowly from side to side, then shrug your shoulders 2 or 3 times.

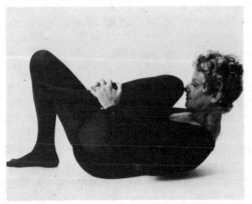 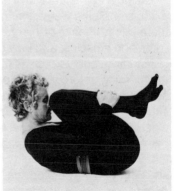

Exercise #2   **Exercise #2**

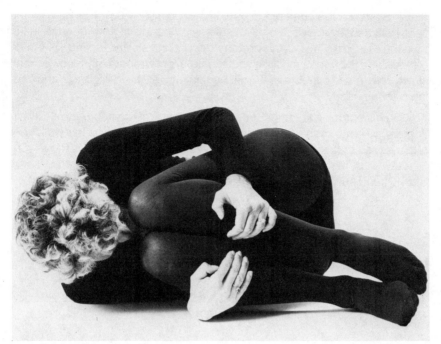

Exercise #4.

#4. Lie on your side and bring both knees towards your chest, and your head down towards your knees. Then still on your side, stretch your body in a straight line, arms towards the head of the bed, feet towards the foot. Alternate flex and stretch, doing each 2 times on each side. Finish by lying on your back and bringing your knees to your chest.

#5. On your back, left knee bent, foot flat on the bed. Keeping your right leg on the bed, try to lengthen it by stretching it towards the foot of the bed. At the same time, reach your right arm up towards the head of the bed. Feel the stretch in the entire right side. Do not overstretch. Repeat on the left side.

#6. This exercise strengthens and tones the buttocks, back of the thighs, and lower back. Lie at the edge of the bed, body supported by the bed, legs hanging down. Slowly lift the right leg until it is in a straight line with the rest of your body, no higher. Slowly lower. Do 2 or 3 times with each leg, building up to 5. When your lower back gets strong, you may lift both legs together, however, do not lift them higher than the bed. The exercise is made harder if it is done with the legs spread apart. Finish by lying on the bed and bringing both knees to your chest to relax and stretch your lower back.

#7. Sitting on the edge of the bed, slowly do a toe touch, reaching for the floor between your legs. Hang loosely, with the top of your head pointing towards the floor. Relax, and breathe deeply and slowly, feeling your body get closer to the floor each time you exhale. Tighten your belly muscles, and slowly roll up one vertebra at a time, beginning with the lower back, and ending with the neck.

#8. This exercise is for the triceps, at the back of the upper arm. Still sitting on the edge of the bed, grasp the bed with your hands and walk your feet away so that you are supported by your arms. The more you move your feet away so that your body is in a straight line, the harder the exercise. Slowly bend and straighten your elbows. Do 2 or 3 times, building up to 8.

Your body is awake and alive, and ready to face the day!

Your in-bed routine and some Yoga deep breathing and stretching may be all you have time for in the morning. Do the rest of your exercises any other time during the day, as long as it is not less than a half hour after a light meal, or an hour after a heavy meal. Let's continue the sexercises with some stretching, which may be done as soon as you get out of bed. I do mine in fresh air. Once you have learned the next exercise, the stomach lift, you can do it easily and quickly as you walk.

This exercise tones and lifts the abdominal muscles and organs, massages and brings fresh supply of blood to the organs and glands, and is supposed to cure impotence. It should only be done on an empty stomach, and not when there is a heavy menstrual flow. Bend forward, resting you hands on your knees. Take a deep breath, exhale, then exhale again, to make certain there is no air in the lungs. Keeping the air out, pull your stomach in towards your backbone, then try to lift it up under your rib cage. When you feel the need to inhale, do so, and let the stomach relax. It may take you a while to get the feeling of this 2 stage lift. When you do, you will feel a suction and a lifting, and there will be a hollow where your gut was once protruding. At that time, tuck your chin in the jugular notch as you hold the position. Do 2 times, holding the position as long as it is comfortable. Contract the sphincter muscles as you hold. If you have high blood pressure, eliminate the neck position and sphincter contraction.

These exercises are for flexibility, the waist, and is an energizer.

#1. Stand with your feet about 3 feet apart, and arms outstreched at shoulder height. Inhale deeply, then exhale as you slowly reach your right hand towards your right ankle. Turn your head so that you are looking at your left hand, which is straight up above you. Hold for 10 seconds or more, and return slowly to the standing position, and repeat on the other side. Do 2 times on each side. If you are very inflexible, or have lower back problems, bend your right knee as you reach for the right ankle: left knee, left ankle.

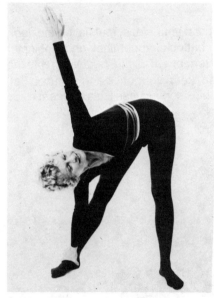

Exercise #1.

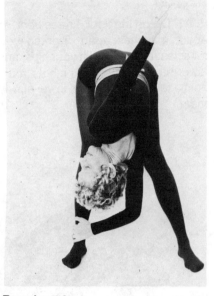

Exercise #2.

#2. Standing in the same position as "#1." Very slowly twist from the waist, and reach your right hand towards your LEFT ankle, looking up at your left arm which is stretched above. Hold for 20 seconds, then slowly return to standing position. Do twice on each side. If you have tight back and hamstring muscles, lift the RIGHT heel as you reach for the LEFT ankle, LEFT heel as you reach with the left hand for the right ankle.

THE RULE FOR THOSE TIGHT OR PAINFUL BACKS IS: ALL FORWARD, SIDE OR TWISTING MOVEMENTS MUST BE DONE VERY SLOWLY, WITH THE KNEES BENT SLIGHTLY.

This exercise is quite beneficial for those with "bad" knees as it strengthens the front and inner thigh, as well as the sphincters:

Sit in a hard chair or on the floor with a straight back and your legs straight out in front of you, touching. Press your legs together as hard as you can, at the same time tightening the sphincter muscles. Hold for 5 seconds. Do 3 times.

For hips, thighs, lower back and abdominals, the following exercises can be performed:

#1. Lie on the floor, knees bent, arms at your sides, feet flat on the floor, about 4 inches apart. Tighten your buttock, abdominal and sphincter muscles, and slowly lift your hips, one vertebra at a time, beginning with the lower back. Lift only as high as you can, keep your back and stomach flat, hold a few seconds, then lower slowly, hips coming last. Relax; repeat twice more.

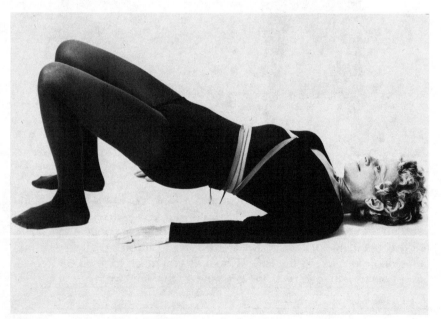

Exercise #1: for the hips, thighs, lower back and abdominals.

#2. This exercise will provide benefits to the abdominal and buttock muscles. When the hips are elevated, lift the right leg slowly. Point to the ceiling, then lower to the floor. Lower your hips slowly, then repeat with the left leg.

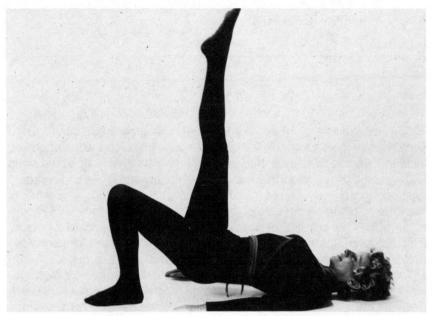

Exercise #2: starting position.

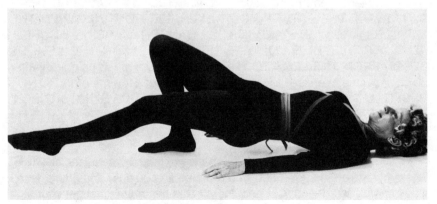

Exercise #2: mid-range position.

Any exercise that reverses the blood flow, such as the head stand and the shoulder stand, sends an extra supply of nourishing blood to the brain.

Any exercise that reverses the blood flow, such as the head stand and the shoulder stand, sends an extra supply of nourishing blood to the brain and all of the glands. Of course, this extra nourishment also goes to the scalp and skin, and the constant downward pull of gravity on tissues and organs is reversed. I once heard a plastic surgeon say that if we could spend half of our lives standing on our heads, we would never need a face lift. Unfortunately, this is not practical or possible. Relaxing on a slant board for twenty minutes as an alternative is quite revitalizing. If your knees are bent, the back is more relaxed, and you can do sit-ups and other exercises.

The head stand is not for everyone, and should be learned from a competent instructor. One of my students, a Yoga teacher, fractured a vertebra in her neck doing the head stand. The shoulder stand can also be dangerous for anyone who is very much overweight, has weak neck muscles, or other pathology involving the cervical spine. In any case, if you feel you can safely do the shoulder stand and variations, IT SHOULD ALWAYS BE DONE SLOWLY AT THE END OF YOUR EXERCISE ROUTINE WHEN THE MUSCLES ARE WARM AND IN LESS DANGER OF BEING INJURED. ALSO, AT THIS TIME YOU ARE HELPING RETURN THE VENOUS BLOOD FROM THE LEGS TO THE HEART. Never stand up quickly after doing a reverse exercise. Always rest your back for a few minutes. DO NOT PERFORM THIS EXERCISE IF YOU FEEL PRESSURE ON YOUR NECK. BEGINNERS SHOULD REST ON THE UPPER BACK, NOT THE SHOULDERS.

#1. Lying on your back, using your hands to help if necessary, slowly lift legs and hips off the floor, until you are standing on your shoulders. Don't worry if you can't get on your shoulders in the beginning; just get your hips up, using your arms for support. If you can get up on your shoulders, press your chin into the jugular notch as you hold your shoulder-stand position, doing slow abdominal breathing. Hold for several seconds in the beginning, gradually building up to 2 or more minutes. Using your hands to help, slowly lower your body to the floor, and rest. If your neck feels tense, relax it by bringing your knees to your chest.

#2. While in the shoulder-stand, hips supported by your hands, bicycle 10 times. Again, lower slowly.

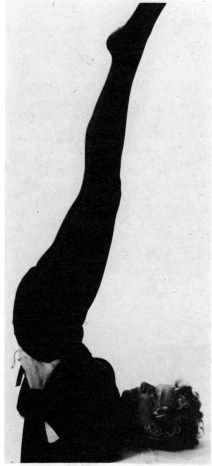

Exercise #1.

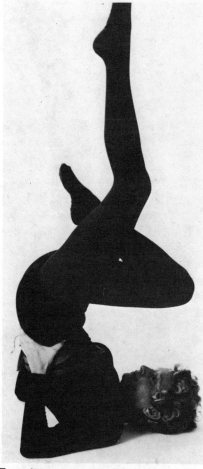

Exercise #2.

#3. In the shoulder-stand position, slowly lower alternate legs to the floor behind you. Now try both legs. If your back or hamstrings are tight, bend your knees slightly. Never let anyone try to push your feet towards the floor, as you can severely strain your lower back. Again, come out slowly, rolling down one vertebra at a time. Touching the floor behind you is not important. Getting a stretch is the goal, one that will be reached at a different point for everyone.

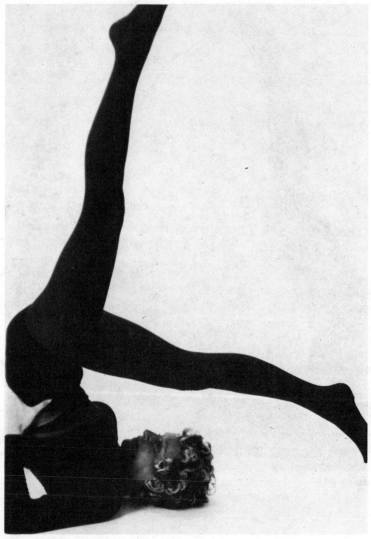

Exercise #3: starting position.

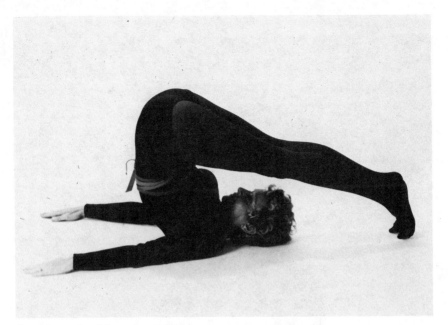

Exercise #3: mid-range position.

It is not necessary to do all of the exercises. You may choose one or two from each group and add them to your regular program. You can tighten your thigh, abdominal, buttock and sphincter muscles any time or anywhere, and no one need be the wiser. However, once you really learn to contract the gluteus maximus (the muscles you're sitting on), your body will rise slightly, a fact you may want to keep in mind when you are practicing in public. Many of the exercises can be done any time you are sitting or standing, such as talking on the phone or watching TV.

No matter how "good" either of you may be in the art of making love, the object is not technical perfection, but the satisfaction and pleasure you give to each other. The aspect of love adds a special atmosphere, but obviously, it is not there for everyone at all times. Most women today expect to get, as well as give, sexual satisfaction. Tightening the vagina during intercourse, especially on the "in" stroke will help achieve this, and a strong, flexible, healthy body enhances all pleasures.

On the first day of exotic class exercise I always jokingly asked the women to bring a note from their husbands (or lovers) on the last day, saying there was improvement. One group of women got even with me for that. They brought in a long, explicit letter, mentioning them by name, and signed "a grateful neighbor."

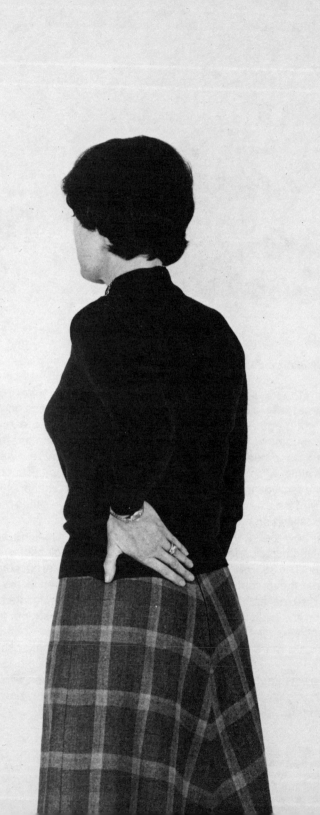

14
OH, MY ACHING BACK!

Backache is one of the most common ailments in this country. One in three will have a severe backache at least once in their lives, and an estimated 30 million suffer chronically.

Corporate America loses over a billion dollars to common backaches each year. Why? Some blame it on our bipedal stance; yet animals, like the Dachshund, are also afflicted. "I have a weak back" is a complaint I've heard many times. In fact, in most cases, the back is not weak at all.

According to Dr. Hans Kraus, leading psychiatrist and medical consultant to the President's Council On Physical Fitness and Sports, at least 83% of all back problems are not organic, but are caused by tension and muscular imbalances, inflexibility and weaknesses. Other causes are referred pain. The back hurts because of a dysfunction, irritation, or weakness in another part of the body.

Let's look first at referred pain. Common causes of backache for women are pre-menstrual pressure, the menstrual period itself, pregnancy and menopause. Although not as common, I have known women who had backaches only during ovulation. At these times, the colon and belly muscles may lose tone, contributing to the backache. A prolapsed uterus, uterine tumors, the IUD, tampons and the diaphragm may all cause back pain.

An imbalance in the endocrine system can create muscular weakness and pain, and almost every mother experiences some post-natal backache. (This responds well to abdominal strengthening exercises, and proper lifting and carrying of the child so as to place minimal strain on the back.)

Other causes of referred pain are diseases of the heart, lungs, stomach, kidneys, colon, ovaries and fallopian tubes. Malformations, such as a short leg, or even a dysfunctioning mandible, can cause pain in the back. An undetected cancer or tuberculosis can cause backache, and must be ruled out as a possible cause of chronic pain.

In most cases, there is no underlying disease, and X-rays rule out fracture, ruptured disc, arthritis, and osteoporosis. The sufferer is usually in good general health, except for pain in the back, which is making life miserable.

If you suffer from backache most likely you are a victim of the modern curse of too much tension and too little exercise. You may not even be aware of this tension, but your body is responding to it with muscles that tense, stiffen, become painful and eventually go into spasm. The muscles are altered, lose their elasticity, become shortened, stress the joints, and develop trigger points.

This syndrome can take place because you hate your job, your boss or your husband. Common everyday irritations, such as traffic jams, long waits in check-out counters, the telephone, noisy children and dogs, and time pressures can cause a painful bout of backache. The pain is not "in your mind," any more than are tension-induced heart attacks or ulcers. If left uncorrected, permanent changes in the musculoskeletal system can result. Add incorrect posture and improper use or over-use of body, and you have a prescription for pain.

Tension wreaks the most havoc on muscles that are already stiff and weak. The spine depends on "guy wires" to support it: abdominal, hip, buttock, thigh and back muscles. When they are not exercised, they require progressively less blood and other nourishment. The capillaries begin shriveling, and muscles shrink or atrophy. Add tension, and perhaps cold, and muscles can go into spasm, an involuntary contraction, or tension.

A sporadic burst of exercise, without first properly warming up or relaxing the muscles first, can cause a painful spasm. "Week-end warriors," who take part in strenuous sports on the weekend and do nothing but sit during the week, often end up in the doctor's office on Monday morning. Doctors themselves make the same mistakes everyone else does. A friend, a pediatrician in his late thirties, spends much time with his orthopedist as a result of week-end strains, sprains and injuries. He was told that because of his age, his muscles and joints had lost elasticity, and he should do flexibility exercises every day of his life. (I give this advice to everyone, whether he or she takes part in sports, or is just plain sedentary.) My friend claims he has no time for daily exercise; yet flexibility exercises for the muscles and joints take so little time, it is a small price to pay for health.

After the age of 30, we begin losing muscle as part of the aging process. Often this is replaced with inelastic connective tissue, some caused by old injuries. There may also be sensitive trigger points, all of which may lead to pain in areas that were injured years ago. Add tension from muscles that are thwarted in their readiness for "fight or flight," and you have chronic pain or tension related illnesses.

Tension backaches may be anywhere from the neck to the lower back.

Oh, My Aching Back!

People and situations can give you a real "pain in the neck." You may be related to, or work with one. The more tense and in pain you are, the more tired and unable to cope you become, resulting in more pain and tension.

If you are suffering from a severe tension backache, your doctor will probably prescribe muscle relaxants (some doctors no longer prescribe them routinely), pain killers, heat and rest. The idea is to stop the cycle of pain causing spasm from causing more pain. In some cases, psychotherapy will be suggested. These therapies will see you through the acute phase, but what about the chronic tension you live with, day in and day out?

Before I go into therapies for tension reduction and exercises, let's look at what is causing tension pain. It is crucial that you are aware of your body, and able to relate a pain to a triggering cause, whether it be physical or emotional. If a certain person causes muscles to tense in an unrequited desire to hit, you need to be aware of your response, consciously relax the tense part, and if possible, stay from that person. If this trouble is caused on the job and you cannot effectively handle the pain response, think of looking for another job.

Relaxing, and stretching tight muscles and strengthening weak ones helps. So does proper posture and body mechanics. We need to stop thinking of our minds as separate entities, and view ourselves as a whole, body affecting the mind, and mind causing a response in the body.

Moshe Feldenkrais **(Body and Mature Behavior,** and **Awareness through Movement),** reeducates body and mind. In his "Awareness Through Movement Groups," he seeks to undo societies' suppression of our vital impulses. He teaches a new way of action: awareness and self-esteem through movement.

Functional integration through manipulation is done with individuals. Relief of back problems is only one of the benefits. The techniques change the deformity in the brain as well as the vertebrae; so the student has a new, more useful, pattern of response. Students learn to become aware of the skeleton itself and its orientation and movement in space.

Another mind-and-body method of treating back and postural problems is the Alexander Technique, developed 75 years ago by Mathias Alexander. The goal is to break the cycle of emotional and physical tension by changing the response to tension-producing circumstances.

The Technique takes time to learn, as it requires first, that you be aware of how you use your body, and second, changing habits that hold tension to ones that release tension. This mens correct posture and use of the body, or alignment and mechanics. Since our minds and bodies are inseparable, it is imperative that we become aware of our physical reaction to emotional stress. (See the chapter on stress).

Common reactions are tense and lifted shoulders, rigid neck and spine, clenched jaws and fists, rapid breathing, forward-thrust head, and a slouch. One of my "back" students showed me a strange slouching posture he assumed when pressures at work became unbearable. He was aware of it — the important first step — and likened it to a dog tucking its tail under. Together we worked out a posture that would take the strain off his lower back.

Once you feel the alterations in your body, you can work to change and correct them, mentally and physically. You will be able to instruct the tense part to relax, and feel it immediately do so.

In the meantime, use any of the tension-reducing techniques in the chapter on stress. Some that are helpful to people with back problems are: inhale and exhale as deeply and slowly as you can; clench your fists as hard as you can once or twice, then let them go limp; lift your shoulders towards your ears, then let them drop and relax; tense any muscle, let it relax. Do each two or three times, or as much as needed. If you can, go for a brisk walk or short jog, and breathe deeply.

In my "Relax Your Back" classes, we relax and release tension before we begin to exercise. The music is slow and relaxing, and lights are dim. All exercises are done slowly, with awareness. Many students who have suffered chronic back pain graduate into a Dynamotion Exercise class, and with some modifications, do well.

There are many ways to relax tense muscles. A massage is marvelous. A warm (not hot) bath soothes and relaxes muscles, promotes healing, and relieves pain and spasm. When my muscles are tense or overworked, I use mineral salts, such as Batherapy, which can be purchased at health food stores, soak for twenty minutes, and get into bed.

A shower massage is especially good for relieving tension and pain in the neck and upper back. Do your neck and shoulder exercises with the warm, vibrating water running down your back.

Exercise can release tension in specific muscles, but the sudden relaxation of very tense muscles can be painful. Relax and release muscular tension gradually, and listen to your body. Pain will tell you if you are going too fast.

People and situations can truly give you a "pain in the neck." The neck is one of the most common sites of tension, stiffness and pain, both in the neck and head. Often the tension can be felt in the form of knots or pain in the trapezius chain of muscles, which begin in the upper back, go above the clavicle, and overlay the splenius cervicus and splenius capitis muscles imbedded in the back of the neck. These are common sites for "trigger points," sensitive areas that orthopedic physicians often treat with injections.

You can observe tension in a person's neck if the head juts forward, the muscles or veins bulge, if there appears to be no neck at all, if there is difficulty in head rotation or looking up, if there is bruxism (grinding of the teeth), clenching of the jaws, an unnaturally high, squeaky or breathy voice, or a constantly tilted head.

Test yourself for neck tension: Sit or stand comfortably. Starting with your head on your chest, roll your head to the sides, back and front as far as you can. If there is pain while rolling, your neck is tight. Do this movement **once only** as a test. You may have seen this as an exercise in a yoga book, but it is potentially harmful to the over-forty neck, as it compresses the cervical vertebra and can irritate spurs you didn't know you had. Another test is to take the back of your neck and squeeze it hard. If thee is pain, or you want to hunch your shoulders, there is tension. Tension can be found in the outer muscles of the neck, or deep chronic spasms, which are serious and need medical attention.

What are the causes? First, emotional tension, and especially in the neck; repressed emotion, which can be reflected as tension in the throat or deep neck muscles. Other causes are whiplash or other injury, poor posture, unnatural positions such as those held by models, dentists, or secretaries, throat singing and unnatural breathing habits. Cold, or a chill breeze, commonly causes a stiff neck, and so do foam rubber pillows.

What can be done about it? If you can get out of a chronic situation that is causing you tension, without creating worse tension, then do so. The following exercises will help, BUT DO NOT DO THEM IN CASES OF NECK INJURY.

RELAX YOUR NECK

- Sit or stand with head erect and back straight. Let your head and neck muscles relax, and your head drop forward freely. Rest there. If the movement causes pain, there may be too much tension to be released quickly, so modify by not letting your neck drop as far or as fast. This relaxes muscles in the back of the neck. Do 5 to 10, several times a day.
- Make a circle in front of you with your face. (Do not tilt your head back so you are looking at the ceiling.) When you reach the bottom of the circle, let your head drop and rest there a few seconds. Twice in each direction.
- Stand with your feet about two feet apart. Bend your knees so they go directly over your feet. You should be almost in a half-squat. Bend forward from the hips, and let your body hang limply, top of the head pointing towards the floor. Lift your head as though you are trying to look across the room; then let your head drop to its original position. As it relaxes, it will bob or bounce once or twice before it hangs still. There is usually a lot of tension or stiffness if the neck does not bounce at all.

Stiff and tense necks can be caused by arthritis as well as tension and trauma. Keeping the neck warm helps, no matter what the cause of pain. Often oil of wintergreen or some other counter-irritant brings relief, especially when used at bedtime. Do not sleep or lie with your head propped up on large pillows, or hanging down with no pillow at all. Keep your spine level with a small pillow under your neck.

STRENGTHEN YOUR NECK

- Look straight ahead with your head in a normal front position. With your fist held firmly under your chin, press down hard with your chin as you resist with your fist. Hold five seconds, exhaling as you do so. Do three times. This one is the best, as it provides traction.
- With your head looking forward, put your fist on the right side of your jaw. Try to rotate your head to the right as you resist with your fist. Hold for five seconds, exhaling as you do so. Do two times in each direction.
- Clasp your hands behind your head. Press back against your hands as you resist. Five seconds, twice.

Do not do these exercises if they cause pain; however, you may create pain simply by pushing too hard. There is no movement in the head or neck, only resistance by the hands.

It is difficult to relax your body when your mind is preoccupied with the source of your tension. It is useless to say "I won't think about it," because, of course, you do. Instead, mentally re-create a situation or place you once found beautiful and tranquil. It should be the shore, a lake, or the mountains, whatever you consider peaceful. Retreat there when you are trapped in traffic, when the pressures are unrelenting, and when you are doing your relaxing exercise.

The following exercises relax back muscles and increase flexibility. Back muscles won't relax completely when the legs are fully extended—one reason your back hurts or gets tired when you stand for long periods of time. To avoid this, use a footstool if possible. If not, get relief by bringing one knee, and then the other towards your chest. Do it standing or sitting if you can't lie down.

RELAX YOUR BACK

ALL EXERCISES ARE TO BE DONE SLOWLY AND UNHURRIEDLY

- Lie on your back with a small pillow beneath your neck and a larger one beneath your knees. Loosely shake and wobble your entire body. Let it feel heavy as it rests against the floor.
- Take a deep breath, and exhale slowly and completely through your mouth. Take another deep breath, and this time tighten every muscle

in your body, hands, legs, feet, fists, face, while you exhale for five seconds. Release the tension SLOWLY. Take another breath and another contraction as you exhale, but this time lengthen and contract every muscle in your body. Your fingers will be stretched wide, your legs lengthened, your mouth and eyes opened wide. Again, hold for five seconds, and relese the tension slowly. Be aware of a big difference between tension and relaxation.

- Lie on your back, arms at your sides, feet flat on the floor, knees bent. Slide your right foot forward and let your leg fall to the floor. Do the same with the left leg.
- Same position. Slowly roll your head both right and left, till you feel a stretch (but not pain) in each direction. Roll three times to each side.
- With both knees bent and together, roll your knees to the right and left several times. Do not let your spine retract.
- On your back, knees bent, feet on the floor. Reach around your body so you are grabbing your upper back, the scapula, if you can reach. Holding your lower body still, roll your upper back from side to side several times.
- On your back, both knees bent, feet flat on the floor. Exhale as you bring your right thigh towards your chest. Hold for a few seconds, lower the foot SLOWLY to the bent knee position, then do the same with the left thigh. Do three with each leg, then GENTLY use your hands to help pull your thigh towards your chest. Do not pull on your kneecap, or directly beneath your knee.
- Lie on your right side, knees and hips bent. Bring your left thigh towards your chest, holding it there for a few seconds. It helps to exhale as you bring your leg towards your body. You should feel a stretch in the lower back and hip area, and a contraction in the abdominals. Three times on each side, then try bringing both knees towards your chest and your head towards your knees.
- On your back, knees bent: Tighten your buttocks and abdominals. Feel your pelvis rotate, and your lower back touch the floor (Pelvic tilt). Do several times, and as often during the day as you can. You can do this exercise standing or seated, as well as lying.
- To strengthen your abdominals: On your back, knees bent, hands on thighs. With your head coming first, exhale as you roll up half way, hands reaching the knees. Keep your mid and lower back flat on the floor.
- To stretch the leg and hamstrings: On your back, left knee bent. Slowly lift your right leg straight overhead; hold for a few seconds, then lower slowly. Do three times with each leg, then three times lowering your leg with your foot flexed (toes pulled towards the face).

- Sit in a chair, feet flat on the floor, and apart. Drop your chin to your chest, then roll down slowly so that you are touching the floor between your feet, the top of your head pointing towards the floor. It helps to exhale and tighten the abdominals as you roll down. Hold the position with your head and arms hanging loosely. Roll up slowly, one vertebra at a time, keeping your chin tucked on your chest until you are all the way up.
- On your back, both knees bent. Roll your right knee out to the side, hold a few seconds, then go back to original position. Do two times with each leg. In the same position, lift your right foot off the floor, and move your knee in large circles both clockwise and counterclockwise, twice with each leg. The movement is in the hip joint, not the knee.

CHECK WITH YOUR DOCTOR BEFORE EXERCISING. YOU MAY BE ABLE TO DO SOME, BUT NOT OTHERS. EVERY BACK IS DIFFERENT.

Do all exercises slowly, with a pause between each. If you are in a hurry, or if it hurts, forget it!

There are many ways to get rid of muscular tension, but not all are suitable for people with back problems.

For instance, if your problem is simple tension or muscular inflexibility, stretching and running may help. Deep breathing and slow stretching will help relax tension and can be done at any time. Sometimes just moving brings relief, as muscles "gel" and stiffen when not moved. Gentle bending to the sides and front, (knees well bent), or shaking vigorously your arms, legs, or whole body, and moving joints through their range of motion all relieve pain and stiffness.

Muscular pain can be caused by overwork as well as tension. Food allergies, chronic strain from poor body positioning, and repetitive movements without rest also cause pain and spasm. Often the cause of pain is not identified, but relief is still attained through rest, heat, relaxation and exercise.

Simple misuse of the body causes back pain and injury. It is important to keep a straight back.

The most common misuse is lifting incorrectly, and can actually cause a "slipped disc." The lumbar vertebrae, (particularly L5) withstand hundreds of pounds of pressure when you lift, even your own body. First of all, don't lift something that is too heavy; wait for help. When you lift, bend your knees, bring the object close to your chest, and lift with your thigh muscles.

Avoid a swayback. Stand with one foot on a footstool, or your knees bent to keep your back straight. If you sit for long periods of time, use a footstool so your knees are slightly higher than your hips. Don't cross your legs, and have your lower back supported. Keep your car seat forward, so your knees are higher than your hips. Sleep on your side with a small, soft pillow under your neck, and your knees and hips flexed slightly. Never sleep on your stomach.* If you sleep on your back, keep a pillow beneath your knees. Hard mattresses encourage you to change positions during the night in order to prevent stiffness. If your mattress is not firm, use a piece of plywood under it to give support. Avoid leaning forward and arching your back, wearing poorly fitting, high heeled or platform shoes.

If you do get a backache from misuse, lie on the floor and rest the calves of your legs on a chair. Stay there for a few minutes, or squat down and hug your knees. If your heels come off the floor, hold onto something for support, but get your fanny down!

Before we consider spinal diseases, and whom to consult, let's take a look at the spine itself.

In the normal back, the vertebrae sit one on top of the other, forming a gentle "S" curve. The vertebrae are separated by discs that act as shock absorbers, and the flexibility, balance and utility of the spine is maintained by guy wires: muscles, tendons, and ligaments.

The first seven vertebrae are the cervical, or neck, vertebrae. One and two, the Atlas and the Axis, are involved in forward and backward movement and rotation.

There are twelve thoracic, or dorsal vertebrae, and five lumbar, or lower back vertebrae. In adults, the five sacral vertebrae are fused to form the sacrum, and the four fused vertebrae beneath form the coccyx.

Although people often talk about their slipped or ruptured discs (some of the disc gel has squeezed from its capsule), as few as 5% actually have this condition.

Any number of other problems can cause the "pseudo-disc syndrome." In addition to weak or tense muscles, there can be spasm, or torn or inflamed muscle, tendon or ligament putting pressure on a nerve.

The normal (I question what is "normal") process of aging causes back pain because gel in the disc becomes stringy and less elastic, muscles weaken and atrophy, and there is a loss of bone calcium (osteoporosis), especially in women. Much needs to be learned about osteoporosis, which often begins around the age of thirty and predominantly afflicts light skinned people. Some of the possible causes are alcoholism, lack of exercise, too little calcium (or improper absorption) or vitamin D in the diet over long periods of time, and excess protein and phosphorus consumption. Severe osteoporosis should be treated by a physician, as hormonal and other therapy may be required. The RDAs for protein for women have been lowered to about 45 to 50 grams per day; so be concerned if you are on any kind of a high protein diet or drink diet sodas (high in phosphates).

*If you must sleep on your stomach, put a small pillow under your hips. Women with "pot bellies" can get away without the pillow; however, pots put a strain on the lower back.

EXCESS amounts of vitamins A and D may cause bone demineralization, and extra calcium is needed if you drink cranberry juice.

Although inadequate calcium intake may contribute to osteoporosis, once it exists, supplementing may or may not help. Exercise and general activity help both as prevention and therapy. (Foods high in calcium are dairy products, leafy green vegetables, almonds, oatmeal and beans. Supplements include calcium lactate and dolomite.)

What can we do when the process of aging causes the spine to shorten and compress, and alters the bones and discs? What is left? Muscles! Exercising for relaxation, strength and flexibility is more important than ever.

When pain is acute or chronic, and doesn't respond to home therapy, you need to consult a specialist. But, who? Usually you call your internist or family physician first. He or she may be able to treat you effectively, or may refer you to an orthopedist, a neurologist (nerve specialist), or a physiatrist (a doctor who specializes in physical medicine, or exercise). Often a diagnosis of ruptured disc is incorrect; always get another opinion.

If X-rays and other tests, such as the mylegram, confirm a ruptured disc, conservative treatment is usually the first course of action. Total bedrest, with or without traction, is most often prescribed, and can be accomplished at home or in the hospital. Eventually, limited exercises are included, no matter what the original treatment, even if there has been surgery. There has been some experimentation with the injection of chymopapain (an enzyme from the papaya plant) to dissolve the damaged disc material. This is a controversial treatment about which you may want to inquire if your only other recourse is surgery.

What about surgery? Certainly it should be a last resort, and its necessity confirmed by more than one doctor. Disc surgery, or laminectomy, involves removal of the extruded disc jelly that is causing pressure on a nerve. Eventually, scar tissue fills the empty space. Sometimes a spinal fusion is done, which connects the vertebrae with a bone graft on either side of the missing disc.

New "microsurgery" procedures are being used by a limited number of surgeons with improved success rates. The operation, "micro-lumbar disectomy," uses a one inch incision, tiny instruments guided by a microscope, and eliminates large cutting of the bony plate.

The chances are that you are one of the majority of back patients who are not suffering from a slipped disc. Other conditions are kyphosis (round upper back), lordosis (sway back), and scoliosis (lateral curvature). I have seen women diagnosed as scoliotic who were well into their middle years. Today, because of parental awareness and a screening program in many junior high schools, it is diagnosed early so that permanent structural damage is avoided. Any of these conditions respond to exercise if the problem is muscular, rather than structural. Even when structural, exercise helps relieve pain and inflexibility.

Scoliosis can be a congenital malformation, but usually the cause is unknown, although the tendency runs in families. It shows up in children and becomes acute during the adolescent growth spurt. Early detection and treatment (bracing and exercises) are crucial.

Other spinal diseases are spondylitis, a bacterial inflammation of the vertebrae, tuberculosis of the spine, or Pott's Disease, and meningitis. All are serious and require immediate attention.

When all conventional avenues have failed, people will seek relief from a chiropractor or an osteopath.

An osteopath is a medical doctor who has additional training in osteopathy, that is, the use of spinal manipulations to treat a variety of complaints. Unlike chiropractors, osteopaths can prescribe medication.

Chiropractors can do more harm than good, but so can drugs and other therapies. Often they bring relief from many conditions other than back pain, when no one or nothing else has. Today chiropractors practice holistic medicine. They treat the whole person, rather than the part, through nutritional and other means. For instance, vitamin C may be part of the treatment for disc problems.

Because so many people ask me about chiropractors, I will say something about them, both then and now.

Chiropractic was begun 86 yeras ago by Daniel Parker. He helped everything from hearing loss to heart trouble by repositioning the spine. Spinal misalignments (subluxations) cause pressure on the nerves to various parts of the body.

Today there are two types of chiropractors, the "mixers" and the "straights." The straights, who are in the minority, adhere to the fundamental theories of spinal manipulation. They believe that many diseases are caused by subluxations and place no emphasis on preventive medicine.

The mixers concern themselves with diet, exercise, rest, environmental conditions and psychological pressures. Their practice includes vitamin therapy, ultrasound, ultraviolet and infrared light, whirlpool baths, hot and cold compresses, heel and sole lifts, and sometimes accupressure and colonics. They believe spinal disorders can be both the source and the result of problems elsewhere in the body. Most people go to chiropractors for problems involving the musculo-skeletal structure.

Although the AMA considers chiropractors to be "quacks," many patients who go to them after unsuccessful standard treatment have nothing but praise. Officially, the Department of Health and Human Services (H.H.S.) disapproves of them, although I know one H.H.S. executive who drove hundreds of miles to his favorite chiropractor when his back "went out."

Chiropractors take the time to know their patients, something most doctors can't or won't do. Also, being touched is comforting to people in pain. Two studies regarding spinal manipulation are under way at the University of Colorado. One shows that the nerves are extremely sensitive to pressure at the point where they branch out from the spine, and the pressure may produce toxic substances. This could be the result of subluxations, and be relieved by manipulation, or adjustments. My own experiences with chiropractors have been good and bad; however, the last time I went to an orthopedist for neck pain, he gave me a chiropractic adjustment.

A new step has been taken in the field of chiropractic by Dr. Lowell Ward, who calls his science "spinal column stressology." His research has led him to believe that aligning the spinal column to relieve stress, rather than nerve impingement, is the key.

Dr. Ward feels that heavy stress on the body, whether it is traumatic, nutritional, congenital, or emotional, causes the spine to leave its proper position, shifting the center of gravity and draining the body of energy and health. He views the spine as a synchronous unit, and treats it as such, believing it both causes and reflects stress. He also feels that an impact or trauma to one part of the spine will be reflected in the entire spine. He uses measurements and X-rays to determine the spinal position, and a variety of techniques to correct abnormalities not commonly used by chiropractors. His adjustments are made with calibrated devices rather than manually, enabling him to record the intensity of treatment used.

Doctors have seen (and often experienced) so much low back pain that they tend to take the attitude, "so, what's new?" Often they say "It's your age," or "get some exercise" without saying what, when, or how much. Many times they give out a booklet of exercises without showing the patient the correct way of doing them or providing any useful information about the proper use of the body. No wonder people go to chiropractors and exercise! In most cases, they help.

Where does one begin in preventing and relieving back pain, once disease has been ruled out?

First of all, poor physical condition (this includes poor posture, excess weight, and lack of exercise) makes you prone to injury, as well as creating the muscular imbalances about which we spoke. If your abdominal muscles are weak, or if you have a pot belly, you are likely to have a forward curve in your lower back, or swayback. This causes further weakening of the muscles and pain. We should always avoid the swayback position when standing, sitting or lying. Along the same lines, also avoid arching your back, especially prone arching.

Chronic strain is another cause of pain. If your job causes you to sit or stand partly bent over for long periods of time, or much time at repetitive movements without a break, you may be placing excess stress on the muscles, have less resistance to acute strain or sprain, and suffer from general tension, fatigue and weakness.

Changing position as often as possible helps, as do stretching, flexing the knees, and easy forward and side-bending with the knees bent. Relaxation techniques help get rid of tension. Adding competitive and stress-including sports like golf, tennis and running to your exercise routine **won't** get rid of tension. Instead they may make you feel worse. Do your fun activities in an atmosphere of non-competitiveness and relaxation.

Exercise prevents back aches as well as relieving them, but the wrong kind can cause trouble and make existing problems worse. Swimming is excellent, but avoid arching your back when you do the crawl. Have someone observe you to see that you are keeping your back straight. Do sit-ups with your knees bent, and only halfway if they are difficult or painful. Forget double leg lifts and back bends—leave them to the fourteen-year-old gymnasts. Never do fast straight-leg toe touches. Roll up and down through the pelvic tilt with your back round and your knees bent. Always lift (even your own weight) with your knees bent and your abdominals tight.

Lift only light weight overhead. When you stretch up to reach something, make certain your back doesn't arch by tightening your buttock and abdominal muscles. Use a firm ladder or platform, not a shaky chair.

Use lightweight rakes, hoes and shovels, and stand near your work. If you shovel snow, push rather than lift it.

Lifting and twisting, and bending and twisting can strain your back. So can sharply twisting your upper body with your hips and feet firmly planted. Even the "back" exercise of pulling your thighs to your chest can cause a strain if you yank too hard. Listen to your body. Never try to force it to do something for which it isn't ready. Move gently, gradually and carefully, and with awareness.

Know what to do in an emergency where a blow, fall or twist to the head, neck, or back may have caused a fracture. Signs of fracture are severe pains across the chest, abdomen and down the legs, muscle spasms, and weakness or numbness below the injury. Don't move the victim or let him sit, stand, or walk, and call for emergency help immediately if you suspect a fracture.

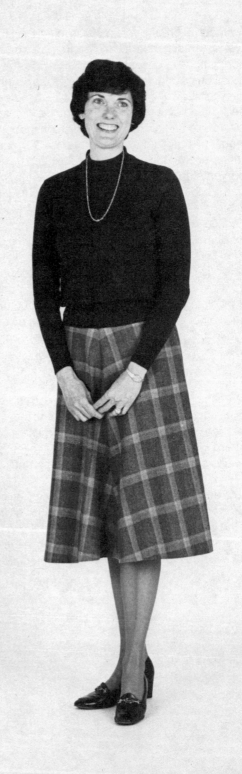

15
POSTURE

Posture, or body alignment, is of primary importance. All of the exercises in the world will be of little value if you place chronic strain on your body by using it in inefficient, unnatural ways.

We are constantly fighting gravity to sit or stand upright. The normal center or gravity goes through the body in a straight line from the front of the ear, past the top of the hip bone, and down the legs, ending around the arch of the foot. Any deviation from the normal body position will create an equal deviation in the opposite direction elsewhere.

Posture begins in the mind. You must visualize correct body positioning before you attempt to hold it or strengthen the muscles that enable you to do so. The importance of body awareness and body-and-mind working together cannot be emphasized enough. When we feel depressed, down, and defeated, our body follows with a slump and forward-hanging head. Constantly holding this type of posture has a negative effect on the mind and emotions. It's a vicious cycle.

Just as slumping can cause you to feel depressed, standing tall can lift your spirits. Obviously, posture and exercise won't cure the mental ills of the world, but in a country where so many women are addicted to Valium and other drugs, its benefits must not be underestimated.

Poor posture not only reflects the way you feel, it affects the way others respond to you. The term "regal bearing" is valid. It not only expresses royalty but self-confidence and the impression that you can handle life's responsibilities. It is human nature either to pity or dump on those who approach us with a hang-dog demeanor. We don't want either!

Poor posture leads to chronic back pain because of uneven pressure on ligaments, muscles and joints. Breathing becomes shallow, resulting in lowered vitality, and organs may shift from their proper positions. The waist, abdomen, hips and upper thighs become larger and targets for fatty deposits.

Posture begins with aligning the skeletal structure. Think of your head, ribs and pelvis as a set of blocks sitting directly on top of each other, joined by the spine. If one segment is out of place, the balance of the entire structure is affected. **Always lengthen your spine; never compress it.** You may even become a little taller.

Imagine that there is a string from the ceiling attached to the top of your head and that the string is constantly lifting, stretching and lengthening your spine. Breathe deeply, and keep your chin comfortably in. Your ribs will be lifted, your shoulders relaxed and down, your waist smaller. Remember— don't arch your back! Standing tall may feel unnatural in the beginning, but as your muscles strengthen, you will not feel comfortable any other way. KEEP YOUR MUSCLES AND JOINTS RELAXED AND FREE FROM UNNECESSARY TENSION.

That takes care of the top half, but the bottom may still be out of line. The correct position for the pelvis is about halfway between a swayback and the pelvic tilt. The lower pelvis is slightly forward, the abdominal muscles are working to support the spine, and excess curvature is removed. You get the pelvic tilt by slightly bending your knees and tightening your buttocks and abdominals so the lower pelvis swings forward. This is an exercise you should do many times a day, but not adopt as your permanent posture. Learn to swing your lower pelvis slightly forward without a hard muscular contraction. (It moves forward and back like a swing.)

Never pull your shoulders back or lock your knees. Keep them relaxed! Remembering that locked knees and stiff thighs makes thighs larger is a good incentive towards relaxation.

When sitting, you may want occasionally to cross one leg over the other to vary position, but don't sit that way for long. Never place the back of one knee on the other, as this can cause varicose veins; instead, cross at the ankles. Sitting with your legs at 90 degrees to your body, feet flat on the floor, is fine for short periods of time. If you have back problems, or you find this is uncomfortable, have your knees slightly higher than your hips.

POSTURE EXERCISES: GOOD FOR EVERYONE, BACK ACHES OR NOT!

• One of the best and simplest postural exercises is deep diaphragmatic breathing. It increases energy as it gently strengthens the muscles of the upper back, ribs and waist. Practice breathing exercises standing, seated, or lying on your back.

When you are learning this technique, it increases your awareness if you place your hands over your ribs, fingertips touching at the sternum. Exhale first to empty your lungs; then inhale deeply and feel your ribs expand outwards. Your hands will separate and your fingers will no longer touch. As you exhale, the ribs will contract and fingers touch again. Do this simple exercise several times a day, whenever you feel the need for an energizing break. It is best to do breathing exercises in fresh air.

• The **pelvic tilt** strengthens the buttock, abdominal and thigh muscles and stretches the lower back enabling us to maintain correct posture. It can be done seated, standing or lying and is the most important exercise you can do. If you've seen a burlesque "bump," you've seen the pelvic tilt. Do this one often, stopping short of stiffness and fatigue. (See exercise 9, back exercises, also "sexercises.")

Get the feeling of the pelvic tilt against a wall. Stand with your back against a wall, feet about six inches apart, heels on the floor, knees bent. Drop your chin to your chest as you try to press the small of your back into the wall. Come to a standing position, keeping your back pressed to the wall as long as you can. This is an exercise, not the way to stand forever.

• Stretching the pectoral muscles helps **correct a round upper back.** Stand about three feet out from a corner. Place one hand on each wall at shoulder level. Keeping your entire body straight, bend your elbows and let your body in towards the corner. (There should be no bend in the back.) If you keep your heels on the floor, the calf muscles and achilles tendon are also stretched. Hold for ten to twenty seconds; repeat two times.

• For the **upper back**: Grasp a towel with your hands about three feet apart. Lift your ribs as you stretch towards the ceiling **without arching your back.** Hold the stretch. Now bring the towel down and behind your shoulders, elbows coming down to your ribs at your sides. Hold a few seconds. Do each three times, working up to six.

• Grasp the towel with hands about two feet apart, arms straight overhead. Bring both arms towards the back of your head as far as they will go. Hold three seconds, repeat four times; then with arms lifted and back as far as they will go, sway them to the right and left.

• The previous exercise **strengthened the upper back.** Finish by **stretching.** With your right hand on the top of your right shoulder, left hand on the left, cross your right elbow over your left as you drop your head. Hold for at least ten seconds; then cross left over right. Twice on each side.

Instead of towels, I use strips cut from old inner tubes. The constant pulling against the resistance of the rubber strengthens the shoulders, arms and upper back.

Always be aware of your posture. Check yourself in store windows and mirrors. If you see a slump or misalignment, correct it immediately. If tension or anger has caused you to lift or hunch your shoulders, or stiffen your neck, inhale and exhale slowly and release the tension.

A warm soak for twenty minutes will relax you and warm up your muscles for exercising. You can do your neck exercises and toe-touch in a long, relaxing shower. Remember, never rush these back or posture exercises, as this will defeat your purpose and may injure a muscle.

Certain conditions require restrictions in your exercise routines as well as your daily life. Only you and your doctor can determine what **yours** may be. That is why it is important to get permission. However, don't become a "back cripple" because you once had a sprain, or you are out of shape and getting older. The more we limit ourselves, the closer we are towards old age and death.

16
ARTHRITIS

What is arthritis, and why does it strike three times as many women as men? Although research is ongoing, drugs being formulated, and new theories regarding causes being expounded, there is no universally accepted "cure" for arthritis. However, the symptoms of pain and inflammation can be treated, thus halting or relieving the degenerating and crippling effects. For this reason it is important to seek medical help before the late stages, which may result in permanent joint changes and chronic disability.

The word arthritis means "inflammation of the joint." There are over 110 types of identified arthritis, not all involving inflammation. Those most commonly affecting women are rheumatoid arthritis and osteoarthritis, also called degenerative joint disease. Many people lump joint pains under the general term of "rheumatism." By any name, it is a real pain in the neck! X-rays would show some form of arthritis in everyone over sixty, even if there were no symptoms. Some put that age as low as forty.

Not all joint pain is caused by arthritis. Tendonitis and bursitis, for instance, can cause similar pain, but require different treatment. Therapy varies according to the type of arthritis; therefore it is important to have a correct diagnosis. There should be an evaluation of symptoms, including past history, observation of any inflammation of the joint, possibly X-rays or an analysis of joint fluid, and lab work including the bentonite test and sedimentation rate. According to Dr. Howard Lutz, Director of The Institute For Preventive Medicine, morning stiffness and pain in the joints (especially the back) can be caused by hyperacidity, rather than arthritis. This has proven true for me. I seldom eat meat, but if I do so late in the evening, my back is stiff and painful the next morning. On the other hand, if I take dolomite before I go to bed, I sleep well, and wake up feeling fine.

Symptoms of arthritis may disappear or go through a remission that lasts for weeks or years; nevertheless, it is a chronic disease, and the doctor may find evidence of it although the patient feels no discomfort. Warning signs of arthritis that require correct diagnosis are:

- Persistent pain and stiffness on arising.
- Pain, tenderness, or swelling in one or more joints.
- Recurrence of these symptoms, especially if they involve more than one joint.
- Recurrent or persistent pain and stiffness in the neck, lower back, knees or other joints.
- Unexplained weight loss, fever and fatigue.

Joints are where bones come together, and most are moveable. The bone ends are protected by a rubbery cushion (cartilage), encased by a capsule of ligaments, which is lined by the synovial membrane that secretes the synovial, or lubricating fluid. Arthritis can cause the fluid to jell, destroy the synovial lining, cartilage, and bone itself. Often the result is bone rubbing on bone, causing pain, restricted motion, and bony spurs. If the arthritic joint is immobile for long periods of time, it can lose its ability to function, fill with inelastic material, and become permanently frozen. Even short term immobility can result in the temporary freezing of a joint. For this reason it is important to find the right combination of rest and exercise. This is individual, and will vary from person to person and time to time, depending on the severity of inflammation.

OSTEOARTHRITIS

Osteoarthritis, or wear and tear arthritis, is the most common kind. We all will get a bit of it if we live long enough. It can be mild to severe and usually does not cripple.

What happens is that the mechanical parts of the joints wear out, especially those under stress such as the weight-bearing joints of the hips and knees, or the elbow of a baseball pitcher. Cartilage can become pitted, frayed, and wear away. Bone ends may become thicker, spurs develop, ligaments thicken, and the structure and shape of the joint changed. The surrounding muscles often become tense or weak or contract. It is not known why some people get osteoarthritis and others don't. Possibly heredity plays a part, or unusual stress, injury, or defects that were present at birth. For example, osteoarthritis of the hip and knee joints is quite common in the overweight.

Doctors separate osteoarthritis into "primary" and "secondary." Primary arthritis starts by itself, without any apparent triggering cause. It is likely to be generalized and hereditary. An example of primary arthritis in women is Heberden's Nodes, bony enlargements of the end joints of the fingers, a tendency that runs in families. Bouchard's Nodes are similar enlargements of the middle joints. Nodes can also form from stress or injury to a finger, in which case it is secondary arthritis, the kind resulting from injury, stress, and strain. Whatever the reason, whether hereditary or environmental, an improperly functioning joint is prone to arthritis.

There are symptoms, although you can have arthritis and be asymptomatic. Most commonly there is pain on movement, and sometimes at rest. Pain may be confined to the joint, or spread to the general area of the part involved. It is caused by irritation and pressure on nerve endings, muscular fatigue, and tension. There may be a loss of mobility, resulting in muscular weakness and postural defects. Usually there is no fever or loss of weight, and the person does not feel sick.
prescribed. A new form dissolves after it leaves the stomach, lessening

What can be done, once it is diagnosed? At this time there are no miracle drugs to cure arthritis. Rest and exercise are used in the correct proportion, sometimes splints or braces, and in extreme cases, surgical replacement of the joint. It is wise to alternate periods of rest with activity, as the joint becomes still when immobile. To keep the joints mobile, take them through their range of motion several times a day. Muscle strengthening exercises can be done every other day. A physical therapist may be needed to assist with the exercises, and weights or springs are useful to build muscular strength. EXERCISE CAN PREVENT CRIPPLING AND DEFORMITY. I have many students who feel better when they exercise, but there are times when exercise is not prescribed, such as when there is acute inflammation and crystals in the synovial fluid. This is why it is important that each case be treated individually. Good posture is crucial, as improper alignment will lead to unnatural stress on the joints, aggravate a pain, and encourage deformities.

Heat is the old standby for relaxing muscles and relieving pain and stiffness. Many doctors recommend a warm tub bath first thing upon arising, when the problems are worst. The bath should be for no longer than twenty minutes, with the temperature around 100 degrees fahrenheit. Warm moist packs, heated wax for the hands, and electric blankets also help. Warm water is so effective that the tub or shower is a good place to do some of your range of motion exercises.

As a rule, morning stiffness with osteoarthritis will not last as long as it does with rheumatoid arthritis.

Although there are new drugs, aspirin is still the most commonly prescribed. A new form dissolves after it leaves the stomach, lessening chances of irritation. To be effective, it is taken several times a day, every day, on the advice of your physician. Drugs such as phenylbutazone and indomethacin cannot be tolerated by everyone. Sometimes a shot of cortisone is given directly into the joint itself. I have heard of the use of niacinamide (not niacin) in the treatment of osteoarthritis, but do not think it is accepted by most physicians. (Large doses of this vitamin can cause side effects.)

A drug you may have been hearing about is DMSO, (dimethyl sulfoxide). The chemical which has been used as an industrial solvent since the forties, is now being touted as the miracle cure for everything from acute muscle strains to chronic arthritis. It is being sold from the backs of trucks because the FDA has given only limited approval for specific conditions, such as the bladder condition known as interstitial cystitis. It has been used for other conditions, and there are side effects, such as nausea, blurring of vision, headaches, diarrhea, and burning on urination. (It is absorbed into the blood stream after being applied to the skin.) Studies are being conducted, and if you are anxious to try DMSO, see if you can take part in a carefully controlled study.

One common form of osteoarthritis manifests as bony spurs on the vertebrae, often accompanied by a narrowing of the space between each vertebra. The cervical spine (neck), and lumber, or lower back, are common sites for spurs. Spurs and compression of the discs may be painful, or there may be no symptoms at all, until you do something that causes irritation, such as aggravating the compression. This problem is so common that I never do certain exercises with people over forty. Neck circling is done with the face looking forward, never reaching the position where you look at the ceiling. (The chin coming down to the chest is all right.) I don't do back arching exercises, either standing or prone. Any exercise that stretches the back is helpful, such as the pelvic tilt, or squatting down and hugging your knees to your chest.

The current enthusiasm for active sports may cause an increase in osteoarthritis, according to Dr. George Ehrlich, director of rheumatology at the Albert Einstein Medical Center in Philadelphia.[1]

Although he admitted his thinking was partially speculative, it reflects current research that links osteoarthritis to early episodes of inflammation. To minimize this risk, he suggests that runners, skiers, and tennis players, who subject their weight-bearing joints to repeated low-grade inflammation, observe certain precautions—such as warming up, wearing proper shoes, avoiding hard surfaces, and rest, and an anti-inflammatory drug if there is pain after exercise. He is not advocating a sedentary lifestyle and concluded by saying . . . "it's probably better to stay fit than to try to totally prevent the disaster."

[1]**The Physician and Sportsmedicine, Sept., 1979.**

RHEUMATOID ARTHRITIS

What causes this potentially crippling disease? There are many theories, and the answers are not in; however, it is felt that one can be genetically predisposed. Some feel that a virus is the precipitator, and that in a derangement of the body's own defense, or immune system, the body produces enzyme antibodies that go haywire and attack the joints. Emotional stress, if not causing arthritis, can aggravate it. Some women find that their arthritis improves during pregnancy. I know of more than one whose ailment began during that time. Whatever the cause, is there a treatment?

Rheumatoid arthritis can affect the entire body, attack connective tissues, and cause weight loss, fever, fatigue, and loss of appetite. Because the whole system is involved, the doctor will treat more than just the joints. Officially, there is no "arthritis diet," but there is special emphasis on good, sound, nutrition. In fact, many feel that patients with inflammatory processes may have somewhat greater nutritional requirements than the average healthy person.

A good doctor will look into the patient's lifestyle, see where physical and mental stress can be reduced, and recommend a balance of rest and special exercises. Most likely an anti-inflammatory drug will be prescribed. There are many, other than aspirin. Phenylbutazone, an older drug, is one, but it may have serious side effects. Newer drugs generically are: fenoprofen, ibuprofen, indomethacin, naproxen, sulindac, and tolmectin. Steroids can have serious side effects, and when they are discontinued, the arthritis returns.

Another new drug, penicillamine, is being used successfully, but like the others, it has potential side effects. One drug that won't work is Tylenol, or aceteminophen. Tylenol is analgesic only, and not anti-inflammatory.

One of my older students showed me her grossly swollen wrists and mentioned the arthritis pain in other parts of her body. The pain was keeping her awake at night, and she was rapidly losing her ability to move. She was being treated by a chiropractor with Tylenol, and he was starting her on niacinamide. He had done no tests to determine the type of arthritis she had, and she was afraid of drugs her family doctor might prescribe. Arthritis is a depressing disease, even when treated "correctly."

Recent studies have shown that zinc sulfate has promising results in the treatment of rheumatoid arthritis. The patient may be deficient in zinc and other minerals; but which came first—the deficiency or the disease—is not known. Nor is it certain whether replacement of the minerals will ameliorate the disease. Studies are being conducted at universities, drug companies, and the National Institutes of Health. Eating foods high in minerals, such as sea food, fruits, and vegetables certainly won't hurt.

Because arthritis is a serious disease with no known cure, there are a lot of fake remedies around. Some do seem to help; perhaps it's the placebo effect. One of my students who is seeing a homeopath says she has been greatly helped by his combination of medications that include bee sting venom. Another is seeing Dr. Lutz, who is treating her arthritis with mineral supplements that include dolomite, alfalfa, perna (a sea mussel), and zinc. She checks the acid balance of her urine daily, keeping the ph between 6 and 7, to aid in mineral retention. She has also been helped.

Dr. Lutz was at one time confined to a wheel chair because of arthritis. He cured it through proper nutrition and the complete removal of all possible food allergens. He has been completely off all drugs for years.*

One thing is certain. **Lose excess weight to reduce stress on the joints.**

Rheumatoid arthritis is not a disease of old people, as it usually begins between the ages of twenty and forty-five. As in all types of arthritis, it is important to balance rest with exercise. Resting the entire body will relieve inflammation; however, staying in one position too long will cause stiffness. In this disease it hurts to move the joints, but it is crucial to do so once the acute inflammation has subsided, to avoid permanent stiffness and loss of motion.

Arthritics can suffer acute pain due to inflammation, which usually responds to heat, medication, exercise and rest. Chronic pain, due to destruction of the joint, is another problem. Many recent strides have been made in pain control. They include transcutaneus nerve stimulation, bio-feedback, self hypnosis, endorphins, behavior modification, acupressure and acupuncture. Pain centers throughout the country are helping many people with chronic pain.

Arthritis patients remain on medication even when there are no symptoms. Although they don't cure the disease, anti-inflammatory drugs slow down some of the destructive processes of the disease.

There is evidence that a small percentage of those with rheumatoid arthritis may be allergic to petrochemicals. We are surrounded by them; they are in our clothing, carpeting, and mattresses, pesticides, synthetic additives, coloring agents and preservatives, in our food, air and water. Sensitivity to these chemicals may cause many diseases of unknown origin, such as colitis, bronchitis, asthma, sinusitis, and vascular-type headaches.

One of the largest of four environmental control units is in Dallas. Staffed by doctors William Rea, a surgeon, Ralph Smiley, an internist, and Robert Stroud, a rheumatologist and editor of the Journal Of Allergy And Clinical Immunology, the unit tests people for chemical sensitivity by isolating them, then reintroducing chemicals one at a time, beginning with water. Their success rate is substantial; 95% of those with migraine and vascular headaches, and 90% of those with arthritis show improvement.

*Milk and beef appear to be the foods most likely to cause arthritis in this country, according to Dr. I.T. Chao in a paper prepared for the annual congress of the American College of Allergists. He says it is a food "incompatibility" rather than strictly an allergic phenomenon.

Chemical hypersensitivity may be a causative factor in some cases of arthritis; if you are one of those, it is worth investigating.

The latest treatment I have heard of is another one of those Chinese cures. My friend swears her arthritis went away by the end of the week. This calls for two cups of cherries the first day, then a cup a day for a week. Maybe it's as worthless as snake oil, but as long as you keep up your regular diet and medication, it wouldn't hurt to try, unless you happen to be allergic to cherries.

ARTHRITIS EXERCISES

Exercises are often prescribed for arthritis patients. **Each individual must be advised by her own physician, as exercise may worsen some conditions, such as acute inflammation.**

Repeat each exercise a few times, **stopping short of fatigue.** Range of motion exercises should be done a few times a day, or any time you feel stiff. When on a long trip, stop at least once an hour and do some easy bending and stretching. In addition to maintaining and restoring joint function, exercise will strengthen and release tension in the surrounding muscles. Many of the exercises can be done standing, seated, or in bed. Even if the joint is splinted, you can still do muscle "setting" or isometrics. ALWAYS HOLD THE CONTRACTION FOR FIVE SECONDS ONLY, EXHALING AS YOU DO SO. LONG-HELD MUSCULAR CONTRACTIONS CAN RAISE YOUR BLOOD PRESSURE AND CAUSE OTHER PROBLEMS.

Before you begin, inhale and exhale slowly and deeply two or three times, feeling your ribs and abdomen expand outwards as you inhale. Slow, deep breathing helps you relax and is an excellent posture exercise. Next, gently shake and wobble your whole body: arms, legs, shoulders, whatever you can move. This relaxes and warms up the muscles, tendons, and ligaments. If your arthritis is acute, you may need someone to help you maintain correct body position to prevent deformity. Aid should be gentle, never forceful. If your arthritis is less acute, do exercises that enable you to maintain your ability to perform your usual activities. If it is very mild, work on increasing strength, flexibility and endurance, for work and recreation.

You may feel mild discomfort, BUT DO NOT EXERCISE BEYOND THE POINT OF PAIN. Taking a warm bath before exercising relaxes the muscles and increases the benefits. Many of the exercises, especially those for hands and feet are BEST DONE IN WARM WATER. **Rest when you feel the need. Overworking the joints can make the condition worse.**

NECK (May be done in the shower).

- Turn your head slowly right and left, as though looking over your shoulders. Keep your shoulders still.
- Slowly turn your shoulders to the right as your head turns to the left; reverse.

- Make a circle in front of you with your nose without tilting your head back. Write your name with your nose from left to right.

WRIST AND HAND (Best done in tub or bowl of warm water.)

Do five times with each hand.

- Make a fist, thumb on top of fingers. Slowly open the hand as wide as possible, spreading the fingers apart.
- Place your hand and wrist on a table, with the fingers spread apart. Holding the thumb in place with your other hand, move each finger individually towards the thumb.
- Touch thumb to fingertips, one at a time.
- With palms on a table, lift one finger at a time, then all together.
- To gently stretch your fingers: Place the palms of the hands on a table, and gently press down, or with your palms together, arms outstretched in front of your chest, bring your hands in towards your body as your elbows move outwards, keeping the palms together throughout.
- With straight fingers, bend your hands at the knuckles and flip a light-weight magazine off the back of your fingers.
- Flick wads of paper, alternating the use of all four fingers with the thumb.
- With your hands in fists, alternate bending the wrists with the fists pointing down, with the wrist upwards and the fingers opening wide.
- With fingers curled lightly, bring your fist upwards while resisting the movement with the other hand.
- Turn a door handle to the left with the right hand, to the right with the left hand.
- Open jars with the right hand, close with the left hand.
- Push against surfaces with the hand flat, as when rising from chairs.

SHOULDERS, ARMS AND UPPER BACK

Begin slowly, working up to six repetitions.

- If your shoulders are very stiff and painful, this is the easiest and allows the most movement:
  Bending forward from the hips, with your arms hanging down in front of you, make circles with your arms, going inwards. Start small, gradually enlarging the circles.
- Lie on a bed, arms at your sides. Keeping your arm flat on the bed, move it up to shoulder level, then over your head, if you can. When your shoulder improves, raise your arm overhead towards the ceiling, then towards the head of the bed.
- Raise your arms as high as you can overhead with elbows straight. Swing them out and down to your sides in as big a circle as you can. When you have regained mobility, try circling your arms up, back, and around, then reversing.

17
BECOME YOUNGER: CAN WE?

"To be seventy years young is sometimes more hopeful than to be forty years old."

Oliver Wendell Holmes

The perennial search for the "fountain of youth" goes on: in the laboratory, in the surgeon's office, at the cosmetic counter, through our way of living and environment. We want to thwart aging, the one biological condition common to all, desiring not only to prolong life, but to be "alive," healthy, active and youthful as long as we live. Sound impossible? Let's look at what is being done both in institutionalized research laboratories, and nonconventional centers.

We have not substantially increased our life span, but simply enabled more of us to live to an old age. Through improved hygiene, food refrigeration and antibiotics, many of the fatal diseases of youth have been practically eradicated. Infectious diseases such as rheumatic heart disease, pneumonia and tuberculosis—which once were fatal to young people—are being replaced by diseases of middle years and old age: heart attack, stroke, and cancer. We are older, but not necessarily healthier or happier. Further, there is some evidence that we were intended to live to 120, an age reached by only a select few. Even this goal is meaningless, if it simply means survival of the organism. Before we look at aging from a cellular level, let's get an overview of the thinking of scientists in the field of gerontology.

The National Institutes of Health has supported research on aging since 1940, establishing an official institute on aging (NIA) in 1974. In 1975 The Adult Development and Aging Branch and Gerontology Research Center separated from the parent group and became the core of NIA. This research center has been conducting longitudinal studies on male (and finally, female) volunteers to gain knowledge of the aging process. It is permanently headed by Dr. Robert Butler.

Finding healthy individuals who are motivated to volunteer for medical studies is not easy. The studies are time consuming, sometimes requiring two and a half days at a time in institutionalized settings. Many of the tests are tedious and demanding, both mentally and physically. Volunteers are people of all ages, living normal lives in their communities, who take a positive interest in the investigation of healthy aging. Their commitment involves returning to the center every two years if they are under 60, at 18-month intervals if they are between 60 and 69, and annually if they are 70 or older.

According to Dr. Shock, retired NIA Scientific Director, the goal of gerontology research is "not to increase the number of years of old age and infirmity but rather to allow more people to reach the presently attainable life span with minimum disability."

The studies involve a constant search for what causes the physiological changes of aging, how we acquire and deal with disease, and how we perform intellectually. These various changes are measured by taking medical histories, physical examinations, X-rays, tests of hearing and vision, metabolism, nutrition, learning, memory and problem solving. There are studies done of the heart, circulation, body composition, kidney and lung function. Much has been learned about aging regarding body cells, glucose tolerance, cholesterol, heart size and performance, alcohol metabolism, problem solving, and memory. Through this research, "norms" are being established for older people that are quite different from those of younger people.

The biological and medical research is on five levels, ranging from molecular and cellular studies to clinical investigations in animal and man, and behavioral and social research. On a molecular level, there is much interest in collagen, the major protein component of connective tissue. Loss of collagen causes a breakdown of many functions, including a loss of elasticity in the skin. A representative of NIA commented that the cosmetics industries are doing more research with collagen facial creams than they are, although the industries' findings may be questioned, considering their bias. (In the meantime, I use collagen creams — just in case they work!)

The study of immunology is another project that is being expanded. It seems that as a person ages the immune mechanisms weaken, leading to a greater susceptibility to infections and cancer. Much knowledge of the immune system comes from mouse studies. There are indications that cellular changes responsible for aging cause a loss of certain immune or infection-fighting cells, an increase in suppressor cells which counteract or inhibit normal immune cell function, and an alteration of the functional efficiency in the immune cells. They found in animal experiments that with the use of dietary restriction there was an increase in life span.

Nutrition is being explored to determine what role it plays in the aging process and in the prevention of diseases that often accompany old age. There is a need to know if nutritional requirements change with age. For instance, one study showed that the protein requirements remain the same for a 65 year old as they are for a 35 year old. The subject of protein itself is of much interest: the RDAs have been lowered to about 45 grams a day for women and 55 for men. Some studies even show that a restriction in protein intake may actually prolong life.

The NIA is also concerned with pharmacology for the older adult. They are looking at drugs — their misuse, actions, and interactions, and the various changes in drug absorption and metabolism that occur with age.

Other alterations that take place as we get older are in the endocrine system. Those under study that are of special interest to us are the ones that occur during menopause. In this case they are looking at the prevention, diagnosis and treatment of diseases, but what about the prevention or delay of the menopause itself? Or do we even want to? It certainly would be nice to prevent some of the changes that seemed to occur at this time, such as osteoporosis, an increased susceptibility to heart attack, depression, and wrinkles.

What has been learned? It seems that we all age at different rates. It is uncertain whether this is caused by environment or genetics. Certainly some of the changes that were once assumed to be a "normal" part of aging, such as loss of hearing, taste, intelligence and sex drive are now found to be not necessarily "typical" or "normal."

Because of the loss of cells in many of the body's tissues, the older person is less able to cope with various environmental stresses such as heat and cold or a sudden expenditure of energy. Since there is evidence that the "stress response" suppresses the immune response (which is already altered due to aging), it is no wonder older people become sick easily.

In my exercise classes, the older people are not worried about competing, and are able to relax and have a good time. This is one of the "plusses" gained with living long enough. If it weren't for this attitude, some of them probably would have been long dead.

In speaking of research, one can't emphasize enough the point that there is a wide range of differences among individuals, and that parallel studies come up with conflicting conclusions. NIA research has shown that there is no adult plateau after which one ages suddenly and rapidly. Rather, the changes are gradual and progressive. An exception is in the ability to handle glucose. There is a decline in the years from the twenties to the forties, a plateau, and another decline in later years. Cholesterol studies showed an increase up to the age of fifty-five, at which it peaks, then is followed by a decrease. High cholesterol is considered a risk factor in heart attack. Under investigation are the causes of the changes in blood cholesterol, such as dietary habits, obesity, and activity.

Studies showed that alcohol was metabolized just as efficiently in older men as in young adults, but there was a greater decline (at the same blood alcohol levels) in memory, reaction time and decision-making abilities.

Some changes observed in the heart itself were an increase in diastolic blood pressure, a thickening in the wall of the left ventricle, and a decrease in the speed at which the mitral valve opens and closes. They found "the size of the heart cavity, the extent of shortening of contractile fibers, and the speed of that shortening do not change much with age."

The studies of sexuality and daydreams (again, of men) show new understanding of sexuality among older people. There is evidence that the frequency of sexual activity slowly declines, and that those who were active during the ages of twenty to forty were correspondingly active after forty.

Now let's look at where aging begins: in the cell. In Baltimore, studies of aging cells were done in vitro, that is, test tubes, where small pieces of skin were taken from upper arms for tissue cultures. It was found that the cells in cultures actually underwent growth and cell division, and that cells from older donors underwent a smaller number of generations of cell division before losing their ability to reproduce. Age differences were also noted in the chemical and structural characteristics of the cells. The question is, are these cell changes intrinsic or environmentally induced, and can they be slowed down, halted, or reversed?

To further these studies, cell transplants, chemicals and diet manipulations (in mice) are being used with some promising and perhaps exciting results. I might add that in speaking to representatives of the National Institute of Aging I keep getting the same answer regarding diet and aging: "We don't know." However, there was also the comment that some researchers were taking vitamin E on their own, "just in case there is something to it."

Other studies on the cellular level are those dealing with the hormone-receptors and their role in aging. These receptors, located both inside and outside the cell, receive signals from hormones circulating in the bloodstream. These signals tell the cell to perform certain functions, such as metabolism of fat. It was found, both in animals and humans, that these receptors decreased with age.

It is thought that if there could be a way to restore the number of receptors in old cells, the anti-aging benefits would be enormous.

The National Institute of Aging has supported the work of Dr. John Marshall of the University of California at Irvine. His theories on aging are based on changes in the central nervous system, rather than a decrease in muscle strength accompanied by an increased accumulation of fat. He found that the brain chemical dopamine provides the necessary "juice" for muscles to function in the normal way. As we age the function is diminished, resulting in certain movement impairments. When Dr. Marshall gave his elderly rats two drugs: L-dopa (a biosynthetic precursor of dopamine) and apomorphine (a dopamine receptor stimulant) there was a dramatic although temporary improvement in the activity of rats. Relating these studies to humans is another thing, as it appears that when dopamine levels rise, so does aggressiveness.

The two basic theories of aging today are: death is programmed into our genes (therefore our cells) and there is little we can do to alter this biological clock; and that cell destruction is due to a series of accidents caused by exposure to free radicals, radiation, and other stressors, some of which can be reduced, resulting in an increase in cell life and integrity.

Dr. Zhores Medvedev, a biochemist whose theories on aging are widely respected in the scientific community, feels that the human organism was built to function for about 90 to 100 years, and there will be no dramatic breakthrough in longevity that will enable us all to reach that magic 100 mark. He does, however, believe it possible for more of us to reach it, by eliminating some of the killer diseases, and by strengthening the systems by which the body protects itself. He feels that evolution did not build years much beyond 100 into our genetic makeup.

Dr. Medvedev was one of the Soviet Union's leading scientists until he disagreed with the establishment, particularly the genetic theories of Stalin's favorite scientist, T. D. Lysenko. He is now attached to the National Institute of Medical Research in London.

His latest paper is calling attention to the problems of trying to explain the mechanisms of aging. Primates have maximum lifespans from 10 to 100 years, with man on the high end of the scale. Why is the speed of aging so different for cells of the same type and design?

His hypothesis is that higher organisms have more back-up genes in their cells to take the place of genes damaged by molecular accidents. Eventually all the genes are used up, and deterioration takes place more quickly where there are few substitute genes.

He is the first to suggest that any organism that synthesizes complex products makes errors. American scientists carried the theory further: when enough errors accumulate, death results.

Medvedev disagrees, believing there are built-in evolutionary safe-guards, enzymes that keep the body functioning by repairing and correcting errors. He feels that if you can activate these enzymes, you can help life itself. He thinks there is no single theory on aging that will explain aging of the different types of cells, for instance, those that live as long as we do, (heart, brain, and liver cells), and those that die and are replenished (called proliferating cells) such as red blood cells.

There are products on the market right now that claim to protect the cell from damaging factors and others that enhance the function of our own enzyme systems to do the same thing. Before we look at these, let's look further into the cell, our basic unit of life.

In the Baltimore center, NIA has been using proliferating cells called fibroblasts, from connective tissue, to enhance knowledge about how cells age. As mentioned earlier, these cells are observed in vitro (in the laboratory) where they undergo a period of rapid proliferation for a number of divisions (usually about forty), then reach a senescent phase where proliferation slows down, and finally stop proliferating after about fifty divisions. Samples were obtained from young subjects aged 20 to 35, and older men of 65 and above.

They found that the behavior of the cells in culture was generally related to the chronological age of the donor. In the older group, cell proliferation ability was greatly reduced, cell population doubling time was longer, the percentage of proliferating cells was lower, with only 2% able to proliferate eight or more times in a two-week period, as opposed to 60% ability of the young donor cells. These differences may actually underestimate the real alterations that accompany aging in vivo (life), as the cultures were taken from healthy, vigorous older people. It might be assumed that those weaker in the general population of older men had already died or were not well enough to submit to such testing.

More research is needed, especially in the areas of age-related changes correlating physiological with psychological studies, and in the field of cell transplant between animals of the same kind but of different ages. Our quest for youth has taken us in many directions, some unfortunate. Monkey gland injection is one, thankfully, that has gone by the board.

I attended a recent seminar on aging. Some of the speakers were clinicians, such as Dr. Murray Susser, who spoke on nutrients that protected the cell from damage. The scientific community may look askance at some of the statements of the speakers, but we certainly need to keep an open mind. The premise that we are undergoing abnormal stress due to our unnatural lifestyles, pollution, both indoors and out, and altered foods is not irrational. The question is not: is there a natural aging process   but, is it being speeded up? And, if it is, can we prevent or even reverse the process?

Cancer, for instance, once thought to be primarily a disease of aging, is now thought, through epidemiological studies, to be at least in part diet-and stress-related. Surely, more people are living longer, and therefore getting cancer, but the incidence is also increasing in the young and middle-aged.

One theory that sees modern technology as a cause of cell damage is called the "free radical theory." A free radical is a chemical entity with an odd number of electrons. (Atoms and molecules consist of protons, neutrons, and electrons.) Normally, electrons exist in pairs. Unpaired electrons may cause random chemical reactions that can produce cell damage, resulting in illness or aging.

Let's look further at the cell, so we can better understand what happens. The cell (other than red blood cells) consists of a nucleus and the cytoplasm surrounded by a sac-like membrane. The nucleus contains DNA, while the cytoplasm contains smaller functional units called organelles (little organs). These include lysosomes, which are sacs containing special degradative enzymes, mitochondria, which is responsible for energy production, endoplasmic reticulum, where protein and steroid synthesis and other processes take place, and others.

Organelles, like the nucleus and the cell itself, are enclosed by membranes composed of lipids (fats) and proteins. These membranes also control what enters and leaves, and contain enzymes involved with cell communication, electrolyte balance, immune reactions, and other processes. The membranes are composed of both saturated and unsaturated lipids, interspersed with protein.

The polyunsaturated molecules are susceptible to destruction by radiation and environmental oxidents such as sulphur dioxide, nitrogen and ozone. By the oxidation process they may be converted to lipid peroxides and eventually break down to form free radicals. These free radicals can then attach to nearby lipids and turn them into free radicals, resulting in a chain reaction and causing destruction of the membranes of the cell.

What happens as a result of this damage? If the mitochondrial membrane is damaged, no energy will be produced, and the cell will die. If the main cell membrane is damaged or breaks, again, the cell will eventually die. If the lysosomes membrane (that carries degradative enzymes) is damaged, these enzymes may spread out and digest the cell and neighboring cells. Further, the function of the lysosome to break down cellular waste may be impaired, because it cannot fully digest lipids damaged by free radicals. Eventually, they become congested, and may contribute to age pigments that accumulate in the elderly.

For over fifty years, scientists have known that the humoral immune response grows less effective with increasing age. Now the same effect is recognized in the cellular immune system. Some of these changes include tissue changes, and a reduction in the number of cells that precede antibody formation, a probable factor in the increased susceptibility of the elderly to infectious diseases. Animal research has shown that older animals have an increased number of cells that inhibit the activities of the body's immune response.

Immunologists are searching for means to enhance the immune response of people of all ages. Again, I cannot make the point strongly enough that EXCESS STRESS causes aging. One of the ways it does this is by suppressing the immune responses, leaving us vulnerable to all disease, including cancer. However, we need some stress; so don't worry about it, or you will handle it poorly. Leadership, and all its trappings, are a predictor of longevity.

Mice studies have shown that animals on a moderately restrictive (especially in the "teen" years) diet lived longer and showed an increase in resistance to some viral infections. The diets were restrictive not only in calories but also in proteins. Although this research is exciting in animals, it may prove to be difficult to translate to humans. Perhaps population studies may provide some missing clues. In any case, the question involving cellular changes still is: are they an intrinsic part of aging, one that is controlled by a biological clock, or are they environmentally induced, perhaps by the formation of free radicals? Or, perhaps, a combination of both?

ANTI-AGING DIET

The "anti-aging" foods mentioned most often are the antioxidents and free radical scavengers, E, C, A and selenium, and the foods containing sulphur amino acids. (You can detect them by their strong odor, such as onions and garlic.)

Vitamin E, an essential nutrient, is a fat soluble antioxident and free radical scavenger. It stops the cell damaging chain reaction by allowing itself to be oxidized by a free radical and capturing it, because it does not form any by-products that continue the chain. Vitamin E and other antioxidents and free radical scavengers are used up in protecting cells, so proper levels must be maintained.

The new U.S. Recommended Daily Allowances set the amount for vitamin E at a low 10-25 I.U. per day. At the time these figures were established, some nutritionists argued that they were too low. Dr. Jack Biery, of the National Institutes of Health, whose research was instrumental in establishing these figures, told me that "no American is deficient in vitamin E because of the high dietary intake of polyunsaturated oils in the form of margarines, etc." (Most cheaper hard margarines are primarily monounsaturates, while the soft, higher-in-oil-content margarines are higher in polyunsaturates.) What he did not mention is that much of the vitamin E is destroyed during processing, and that when one increases the amount of polyunsaturates in the diet, the requirements for vitamin E are also increased, a fact that is mentioned in the R.D.A. The reason for this is that the cell membranes reflect in their lipid content the amount of polyunsaturated fats eaten. It is the polyunsaturated fats that are susceptible to lipid peroxidation.   It has been suggested that those living and exercising in polluted areas need vitamin E supplements to protect their lungs from cell damaging effects. The amount most often recommended is 200-400 I.U.'s daily.

Vitamin C is considered a "youth" vitamin by the Russians. One of the reasons is it promotes the formation of collagen, the proteinous substance that supports and gives elasticity to the tissues. It is an antioxident and free radical scavenger, and works in the water-soluble portion of the cell where free radicals may do damage. Its antioxident quality helps protect the body from damaging radiation and smog. It aids in the formation of bones and cartilage, maintains capillary strength, and helps protect the body against viruses and bacteria.

Vitamin A, a fat soluble vitamin (stored in the fatty tissues and liver), maintains and protects the respiratory tract from nitrogen dioxide, a by-product of industrial and automobile combustion and cigarette smoke. Like vitamin E, it protects us from damage due to ozone, and maintains the cell integrity as an antioxident.

Scientists in India found that vitamin A fed to rats can block normal oxidation that occurs when tissue is exposed to air. When vitamin E was fed along with A, the antioxident effect was even stronger.[1] The FDA for vitamin A was lowered to 5,000 I.U.'s daily. The vitamin can become toxic in large amounts, as it is stored in the body. It is found in yellow and green vegetables, liver, and fish liver oil. It needs vitamin D to be utilized by the body (400 I.U., RDA) which we get from sunlight, fortified daily products, and fish liver oil. Studies have indicated that vitamin A, or carotene (a vitamin A precursor) may prevent some cancer.

Selenium, a trace mineral, is a potent antioxident and free radical scavenger. It is needed to promote the activity of the enzyme glutathione peroxidase, which protects cell membranes from oxidation. Selenium works synergistically with other antioxidents, and is found with natural vitamin E, such as cold pressed wheat germ oil. Selenium is found in fish and grains grown on soil rich in the mineral. it is best utilized by the body when it is in the organically bound form of selenium amino acids, formed by feeding yeast with nutrients rich in selenium. As SELENIUM CAN BE TOXIC IN EXCESS, more than 100 mcg (micrograms) per day are not recommended. Like vitamin A, it has been shown to prevent cancer in mice.

There is one other weapon against superoxide radicals: superoxide dismutase. In 1969, Dr. Irwan Fredovich of Duke University Medical Center identified superoxide radicals, and almost simultaneously discovered a natural body chemical that neutralized the radicals, superoxide dismutase (SOD). The chemical is being touted as an aging preventative and "cure" for some age related diseases such as arthritis. According to a paper submitted in the journal **Experimentia** by Dr. George Bartosz in 1979, "adequate amounts of SOD were found to be life prolonging." In addition, gerontologist Dr. Hans Kugler, author of **Seven Keys to Aging**, cites studies showing that test animals' lives were prolonged with the use of SOD.

It appears that our own production of SOD diminishes as we grow older, and it is now being sold in health food stores. Dr. Lutz gives SOD by injection, as it is destroyed during the digestive process. SOD is found naturally in liver, and the trace minerals manganese and zinc help us to synthesize it in our own bodies. The possibilities sound exciting, and I am looking forward to seeing the results of further research.

In any case, diet does seem to be a factor that affects aging, although studies show conflicting findings.

Dr. Charles Barrows and Dr. Eleanor Schlenker jointly presented papers

---

[1]International Journal of Vitamin and Nutrition Research, Vol. 47, No. 4, 1977.

on Nutrition and Aging at the State of the Art Seminar on Aging Research given at the Gerontology Research Center in Baltimore, Maryland, October 1, 1979. Dr. Barrows discussed the effect of nutrition restriction on lifespan as seen in animals, and Dr. Schlenker presented her findings from research she has done on the nutritional status of older women.

Dr. Barrows found that the life span was increased when animals were on a protein restricted diet, and it was safest and most effectively used when the restrictions were in adult life. However, when the animals were on an extremely restrictive diet, the life span again became that of those "well-fed."

He concluded that there was a reduction in the rate of aging as well as a delay in the onset of disease in the animals with restricted diets, and these findings could have potential significance for humans.

Dr. Schlenker feels that longitudinal studies (long-term studies that follow the same person as they grow older) need to be done to show the influence of nutrients (vitamins, minerals, proteins, carbohydrates and fats) taken in early life on health in later life.

She did a four-year study in California that showed a higher mortality rate among older subjects who had reported lower intakes of vitamin A, niacin and vitamin C. A twenty-four year longitudinal study of women in Michigan showed that the deceased subjects had a lower intake of niacin and vitamin C. The survivors were a significantly "younger" group, and had higher intakes of protein as well as vitamin C. The lower intake of protein in the deceased could be explained by dietary life-long patterns, changes in food patterns with age, or economic restrictions imposed by retirement.

It was found that vitamin C deficiency is a disorder that may be related to aging. It is not always correctible through the use of supplements, as some people cannot either absorb or properly utilize the vitamin. Among subjects with a vitamin C deficiency, those who responded to supplementation had a lower mortality rate than those whose vitamin C levels remained low.

It seems that more research needs to be done regarding the nutritional needs of older people. The ninth edition of the Recommended Dietary Allowances makes special comment on the needs for protein as we grow older. The protein requirements were recently examined by three groups of investigators with conflicting results. One group (Uauy, et. al, 1978) felt that the diet should consist of 12% to 14% protein, as opposed to 10% recommended by the Committee for Dietary Allowances for those over 50. In fact, it is felt that 12% or more may be needed, because there are more recurring diseases and/or surgeries in older people, and convalescence requires extra protein for repletion of wasted tissues. Although studies are conflicting and inconclusive, and more are being done in the labortory and with epidemological and longitudinal studies, there comes a time when we must act on the best available knowledge we have now. I am in favor of vitamin C, from a natural source, so as to get the complete vitamin, not just one selective element. A friend who is a research chemist says he doesn't believe in God or vitamin E. He adds, however, he may find out twenty years from now that vitamin E does serve a useful purpose, and God does exist.

Altering our protein intake may or may not delay aging, but that and other dietary changes—plus exercise—WILL slow the aging process, according to Nathan Pritikin, author of **Live Longer Now** and **The Pritikin Program for Diet and Exercise.** His gospel is preached and practiced in his Longevity Center in Santa Monica, California, where people come to get healthy or stay that way, or sometimes to avoid open heart surgery.

Pritikin claims his diet and exercise program will help prevent the onset of degenerative diseases if you don't have them, and diminish (or end) their symptoms if you do. The way this is accomplished is through the alteration of blood chemistry, which is monitored during a stay at the center.

The diet is low in calories, containing 10% fat, 10% to 15% protein, and 75% to 80% complex carbohydrates (fresh NATURAL fruits, vegetables and grains). Most people lose weight on the eight SIMPLE meals a day and none get hungry. "Simple" means that one meal is just a bowl of soup, another citrus fruit, another a potato. Caffeine and smoking are not allowed. Exercise, for those who can do it, is simply walking or roving, a combination of walking and jogging. Many who cannot exercise when they first arrive at the center find that they can by the time they leave. Drops in cholesterol, triglycerides, blood glucose and blood pressure are usually observed after several days.

The progrm has gained enough respect that some insurance companies are paying for part of the cost. Pritikin's contention that his diet actually re-opens plaque-filled arteries is controversial. At one time the medical community said that once atherosclerosis was begun it could not be reversed; however, new evidence is disputing that. There have been ongoing discussions between Pritikin and the National Institutes of Health as to the benefits of his program, which may eventually result in some of his patients being tested at the NIH to see what, if any, changes took place in the arteries.

If the Pritikin Diet is considered controversial, then what about **Gerovital, H3**, the anti-aging wonder drug?

Gerovital was originally procaine hydrochloride, a substance synthesized from two B vitamins, PABA (para-aminobenzoic acid) and DEAE (diethyl-aminoethanol). Its discoverer and chief proponent throughout the world is 85-year-old Dr. Ana Aslan, who takes Gerovital herself. A reputable Romanian physician and director of the Institute of Gerontology and Geriatrics, Dr. Aslan has treated notables all over Europe, including Nikita Kruschev and Indonesian President Sukarno.

She has tested GH3 extensively, with amazing results that show a reversal of many of the symptoms of aging, such as depression, muscular weakness, arthritis, impotence, loss of hair color and skin wrinkling. It can be taken orally or given by injection, and is sold in most parts of the world "over the counter," but is still not approved by the FDA in this country. The reason given is "insufficient testing." However, when English and American scientists failed to replicate her findings, Dr. Aslan said it was because they used procaine alone, rather than with benxoic acid (a preservative) and potassium metabisulfite (an antioxident) as the Russian and East European doctors who tested it did. They WERE able to confirm her findings.

Dr. Butler of the NIA does not label Gerovital a fraud, although he says it may not be as effective as claimed. He admits that it has been proven useful in treating depression, and for this reason alone one should be able to get a prescription for it. Dr. Alfred Sapse, a Los Angeles physician who interned at one of Dr. Aslan's Rumanian clinics, says he saw people start to pay attention to their physical appearance, get new energy, sleep better, and even become rejuvenated.

Dr. Sapse wanted to get Gerovital approved, at least as an antidepressant for older people. (It is thought that GH3 helps to control an enzyme called monamine oxidase which may go awry in people over 45, leading to depression.) He formed a company to fund research that was conducted by well respected scientists; however, it went bankrupt when the FDA would not approve the drug for sale, asking for more testing. Most of the anti-depressant drugs now on the market are more expensive and may have side effects; so it is difficult to understand why the FDA will not approve a natural substance that has been used safely for years.

No one knows for sure exactly how or why GH3 works. It is thought to improve the oxygen capacity of the blood, thereby toning up all of the cells. PABA works in the glands and intestines and aids the body in blood cell information, protein metabolism and skin functions, and stimulates the production of other B vitamins. DEAE produces mental stimulation and has an antidepressant effect.* Both of the vitamins are part of the body's anti-stress system and work together, rather than singly, towards "anti-aging."

Dr. Aslan believes that all people over 40 would be benefited by GH3. I happened to be just that age when I was in St. Maarten and met a pharmacist who was selling the European product. Having read about it for years, I became even more interested when he pointed out various doctors who had flown in from the States to buy it for special patients and themselves. The pharmacist himself was in his 70's, and despite his island tan, he had soft, smooth skin. I bought some, but it was impounded in customs, and that was the last I saw of GH3. Since then, the state of Nevada has declared itself independent of the FDA ruling, and has allowed the manufacture of Dr. Aslan's product within its borders.

Recently I received literature on, and advertising for two different products which claim to duplicate Dr. Aslan's current formula. One, Procaine vitamins, and Vitamin Creme, also contains the amino acid methionine (a sulphur amino acid) which they claim acts to break down serum cholesterol

*You should not take DEAE orally as it is carcinogenic when combined with nitrosamines which may be present in the stomach.

in the blood and enhance procaine's effectiveness. The other, Gerovital HP comes in a capsule along with other vitamins and minerals. With it you can buy a cream containing soluble collagen, RNA, and vitamin E. I have tried neither and therefore cannot vouch for their "safety and effectiveness."

Dr. Aslan recently spoke again at the NIH. Someone commented to me that she looked older. After all, she is 85 and does not claim Gerovital will prevent aging altogether!

More exciting news! Temple University researcher Dr. Arthur G. Schwartz has artificially produced a hormone he says may one day be used to lengthen life, promote thinness and decrease the likelihood of cancer. What more can you ask for?

The human-produced hormone, DHEA (Dehydroepiandrosterone), decreased the incidence of breast cancer in mice and caused them to lose weight, which he thought was caused by an acceleration in the metabolism rate. The mice also looked younger, with less graying and coarsening of hair.

DHEA is most abundant in young children, decreasing by 90% by the age of seventy. Dr. Schwartz is seeking more money for further research. Let's hope he gets it!

One anti-aging researcher who is working on a cellular level is Dr. Benjamin Frank, author of **The No-Aging Diet**. Another is Dr. Paul Niehans, whose live-cell therapy treatments in Switzerland have seemingly cured and prolonged the lives of many notables throughout the world. I am not sure of the National Institute On Aging's official position regarding Dr. Niehans, but they give little credence to Dr. Frank. I mention this in passing, not as a judgment, considering the government's ultra-conservative desire to stay out of controversial areas.

Dr. Frank's nucleic acid therapies for symptoms of aging are based on the "genetic catastrophe" theory. That is, the DNA (deoxyribonucleic acid) of which genes are made, and RNA (ribonucleic acid), which direct cell activity and the manufacture of proteins and enzymes, are subject to deterioration and a limited number of mutations. Once a certain number of mutations is reached, "genetic catastrophe" occurs, and the cell dies. As we age, cells have a shorter life span, and when enough die, signs of aging become apparent. Theoretically, if we knew what caused cells to die, we could slow down the aging process and increase the life span.

Dr. Frank, a New York physician with a degree in biochemistry, conducted research with nucleic acid and its effect on aging both in the laboratory and in the clinic. He feels that a diet high in nucleic acid and other factors, plus additional vitamin and nucleic acid supplements, can slow down or even reverse the signs of aging. Claimed benefits are a reduction of wrinkles, improvement in skin tone, and an increase in energy and stamina.

Nucleic acids are present in all living cells, therefore in most foods. Sardines are one of the highest sources, and it is abundant in brewer's yeast, seafood, beans, spinach, cauliflower and organ meats. Dr. Frank has combined RNA with the antioxident superoxide dismutase to boost its effectiveness. Both nucleic acids and superoxide dismutase occur naturally in calves liver.

When I visited him in 1970, Dr. Frank did not accept a patient for nucleic acid therapy without first doing a complete physical and blood work-up. Apparently, conditions such as tumors may be adversely affected by the diet. In 1970 the diet included a daily glass of raw vegetable juice, some skim milk, brewer's yeast and lecithin plus vitamin, mineral and nucleic acid supplements. As his research is continuing, I don't know exactly what the diet consists of today, or if the supplements you can buy over the counter duplicate his. You must exercise caution before buying supplements, because you can create an imbalance by overdosing on specific nutrients. Liver once a week won't hurt most people, neither will sardines or **fresh** vegetable juices. (There is a big difference between fresh and canned juices. If you don't have a juicer, go to a juice bar and get the real thing.)

Fighting aging with nutrition seems a safe way to go, but we must enter the arena with skepticism and caution. Unless your doctor indicates otherwise, at least 50% of your diet should consist of whole, natural, raw foods. "Live" foods preserve life. An orange-colored drink with ascorbic acid added is not the same as an orange, nor are potato chips or french fries equivalent to a potato eaten with the skin. If you are already eating 50% of your diet raw, increase it to 80%.

Gerovital and nucleic acid supplements may be unavailable, but you can have a home version by adding brewer's yeast to your diet. Brewer's yeast is a source of protein, nucleic acid, B vitamins and PABA, and can be taken with meals, sprinkled on food or mixed with juice. The powdered form is preferable to tablets, and if you can't stand the taste, try the debittered variety. Some people become "gassy" when they first start taking it; so start with less than a quarter teaspoon a day, and increase slowly. Brewer's yeast is high in phosphorus and should be balanced with calcium and magnesium. Remember, any food can cause an allergic reaction in sensitive individuals.

Other supplements being used for both health and rejuvenation are glandulars, or glandular therapy. Based on the theory that like cells benefit like cells, the cross-species approach transfers glandular cells from young or embrionic calves to humans.

Begun by Dr. Paul Niehans in Switzerland, it is being carried on in this country today usually through the use of capsules, rather than injections. Although radioactive isotope tracings indicate that injected glandular factors are absorbed by the corresponding glands, it is uncertain how much is absorbed when taken orally.

Nutritional therapists I have heard discuss glandulars say that they are gland or organ specific, and the glandular must be raw, that is, not treated at temperatures higher than body temperature, or 98.6°F.

Promising research is being conducted with the thymus gland to bolster the immune system of people with severe illnesses or those whose immune responses are lowered due to aging.

You can buy glandulars, but I would be afraid of them unless they are taken under the advice and supervision of a nutritional counselor. In the meantime, we can eat liver, and heart, etc., but adrenals and thymus require a little more sophistication.

It would be wonderful if we could take a pill and slow down or reverse the ravages of aging, but Nirvana is either unattainable or not yet here. We have many questions and some answers; moreover, some of those answers (such as the question of protein) are contradictory.

In June, 1978, at a N.I.A. nutrition conference, recommendations were made for future research on nutrition and aging. Some of the relationships of food and aging concern the elderly, while other nutrition-related problems such as osteoporosis begin in the thirties. Everyone over forty needs to look at diet, not only in regards to obesity, but how it affects overall health.

Some of the unanswered questions asked at the conference were:

● It is believed that as a person ages there is a decrease in lean body mass and an increase in fat. (This is the reason the Basal Metabolic Rate goes down). Along with this there is usually a decrease in activity, leading to the assumption that we need less calories. The question is: Do we then need less nutrients?

Since this question was asked, research has indicated that older people need the same nutrients that young people do. If we must restrict calories, the food we eat should be of optimal quality and nutritional value to preserve lean body mass and health.

● Degenerative diseases include not only loss of muscle fiber but bone tissue as well. Do we then need more calcium, and if so, how much? The subject of protein is controversial. Some studies indicate we need more, others the same, others less. Regarding calcium, recent studies have indicated that we may need 1200-1400 mgs. per day to treat and prevent osteoporosis, as opposed to 800 mgs. per day recommended. (Some women also need the judicious use of hormones and vitamin D.)

● There is a need to know if diet can affect the decrease in the kidney's efficiency that occurs with aging, and we need also to discover the role of sodium and fluid intake on the weakened renal system.

● Since there is a diminished ability to handle glucose, should the older person restrict sugar?

● Older people suffer from constipation, as well as other G.I. maladies. What foods, other than those with high fiber, are beneficial?

● What is a good diet in the aftermath of prior diseases, and in the presence of concurrent ones?

Comment was made on social and behavioral changes that affect nutrition. Often people are poorer after retirement. Friends or spouse may be gone, and there may be a decreased ability to care for oneself. Women may be trapped in their homes for fear of crime in the neighborhood. Loneliness, grief and depression may cause loss of appetite, and coupled with the lack of desire to cook for oneself, often leads to malnutrition.

It was recommended that further studies be done on the relationship between sodium and hypertension, taking into account sodium and potassium intake, obesity, physical fitness, alcohol and genetic factors.

There is a need to evaluate protein and ascorbic acid intake and how it affects the absorption of iron, calcium, zinc, and other heavy trace metals. Do changes take place in the efficiency and utilization of nutrients, and if so, what alterations should be made in dietary requirements and allowances? We need to learn more about lifelong nutritional patterns and hereditary factors in malnutrition.

There is a need to know answers to one of the questions I am asked the most: What happens to endocrine function as we age; what are the factors that regulate changes in lean body mass, body composition, energy balance and regulation of metabolic fuels? Some answers will be found in studies that look at the roles of diet, weight, and physical exercise in regard to endocrine and metabolic changes that take place as we age.

We need to know more about the effect of excess calorie intake and obesity on older people. Included in the recommendations for further study were the need for investigations into the interrelationships of nutrition, aging and dental health. The problems of periodontal disease, caries, edentulousness, and dentures on diet intake, taste, smell and emotional state would be explored.

Dr. Keyes of the National Institutes of Health has developed a therapeutic and prophylactic program for care of the gums and periodontal disease. It consists of antibiotics (when necessary), and the use of a waterpik with salt water, rubber tip gum massage, and a special gum brush using a paste of bicarbonate of soda and mild peroxide. I am on the program, and it works. Before you agree to gum surgery, find a dentist or periodontist familiar with this method.

Research centers have been established around the country to find some answers to these questions about aging. A new one will be built at Tufts University, whose president is the well-known nutritionist Dr. John Mayer, a former professor of nutrition at Harvard University.

Dr. Mayer cites many fairly new conditions associated with aging that may be nutritionally influenced. Many were recommended for research at the N.I.A. conference, such as dental caries, periodontal disease, hypertension, diabetes, kidney and liver diseases, some forms of cancer, arthritis, osteoporosis, decreasing sharpness of vision, and less acute perception of scents and flavors. Regarding the latter, nutritional therapies being explored are zinc to restore the sense of smell, and vitamin C for taste. It is interesting to note that "bad smells" are individual and may be sex-and culture-related. Children, up to a certain age, do not perceive of anything as smelling bad. A lack of interest in food relates not only to the ability to smell, but that the odors be pleasant.

Of particular interest to Dr. Mayer is the question of dietary allowances for older people. Although they need fewer calories, do they need fewer nutrients? It is difficult to get all you need from a diet of less than 1500 calories even when you are extremely careful. This is one reason why exercise is extremely important for people over forty. He also feels that older people commonly have a decline in digestive secretions and in the intestinal absorption of calcium and perhaps other vitamins and minerals. The answers to these and similar questions are not simple, nor will they be the same for everyone.

Dr. Lawrence Lamb, cardiologist and syndicated health columnist, notes that a calcium deficiency is common in this country. Dr. Mayer mentions iron deficiency anemia, and the fact that a deficiency of B vitamins may contribute to the mental confusion seen in some older people. He also thinks that some may have deficiencies of the fat soluble vitamins, A, D, and E due to a diet high in buns, pastries, cereals and baby food. He is concerned about the problems of lack of companionship and transportation with many of the elderly.

With all the discussion on the role of diet and aging, one would wonder if that is the secret—the answer to staying young, healthy and vigorous. Are we what we eat? If the answer to that question were an unequivocal "yes," solutions would be far simpler. The fact is, we are also what we breathe, think, feel, and do, and what we are born with.

I once heard Dr. Arthur Jay Green comment that it would do us no good to sit in the health food store drinking carrot juice if we spent the time worrying about growing older. Which brings us back to the world's leading expert on stress, Dr. Hans Selye.

Stress, in all its many and varied forms, is the ager, the precursor to illness and death. Dr. Selye points out that a certain amount of stress is both healthy and necessary, and advises us to FIND OUR OWN STRESS LIMITS, and not go beyond. Many of us are not aware of our limits, or are helpless to avoid situations that may take us beyond these limits. Dr. Butler says that a total lack of stress leads to aging and death, and the secret is to NOT WORRY ABOUT STRESS. In any case, many executives and other city dwellers have bought land and gone "back to the earth." This may be the answer for some, but most of us find a lowered standing of living a major cause of stress! (See the chapter on Stress.)

Exercise keeps us young in many ways. If **excess** stress causes us to age, and exercise reduces stress, the correlation is obvious. Exercise relieves tension and depression and helps the body throw off some of the stress-induced toxins stored in the tissues and the heart itself.

For many of us, competitive exercise aggravates stress. You see this on the golf course, tennis courts and running trails. Instead of feeling better, people come away tense, depressed and exhausted. Have fun, be a child, express and enjoy yourself. Run slower, and enjoy the scenery and companionship. Try clogging or square dancing; they're simple and fun. Go where groups and whole towns are playing non-competitive "New Games." Forget your age, and try free-style disco and rock dancing, great for stimulating energy, burning calories and relieving depression. If you feel inhibited, try it at home before you go, and go with someone with whom you are comfortable, perhaps a relative.

Exercise restores youth by toning the cardio-respiratory and cardio-vascular systems, giving us "aerobic" benefits, not the least of which is more energy. It helps prevent and cure many of the degenerative diseases caused or aggravated by sedentary living. Those include heart conditions, osteoporosis, arthritis, and a host of old-age complaints. Exercise stimulates and tones the entire glandular system, and all of us over forty know how important that is. A healthy skin tone due to increased circulation, and a youthful figure are some of the cosmetic youth benefits derived from exercise.

Why do we age? We are learning some answers and hoping, within our lifetime, to achieve the goal of extending the prime of life, not just life itself. It would be wonderful if we could get a little exercise and take a pill and stay young and healthy forever, and although we are learning, it's not that simple.

Consider the pituitary hormone called DECO (decreasing oxygen consumption). The evidence is that as the body ages the gland produces more DECO. Old rats who had their pituitaries removed (they were given other pituitary hormones in their feed) became young and active again. Obviously, we don't want to live without our pituitaries, but the theory has possibilities.

DNA research is exciting, but it is debatable whether eating foods high in DNA and RNA will reverse aging.

Central to DNA research is Ronald Hart, PhD, a gerontologist who is professor of radiology and pharmacology at the Ohio State University College of Medicine. He believes that aging, like cancer, is a degenerative disease associated with damage to the DNA which is caused by many things both inside and outside the body. Some of these are ultraviolet rays, ionizing radiation, natural and synthetic chemicals, heat, etc., which can cause DNA damage, creating mutations when the cell replicates itself. The cell has a number of repair mechanisms, and when there is a lack of repair, or misrepair, damage (aging) takes place.

Dr. Hart, and cancer researcher Richard Setlow, PhD, are working on the theory that there is a correlation between the lifespan achievable for a species and the ability of its cells to repair genetic damage. They feel that the repair capacity is the factor that controls the rate at which damage accumulates, and if that were modified, there could be protection from some of the ravages of life.

Joan Smith-Sonneborn, PhD, has actually doubled the lifespan of the tiny paramesia by stimulating its repair mechanism to repair damage done by ultraviolet light. That brings us into the realm of truly reversing the aging process by manipulating the repair systems of the body, some of which are yet unknown.

Perhaps if we increased our productive years on earth we would finally solve some of our age-old problems. It could be that there would also be an increase in intelligence, happiness and creativity, as well as productivity.

Let's return from speculation and theory to "facts" as reported in a **Special Report On Aging: 1979** put out by the National Institutes of Health. Some of the studies show that old animals can compensate for nerve cell loss. Brain cells have the capability (functional plasticity) to change their function. Compensation was made in old and young animals for nerve cells lost to strokes, tumors or senility. If we knew how to enhance the proper regrowth of brain circuits, we could reduce the damage caused by degenerative changes.

The NIH report indicated that the major cause of lack of taste in older people is actually a decline of smell sensitivity, and that strong odors made food more flavorful to the elderly. The continued use of smell over a person's lifetime (perfumers, for example) decreased the loss of the sense of taste.

It was suggested that food flavor be enhanced by adding amino acids with sweet or salty components to the diets of the elderly, thus lowering the sugar and salt content, and increasing the protein intake.

If we stop salting our foods, we learn to detect and enjoy their true flavors. Perhaps by doing this, and enjoying our sense of smell, we can eliminate the loss of taste that may occur with age.

The NIH findings indicated that people with **mildly** elevated blood pressure were not so likely to show a decline in intellectual performance.

Note the emphasis on **mildly** elevated. High blood pressure (hypertension) can lead to strokes, heart attacks and kidney diseases. It is estimated that 80% of older people diagnosed as "senile" are actually suffering from two irreversible conditions, multi-infarct dementia (many small strokes) and Alzheimer's Disease.

Alzheimer's is the most common, and as yet its cause and cure are not known. Once thought to be rare, it is now believed to affect between 500,000 and 1.5 million Americans of all ages, and leads to death within five to ten years.

Research has looked in many directions for a cause. One is the relationship of aluminum to Alzheimer's. There appear to be high concentrations of aluminum in the brains of people suffering with this disease, and it is thought that it may interact with DNA. Although officially there is no "cure," some people have experimentally been treated successfully with the brain enzyme choline acetyltransferase, which stimulates the production of acetylcholine, a chemical compound that helps transmit nerve impulses. Foods such as eggs and lecithin (found in eggs and soybeans) contain choline, however, not in the potent form used therapeutically for Alzheimer's.

There was a final word about sex and longevity. If sex helps us by reducing stress and enhancing chemistry, will it not also prolong youth? Not necessarily so, according to rat studies. Breeder rats, those forced to copulate and breed often, suffer from more life-threatening disorders, such as hypertension and blood and arterial problems. This does not say it is healthier to be celibate; it merely indicates that it may not be wise to have many children by many partners, a fact that has small relevance for most of us.

In fact, according to Dr. Butler, a partner may be crucial to survival. It may be the emotional involvement that keeps people alive, or someone to care for you when you are sick. People with social ties and relationships have lower mortality rates than those without ties, and it seems that divorce and loneliness are harder on men than women.

Leaders, and those with lives of substance and goals which they pursued live longer, as do those who are happy in their marriages and with their lives in general. Maintaining a continuing involvement—activities, clubs, daily and long-term objectives, keeps us alive.

Dr. Butler feels that physical fitness is important, as are flexibility or resourcefulness, and the ability and desire to keep learning. Exercise is for the mind as well as the body; you lose what you don't use.

The age of our parents is important in longevity, but we can undo the benefits of good genes by poor self-care, and overcome genetic shortcomings by taking good care of ourselves.

What does Dr. Butler do for himself at age 63? How does one live who has all the latest information on longevity? He eats an almost exclusively vegetarian diet high in complex carbohydrates and fiber; never adds salt or sugar to his food; takes a multivitamin daily; seldom drinks alcohol; jogs about two miles, five times a week; doesn't smoke; drinks skim milk and rarely eats high fat foods; keeps his weight down; is outgoing, optimistic and committed to his work.

One thing undisputed is that the QUALITY, NOT THE QUANTITY OF LIFE IS IMPORTANT. For me, quality is health and the ability and energy to enjoy simple things. Today I felt as young and happy as a chld as I walked through the winter woods. I derived great pleasure from nature and the feeling of strength, health and happiness, and freedom from pain and depression. I saw, as though for the first time, the white tails of deer running through the meadows, and the sunlight glistening on snow as it fell through the trees to the green ground pines. I heard the wind roaring like the ocean in the treetops, and the symphony of the rubbing branches. I felt and smelled the sweet, clean air, and truly became new, younger, and alive.

More than a time of life, youth is a state of mind.

18
THE ALPHA
AND OMEGA

Where should you begin, and is there an end? Start where you are, right now. Put the book down and stretch, or do pelvic tilts while you are reading. There is no end; fitness is a lifetime personal commitment that YOU can live with. This doesn't mean you can never step off the straight and narrow. You do so guiltlessly on occasion, and go right back where you left off.

It is not difficult to make reasonable changes and to feel good about yourself while doing so. For instance, if you want to lose a pound a week, you will need a caloric deficit of about 500 per day; two pounds a week, 1,000 a day. Do it the easy way by decreasing your intake AND increasing your activity.

Don't destroy your marriage by becoming overly competitive with your husband. It is helpful if you share a diet as well as exercise, keeping in mind that a medical evaluation is recommended for those over 35 who are beginning a vigorous exercise program. Don't feel cheated if his exercise heart rate is lower than yours. His heart is larger and doesn't have to work as hard.

Interest in fitness will increase your awareness of related health facts. For instance, many insurance companies charge additional premiums if you suffer from hypertension, and will reduce the premiums (if asked) if your blood pressure returns to normal. Women's health care is often not as good as men's. We are still sometimes taken frivolously, and given the advice to "Take a little Valium, honey."

Go to health seminars, inquire, read, and keep an open mind. All of the facts are not in, and probably never will be until the day comes when we are cloned! Listen to the experts who say "we don't know." That is the truth.

I recently attended a fitness seminar, where a cardiologist spoke on the cardiovascular benefits of exercise. He said exercise will not GUARANTEE you immunity from heart attack, nor will it cure a heart condition. He, however, is a runner, and pointed out the cardiovascular and other benefits of exercise, such as beneficial changes in blood viscosity, a defusing of the stress reaction, and perhaps, better sex. He acknowledged that we don't know all the determining factors regarding cardiovascular diseases, although genetics, obesity, smoking, high blood pressure and cultural factors are generally considered important.

At question are the explanations of statistics. We have a much higher heart attack rate than Orientals; why? Is it our diet, genetic code, or stressful lifestyle? High cholesterol levels have been linked to heart attacks, yet there are many unanswered questions. Although it is considered prudent to lower your cholesterol and saturated fat intake, especially if you fall into the high risk of heart attack category, some feel it is fat and not cholesterol that makes the difference. A widespread theory is that the blood vessel becomes damaged and fatty plaques form, no matter what the cholesterol level. Another theory is that a deficiency (I have heard magnesium and B6 mentioned) predisposes one to atherosclerosis. Even the statement that type A behavior increases the risk of heart attack has been questioned. We must consider the individual, and **all** factors.

There was another speaker at the seminar, a local sportsmedicine authority whom I have heard many times. I endure his rantings, because some of what he says is true some of the time for some individuals. But that is not the way he presents it. Although his opinions have changed through the years, he offers as gospel his CURRENT thinking, leaving no room for argument. Almost always another doctor in the audience disagrees with him, at times to the point of fighting. This is good, because it allows people to hear other expert opinions. No one is right all of the time, but most of us are not in the position to judge.

On this occasion he stated unequivocally that obese people eat no more than slender people; their metabolic functions are simply slower. He cited as an example that the sodium pump works harder in thin people (thereby using more energy). I have read of similar studies, one using the movement of red blood cells as an indicator. His solution for speeding them up was exercise that maintains a heart rate of 120 beats per minute, 30 minutes, 3 times a week. I agree with him regarding THESE PARTICULAR PEOPLE, and recently I gave similar advice to my hairdresser, who needs to be on a starvation diet of 350 calories to lose weight. (It is to be hoped that the exercise would allow her to eat more.)

Despite his dogmatic statement, the fact remains that **most** obese people DO eat more food than thin people, more of the wrong foods, and they eat it faster. That is one reason behavior modification has been successful, although it, too, is only part of the story. I will never argue against exercise, but it is a gross injustice to misinform people about the benefits of diet. He also flatly stated that all diets are harmful, citing as examples the Scarsdale Diet and the Linn Diet. That's like saying that everyone who flies will be a victim of a skyjacking.

Here's a typical example of how diet effects obesity: I recently lunched with one of my students who is at least 75 pounds overweight. At her suggestion we went to a salad bar. She ate quickly and filled her plate to overflowing again, taking second servings of both potato and macaroni salads. I ate neither of these, knowing that mayonnaise is one of the most fattening foods; she ate no bread, thinking that carbohydrates, in the form of bread, are what puts on the pounds. I had enough time to eat only one dish of food. If all other things had been equal, she would have eaten twice the number of calories because she went back for seconds. However, she also dumped on the dressing. You can easily consume 2,000 calories if you eat the wrong foods at a salad bar!

This woman blames her obesity on the fact that she snacks all evening. Certainly that is a factor but not the whole story. She IS exercising, but because of her weight she can't run or jump. Bicycling and swimming are good for her, as long as she gets her heart rate up to at least 120. SHE ALSO NEEDS TO BE AWARE OF HER DIET!

Examine YOUR possible hidden psychological causes of overeating. Are you fat because you really don't want to bother sleeping with your husband? Or are you eating because you can't stand the hassles and competition of the singles dating game? Group therapy may be helpful in recognizing and dealing with your feelings and relationships with others.

FEEL GOOD ABOUT YOURSELF! The myth of male superiority is just that: a myth. It was begun by men and carried on by religious and social traditions. For example, the highest suicide rate is among single men. Women's life expectancy is almost eight years longer than men's. Although it is estimated that between 130 and 150 males are conceived for every 100 females, more male fetuses are miscarried, bringing the birth ratio down to 104-107 for every 100 females. Furthermore, the death rate for males is higher in the first month of life, and women have the advantage for the rest of their lives.

Part of this advantage is because of a social conditioning that encourages violent behavior in males, and part caused by the toll the male hormones exact on the heart and circulatory system.

More women than ever are smoking, and starting younger—stupid choices on our part. We do not have to choose between smoking or being fat. We can choose to do neither!

In the December, 1980, Health and Human Services Annual Report, then

Surgeon General Dr. Julius Richmond said that with some exceptions, American's health had never been better. Some of his conclusions were:

- Life expectancy is up 2.7 years, to 73.3 years.
  Although still the number one killer, the death rate from heart disease declined 20%, stroke, 33%.
- Fewer people under 49 are dying of cancer, because of reduced lung cancer in younger men, and advances in the treatment of breast cancer, Hodgkins's Disease, and childhood leukemia.
- Infant mortality rates dropped 47% since 1965, to 13 for every 1,000 births.
- The incidence of childhood infectious diseases has fallen. Some minuses were reported.
- The death rate is rising for Americans between the ages of 15-24, because of accidents, drugs, and violence.
- Deaths from motor vehicle accidents are up.
- There may be too much unnecessary surgery. Fifteen percent of all births are by Caesarean, up 3 times that of 10 years ago.
- Health care costs now exceed 212 billion dollars a year.
- Blacks and the poor still have higher rates of illness and worse health care than whites and the rich.

We can only hope that the statistics will improve in all areas, as women assume more active roles and we reevaluate our social standards.

If you think the road to change is too difficult, look at Paul Kimmelman. According to the Guiness Book Of Records: "The speed record for slimming was established by Paul M. Kimmelman, 21, of Pittsburg, Pa., who, from December 25, 1966, to August 1967, went on a crash diet of 300 to 600 calories per day to reduce from 487 pounds to 130 pounds, a total loss of 357 pounds."

Paul says the figures aren't quite correct. He went from 530 pounds on New Year's Day in 1967 to 130 pounds seven months and three days later!

The Guiness Book does not mention that Paul did it on his own, with no doctors, clinics, or pills, and that he almost lost his life along with his weight. He has since attained a normal weight, diets and exercises sensibly, feels fine, and what's most important, has maintained this weight for fourteen years.

The alternative to gorging is not starvation, nor is marathon running the only way to exercise. The first step is from where you are right now.

Consider the fact that the United States has the largest older population in the world and that you may live to be eighty or more. Active people look and feel younger, have more energy, and earn more money by being able to work longer and harder. More important, they can spend some of that money on things they **enjoy** rather than on doctor's bills.

ENJOY is the key word, not endurance. We need endurance to have the strength and energy to be able to do the things that we enjoy, but fitness is a means as well as an end. Getting fit is as much fun as being fit.

Exercise for recreation, and recreation for exercise. Eat low calorie foods that you like. Food that is hated is not sustaining. If you indulge on occasion, do so with enjoyment, not guilt. Think of getting in shape as buying a high interest, long-term certificate of deposit. It's fun to be able to buy it, it's there when you need it, and its value increases with time.

Find pleasure in the journey, and you WILL get there. We don't know where or when our travels will end; so live every moment along the way. Surround yourself with happy, lively, stimulating people and places.

I don't understand why people travel great distances to the ocean, and then lounge around a pool without even bothering to swim. Pools and cement are dead; the ocean is vibrantly alive. It affects both "psyche" and "soma" and awakens the pleasures of all the senses. Absorb life from the ocean. Fine-tune your whole being so you are **alive** all of your life.

Listen to the many sounds of the surf and birds. Watch the colors change from sprinkled diamonds to a veneer of deep violet. Smell and taste the air and water; feel the wind and spray on your face, and the surf under your feet and over your body. Know the ocean when it is warm and when it is cold, when it is calm and when it is frenzied.

Let the ocean relax or excite you. Stay until you feel it surging and ebbing through your body. Walk the shore when the sky is brilliant and when it glowers. Go in the early morning and at sunset, and again when the moon rises. Walk alone in the winter, and gather gifts from the debris at your feet.

Ralph Waldo Emmerson said:

"Each moment of the year has its own beauty . . .
A picture which was never seen before and shall never be seen again."

Life itself seems to pass as rapidly as my three favorite months, April, May and June. No two springs are alike, and I wouldn't miss one moment of any season that is given to me. Each year I celebrate the exciting emergence of new life.

Celebrate YOUR gift of life with fitness!

BIBLIOGRAPHY

Adams, John. "Improving Stress Management." *Social Changes, NTL Institute,* Vol. 8, No. 4, 1978.

Agriculture Handbook No. 8. Department of Agriculture, Washington, D.C. Gov't. Printing Office, 1975.

Alzheimer's Disease, Q. and A. Dept. of Health, Education and Welfare, Nat. Inst. of Health pub. no. 79-1646. Sept., 1979.

Arthritis: The Basic Facts. Arthritis Foundation. Atlanta, Georgia, 1978.

Arthritis Forum. Arthritis Foundation. Vol. 5, #3. Atlanta, Georgia. Fall, 1979.

Arthritis Forum. Arthritis Foundation. Vol. 5, #2. Atlanta, Georgia. Summer, 1979.

Bailey, Covert. *Fit Or Fat?* Boston: Houghton Mifflin Co., 1977.

Berland, Theodore, and editors of Consumer Guide. *Rating The Diets.* 1979; 1980 NAL

Benjamin, Ben. E. *Are You Tense?* New York: Pantheon Books, 1978.

Benzaia, Diana. "Rejuvenation, 1980s And Beyond." *Harper's Bazaar,* July, 1979, pp 280-244.

Black, Johnathon. "The Brain According To Mandel." *The Runner,* April, 1979, pp 79-83.

"Body: Megavitamin Therapy." *People,* 15 Dec., 1980. pp 115-121.

Bourne, Lydia. "Lifestyle Changes: How You Can Stay Healthy." *Group Health Asso. News,* April, 1980.

Calories And Weight. Agriculture Bulletin #364. Washington, D.C. Govt. Printing Office, 1976.

Cells And Aging. Nat. Inst. of Health Pub. #79-1860. Sept., 1979.

Changes. Dept. Health, Education and Welfare Pub. #78-85. Washington, D.C.: U.S. Govt. Printing Office.

Conoley, Gillian. "Living May Be Hazardous To Your Health". *American Way,* Feb., 1980, pp 36-44.

Cooper, kenneth. *The New Aerobics.* Bantam, 1970.

Cureton, Thomas Kirk, PhD. *Physical Fitness and Dynamic Health.* Dial, 1975.

Current Food Consumption Practices and Nutrient Sources In The American Diet. U.S. Dept. of Agriculture. Washington, D.C. Govt. Printing Office, June, 1980.

DuPrau, Jean. "My Aching Back: Relief Through The Alexander Technique." *Journal of The Nutritional Academy.* Vol. 2, #1, pp 41-43.

Ellwood, Catherine. *Feel Like A Million.* Pocket Books, 1956.

Ellwood, Catherine. Unpublished lectures. Montgomery Coollege, Takoma Park, Md., 1971.

Epps, Garrett. "Brains And Ambition." *The Washington Post Magazine.* 11 Nov., 1979, pp 32-40.

"Exercise and the Cardiovascular System." A round table. *The Physician and Sportsmedicine.* Sept., 1979, pp 54-71.

Fats In Food And Diet. U.S. Dept. of Agriculture. Ag. Bulletin #361. Washington, D.C.: U.S. Govt. Printing Office, 1974.

Fast Foods. U.S. Dept. of Agriculture. Washington, D.C.: U.S. Govt. Printing Office.

Fitness For The Fun Of It. Fitness Ontario, 1979.

Feldenkrais, Moshe. *Awareness Through Movement.* Harper and Rowe Publishers, 1972.

Food. U.S. Dept. of Agriculture no. 0-302-627. Washington, D.C., U.S. Govt. Printing Office, 1979.

Gallo, Nick. "The New Age of Structural Therapy." *Journal Of The Nutritional Academy* vo. 2, #1, pp 24-27.

Garr, Doug. "Getting Drugs: By Hook Or By Crook." *Family Health*, Nov., 1979, pp 34-40.

Getchell, Bud, PhD. "The Calorie Costs of Rope Skipping and Running." *The Physician and Sportsmedicine,* Feb., 1980, pp 56-60.

Goldwag, Elliot, PhD. et. al. *The Joy Of Life.* London: Octopus Books, Ltd., 1978.

Gottleib, Bill. "Vitamin E When It's Sink or Swim." *Prevention,* May, 1979, pp 132-136.

Gottleib, Bill. "A Lifetime Of Fitness." *Prevention,* Dec., 1980, pp 53-59.

Gorner, Peter. "The Optimistic Tiger." *Success Unlimited,* Jan., 1980, pp 28-31.

Grant, Lillian. "The Key To Physical Fitness At Any Age." *Bestways,* March, 1978, pp 52-53.

Gross, Iris. "Are Unnatural Fats Linked To Jewish Cancer Rates?" *Ha-Koach.* University of Maryland, Nov., 1979, p 8.

"How To Have A Longer Life And Enjoy It More." *U.S. News and World Report,* 12, July, 1976, pp 29-32.

Human Nutrition, Report Number 2. U.S. Dept. of Agriculture, Aug., 1971.

Iyengar, B.K.S. *Light On Yoga.* Schockan Books, Inc., 1966.

Jones, Susan Smith. "The Effects Of Supplements On Athletic Performance." *Bestways,* March, 1978, pp 35-37.

Julian, James, M.D. "The Quest For Youth and Vitality." *Body Forum,* Nov., 1980. pp 9-22.

Kahn, Carol. "The Happiness Hormone." *Family Health,* Dec., 1978, pp 48-51.

Kahn, Carol. "Why We Age: The Toughest Puzzle Of All." *Family Health,* April, 1979, pp 49-54; May, 1979, pp 36-48.

Katch, Frank, and Wm. D. McArdle. *Nutrition, Weight Control and Exercise.* Boston: Houghton Mifflin Co., 1977.

Kraus, Hans. *Backache, Stress and Tension.* Publisher and Date unknown.

Kraus, Hans. *Clinical Treatment Of Back And Neck Pain.* McGraw, 1970.

Krucoff, Carol. "Coping: The Plight Of Women In a Graying America." *The Washington Post,* 6 May, 1980.

Krucoff, Carol. "Gray Power: Sex After Sixty." *The Washington Post.* 26 March, 1980, p E 5.

Kugler, Hans, PhD. "The Healing Properties Of Cell Therapy." *The Body Forum,* Dec., 1979, pp 23-53..

Lesser, Michael, M.D. *Nutrition and Vitamin Therapy.* Grove Press, Inc. 1980.

Letvin Maggie. Maggie's Back Book: *Healing The Hurt In Your Lower Back.* H.M. 1977.

Levine, Jack, M.D. "Chondromalacia Patella." *The Physician And Sportsmedicine,* Aug., 1979, pp 40-49.

Lutz, Howard, M.D. Unpublished Lectures, Berkeley Springs, West Virginia, 1980.

Mayer, Jean. "Nutrition: The Secret Ingredient In Graceful Aging." *Family Health,* May, 1979, pp 48-54.

McCauelay, Carole Spearin. "Endorphins." *Self,* Dec., 1979, pp 72-73.

Morehouse, Lawrence E. PhD. and Leonard Gross. *Maximum Performance.* Pocket Books, 1977.

Morgan, Wm. P. "The Mind Of The Marathoner." *Psychology Today,* April, 1978, pp 38-49.

National Institute On Aging. Dept. of Health, Education and Welfare publication #78-1129.

Nicholas, James, PhD. "Orthopedic Problems In Middle-Aged Athletes." *The Physician and Sportsmedicine,* Nov., 1979, pp 37-46.

Nutrient Levels In Food Used By Households In The U.S., Spring, 1977. U.S. Dept. of Agriculture, Jan., 1981.

Nutritional Value Of Food. U.S. Dept. of Agriculture, Home and Garden bulletin #72, 1970.

Nutrition And Aging. Testimony before the Senate Select Committee on Nutrition And Human Needs, Sept. 23, 1977. Dept. of Health, Education and Welfare #(NIH) 79-325.

Nutrition And Aging. National Institutes Of Health pub. #79-1409. Washington, D.C., Govt. Printing Office. July, 1979.

Olds, Sally Wendkos. "How To Calm A Stress Sensitive Stomach." *Self,* Dec., 1979, pp 70-72.

Pate, Russel R., PhD. "Dietary Iron Supplementation In Women Athletes." *The Physician and Sportsmedicine,* Sept. 1979, pp 81-89.

Parrish, Louis, M.D. "Finding A Solution To Sexual Impotence." *The Body Forum,* Dec. 1979, pp 13-49.

Pekham, John. "Secrets Of Eternal Youth." *The Washingtonian,* May, 1980, pp 115-123.

Pines, Maya. "Food For Thought: A Safe Memory Pill." *The Washington Post,* 7 Sept., 1980, pp D1-D4.

Pritiken, Nathan. *The Pritikin Program For Diet And Exercise.* New York. Grosset and Dunlop, 1979.

"Proven Diagnostic Tool Not Accepted In U.S." *Nutrition Health Revue,* Spring, 1980, p 4.

Prudden, Bonnie. *How To Keep Slender And Fit After 30.* New York. Pocket Books, 1970.

Recommendations For Future Research In Nutrition And Aging. National Institute On Aging Nutritional Conference, June 5, 6, 7, 1978.

Recommended Dietary Allowances. The National Research Council. 9th Edition, 1980.

Research Programs of the National Institute on Aging; Robt. N. Butler, M.D., From Public Health Reports, U.S. Dept. of Health, Education and Welfare, vol. 92, no. 1, Jan.-Feb., 1977. pp 3-8.

Rogers, Jean. "How To Say Yes To Yeast." *Prevention,* Jan. 1980, pp 120-125.

Rovner, Sandy. "The Rhythm Of Life." *The Washington Post,* 12 Oct. 1979, p B5.

"Senility." *Harvard Medical School Health Letter,* May, 1980.

Schultz, Paul. "Flexibility: Day of The Static Stretch." *The Physician And Sportsmedicine,* Nov., 1979, pp 125-128.

Schuster, Karolyn. "Equipment Update: Jogging Bras Hit The Streets." *The Physician and Sportsmedicine,* April, 1979, pp 125-130.

Sheehan, George, M.D. *Dr. Sheehan On Running.* World Publications, 1975.

Shyne, Kevin. "Thomas K. Cureton, Jr.; Sportsmedicine Pioneer." *The Physician and Sportsmedicine,* Nov. 1979, pp 125-128.

Skinner, Mike. "Sex and Nutrition." *Body Forum,* Nov., 1980, pp 44-50.

Special Report On Aging: 1979. U.S. Dept. of Health, Education and Welfare. National Institutes Of Health Pub. #79-190S, Sept., 1979.

Stauth, Cameron. "Spinal Stress." *Journal Of The Nutritional Academy,* Vol. 2, #1, pp 16-23.

Stearn, Jess. *Yoga, Youth and Reincarnation.* Doubleday and Co., Inc. 1965.

Subotnick, Stephen I.D.P.M. "Variations In Angle Of Gait In Running." *The Physician and Sportsmedicine,* April, 1979, pp 110-115.

Subotnick, Steve, M.D. "Shoes and Feet." *Runner's World,* Aug., 1979, pp 137-138.

The Baltimore Longitudinal Study of the National Institute On Aging. Dept. of Health, Education and Welfare Pub. no. (NIH) 78-134.

"The Bran Hypothesis"—A Grain Of Truth?" *Harvard Medical Health Letter,* Vol 5, #11, Sept., 1980.

Ullyot, Joan. *Women's Running.* World Publications, 1976.

"Weight Control." *Harvard Medical School Health Letter.* Dec., 1980.

Williams, R.J. *Nutrition Against Disease.* New York: Pitman Publishing, 1971.

Yates, John. "A New Pathway To Longer Life." *Prevention,* Dec., 1980, pp 95-98.

Yenckel, James. "Self Help: Being Your Own Therapist." *The Washington Post,* 15 May, 1980, p F5.

Yenckel, James. "Careers: The Working Tense." *The Washington Post,* 2 July, 1980.

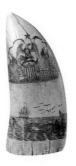

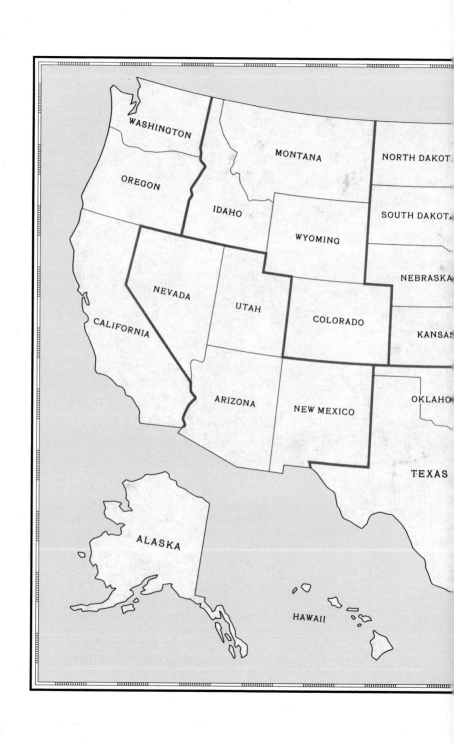

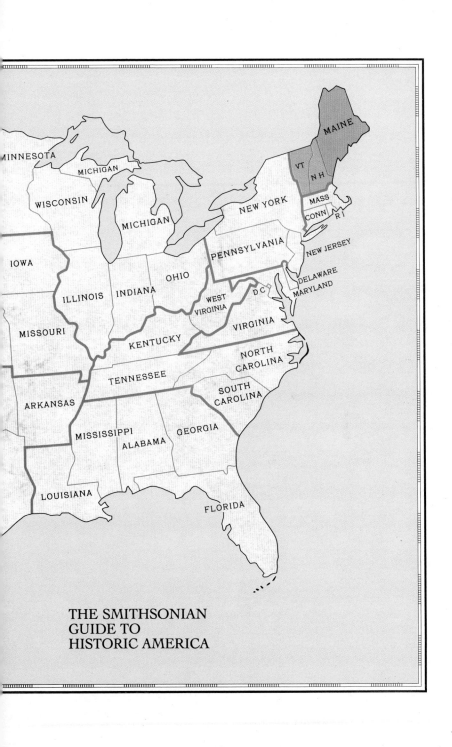

MINNESOTA

MICHIGAN

WISCONSIN

MICHIGAN

IOWA

ILLINOIS INDIANA OHIO

MISSOURI

KENTUCKY

ARKANSAS

TENNESSEE

MISSISSIPPI ALABAMA GEORGIA

LOUISIANA

FLORIDA

NEW YORK

PENNSYLVANIA NEW JERSEY

DELAWARE
DC
MARYLAND

WEST
VIRGINIA

VIRGINIA

NORTH
CAROLINA

SOUTH
CAROLINA

MAINE

VT
N H

MASS
CONN
RI

THE SMITHSONIAN
GUIDE TO
HISTORIC AMERICA

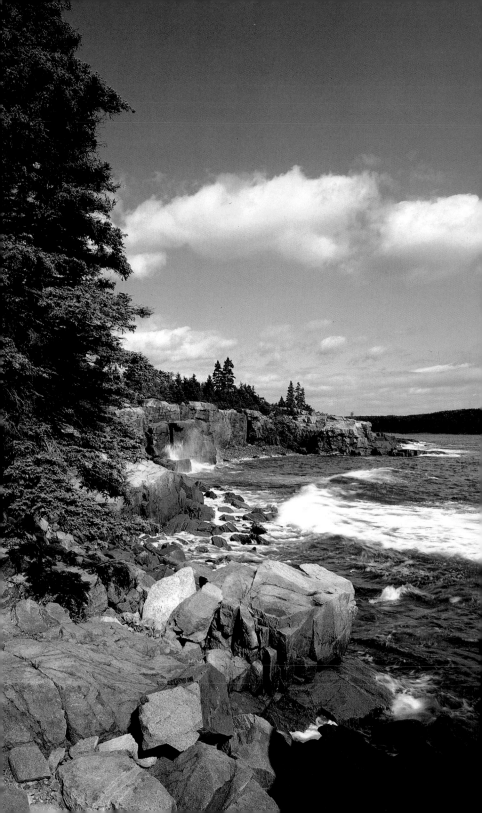

THE
SMITHSONIAN
—— GUIDE TO ——
HISTORIC AMERICA

NORTHERN NEW ENGLAND

TEXT BY
VANCE MUSE

SPECIAL PHOTOGRAPHY BY
PAUL ROCHELEAU

EDITORIAL DIRECTOR
ROGER G. KENNEDY
DIRECTOR OF THE NATIONAL MUSEUM
OF AMERICAN HISTORY
OF THE SMITHSONIAN INSTITUTION

Stewart, Tabori & Chang
NEW YORK

Smithsonian Books
WASHINGTON, DC

Published in 1989 by Stewart, Tabori & Chang, Inc., 740 Broadway,
New York, NY 10003.

FRONT COVER: Waits River, VT.
HALF-TITLE PAGE: Scrimshaw, Shelburne Museum, VT.
FRONTISPIECE: Acadia National Park, ME.
BACK COVER: North Ferrisburg, VT.

SERIES EDITOR: HENRY WIENCEK
EDITOR: MARY LUDERS
PHOTO EDITORS: DAVID LARKIN, MARION PAONE
ART DIRECTOR: DIANA M. JONES
DESIGNER: PAUL P. ZAKRIS
ASSOCIATE EDITOR: BRIGID A. MAST
PHOTO ASSISTANT: BARBARA J. SEYDA
EDITORIAL ASSISTANT: MONINA MEDY
DESIGN ASSISTANT: KATHI R. PORTER
CARTOGRAPHIC DESIGN AND PRODUCTION: GUENTER VOLLATH
CARTOGRAPHIC COMPILATION: GEORGE COLBERT
DATA ENTRY: SUSAN KIRBY

LIBRARY OF CONGRESS CATALOGING-IN-PUBLICATION DATA

Muse, Vance
    Northern New England.

    (The Smithsonian guide to historic America)
    Includes index.
    1. New England—Description and travel—1981-   —Guide-books.
2. Historic sites—New England—Guide-books. 3. Maine—Description and travel—1981-
    —Guide-books. 4. Historic sites—Maine—Guide-books. 5. Vermont—Description and
travel—1981-   —Guide-books. 6. Historic sites—Vermont—Guide-books. 7. New
Hampshire—Description and travel—1981-   —Guide-books. 8. Historic sites—New
Hampshire—Guide-books.
    I. Rocheleau, Paul. II. Kennedy, Roger G. III. Title. IV. Series.
F2.3.M8 1989   917.4   88-33092
ISBN 1-55670-066-0 (pbk.)   ISBN 1-55670-049-0

Distributed by Workman Publishing, 708 Broadway, New York, NY 10003

Printed in Japan

10 9 8 7 6 5 4 3 2 1
First Edition

CONTENTS

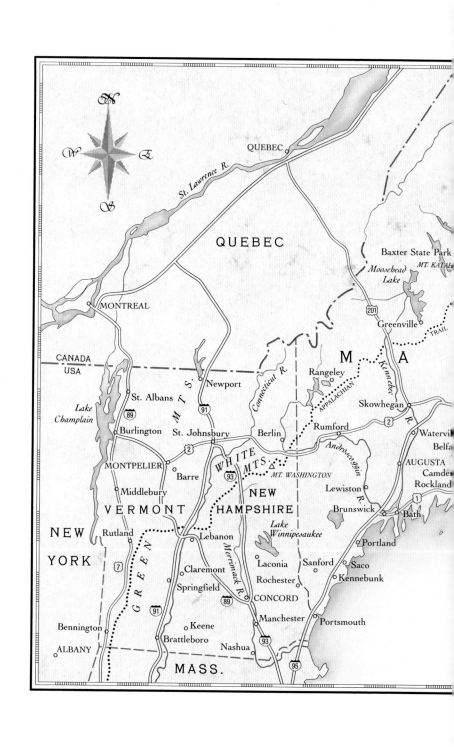

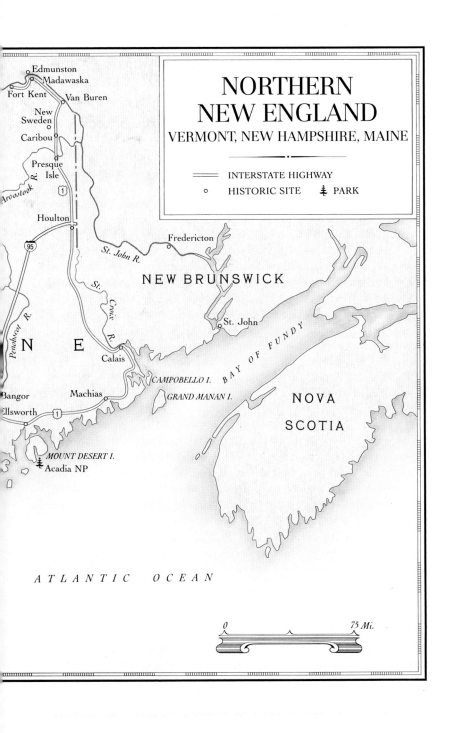

NORTHERN
NEW ENGLAND
VERMONT, NEW HAMPSHIRE, MAINE

══════ INTERSTATE HIGHWAY
○ HISTORIC SITE   ⚘ PARK

Edmunston
Madawaska
Fort Kent   Van Buren
New
Sweden
Caribou

Presque
Isle
Houlton

Fredericton

NEW BRUNSWICK

St. John R.

St. John

St.

Croix

R.

Calais

Penobscot R.

N   E

Bangor
Ellsworth

Machias

CAMPOBELLO I.

GRAND MANAN I.

BAY OF FUNDY

NOVA

SCOTIA

MOUNT DESERT I.
Acadia NP

ATLANTIC   OCEAN

Aroostook R.

0   75 Mi.

INTRODUCTION

ROGER G. KENNEDY

The Northland is irreconcilable, an Old Testament place of absolutes: sky and sea, rock and marsh. Ambiguities and meadows are luxuries for summer people. This is an unforgiving land; the scars men make last almost as long as they do in the desert. The "duff" holds together grass and moss and pine needles in a poultice, but when it is ripped by a hiker's boot a tear opens that the wind will worry until all that is left is the gray-rock platform upon which northern New England is built. The miracle is that between the dark spruce forest of the far north and the hardwoods of Massachusetts so many tall pines managed to grow, finding nutriment and anchorage in crevices, to rise above 160 feet on trunks six feet across at the base. When loggers climbed a pine they would drop a spruce diagonally against the trunk to use as a ladder to the first pine branches, sixty feet up. The first Europeans to search for the big pines wanted a few of those branchless trunks, entire, for the making of masts; it was only much later, in the 1820s, that the great lumber booms began, and sliced pine became a great commercial crop.

Whatever their ultimate destination, whether for fleets, floors, or furniture, the pines have mostly gone. Paul Bunyan, the mythical logger, left large footsteps. Some say they are the chains of elliptical lakelets of the north, but more likely, the record of his passage is in patches of desolate stumpage, slowly, slowly healing.

Inland Maine and New Hampshire were depicted as a vale of ease only by those who had an interest in selling pieces of them: Sir Ferdinando Gorges and Sir John Popham, who thought of Maine as a fine place to colonize with English Catholics, and French entrepreneurs who, in 1604, established the first European agricultural colony in North America and thought it ideally situated to receive French Protestants. In southern New England there was Indian agriculture to poach upon, and in its hardwood forests a profusion of deer and small animals browsed upon the berries, nuts, acorns, edible bark, and tender understory. Massachusetts was a hospitable wilderness. But Maine, though bracing, is only intermittently salubrious. The growing season is short, and in the gloom beneath the giant pines one might walk for days without seeing a deer or turkey. The northern spruceland is treacherous with unexpected bogs and disrupted by sudden granite mountains, such as Katahdin, so uncompromising that their slopes will have nothing to do with trees or even bushes.

The Saco River has always divided this difficult terrain from the more fertile portions of New England and has divided occupations for so long that the woodland Eastern Abenaki spoke one set of dialects and the agricultural Western Abenaki, who commanded much of New Hampshire and Vermont, spoke another. The eastern cousins knew as much about fishing as the western knew about corn and squash, beans and tobacco; accents and occupations still are divided roughly along those ancient lines.

The Abenaki were fierce fighters; they first held the English to a few starveling settlements along the coast and then drove them out of Maine entirely. Until European diseases and intertribal warfare weakened them, they also held their villages and fields along the Connecticut River. When the remaining Abenaki ultimately retreated northward to take shelter with their French allies, they left those terraces to be assumed by the English, who simply continued to plant as the Indians had done.

Along the Connecticut River Valley there are architectural vestiges of the great merchants, called "the River Gods" by their contemporaries, who occupied the valley once the Indians had receded. These vestiges are the famous "Connecticut River doorways," bold statements, curving into mannerist, with overscaled celebrations at the top. In their most magnificent versions, they are supported by piles of simulated blocks up the side that frame the door opening. Headstones in valley cemeteries took similar forms at the end of the eighteenth century. Deerfield, in Massachusetts, has the most famous of these artifacts, but there are examples to be found all the way up the river to the point where the moose and the wild-rice meadows take over.

Architectural form is an eloquent evoker of character: The Connecticut River doorways and headstones display a strutting bellicosity. This is the noisy, passionate side of the English character, the Shakespearean side. The River Gods had only a brief reign; toward the end, in the 1780s, their doorways shut out an increasingly disrespectful outside world. Their headstones, full of pride, were entryways from a revolutionary world into the silent order of the grave.

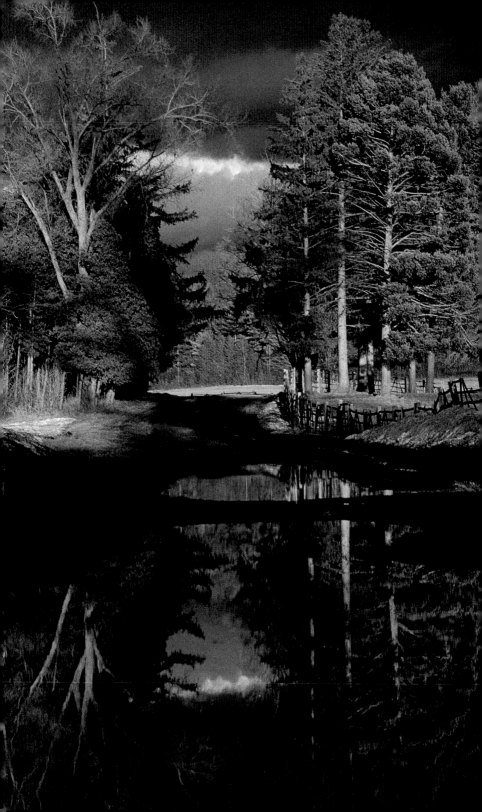

Northern New England was a landscape dominated by huge landholdings. Maine was a proprietary colony: Its people owed fealty to courtiers of the king who held the land grants to their settlements. Between 1690 and 1750, western Vermont and much of New Hampshire had been organized into "seigneuries" by French colonial officials and two English governors, George Clarke of New York and Benning Wentworth of New Hampshire. These two shrewd politicians made use of their posts as the chief representatives of the Crown to swell their own fortunes, distributing the best land to themselves and their supporters. The Wentworths ultimately owned nearly 100,000 acres—the reach of Benning Wentworth's aspirations is disclosed by the very name of Bennington, Vermont—and the Clarkes came to own 120,000 acres, some of it in the Green Mountain State.

The Clarkes and their "Yorkers" were opposed by the redoubtable brothers Ira and Ethan Allen. Ethan had already given Vermont its patriotic text in an altercation with the Clarkes' lawyers: "the gods of the hills are not the gods of the valley"—a deliberately ambiguous utterance that might be loosely translated as "come and get me." Ethan Allen's Green Mountain Boys were first organized in 1770, not to gain independence from Britain but to rid themselves of the Clarkes and their rent-collectors. From 1770 onward there was a small-scale civil war in Vermont between the Green Mountain Boys and the settlers from New York, marked by beatings, burned-out farms, and the rough expulsion of New York sheriffs. Later, Ethan Allen moved to wrap himself in larger causes and to unhorse the Portsmouth landlords, the Wentworths, by leading the Green Mountain Boys against the source of all royal titles, the British Crown. They captured Fort Ticonderoga from the British in 1775; Allen was captured by the British later in that year.

His followers, however, proclaimed Vermont to be independent of everybody in 1777; some New Hampshire towns on the eastern side of the Connecticut enthusiastically applied to join, which enraged the patriots of New Hampshire and encouraged Massachusetts to claim a portion of the new republic for itself.

Between 1779 and 1783 Ethan Allen, released with suspicious ease from his Canadian jail, negotiated on the part of the republic of Vermont with the governor-general of Canada—perhaps the

OPPOSITE: *Shelburne, Vermont, after an autumn rain.*

Green Mountain State might become re-attached to the British Empire, under the right conditions. But Lord Cornwallis surrendered at Yorktown, and the British conceded Vermont to the United States in 1783. Though its neighbors punished its ambiguities by denying it membership in the original thirteen states, Vermont was not quite done with its Balkan politics: As late as 1796, Ira Allen had 20,000 muskets and 24 cannon on board a ship from France to provide for a new revolutionary army, this time to create "New Columbia." Northern Vermont supplied most of the provisions that fed the British armies of the north during the War of 1812. Southern Vermont settled into the United States with greater equanimity as the seigneuries and the great Clarke and Wentworth landholdings came apart.

After independence, the distant aristocrats and oligarchs were replaced by merchant speculators. Maine, especially, was hustled by land-merchants of genius: William Duer, who coupled Old Etonian charm with a total absence of scruple; William Bingham, the "Golden Voyager" with three million acres to dispose; and Alexander Baring, who, as Lord Ashburton, held a million acres of timberland and negotiated its borders with the government of the United States, under whose jurisdiction it came. Bingham's landholdings came as a purchase from Duer, who had bankrupted himself in a frenzy of avarice, devouring confiscated Tory holdings. They constituted the largest holdings east of the Appalachians still remaining under one man's dominance after American independence, and his heirs held on to some bits and pieces until the 1960s.

Traces of these patterns of landholding persist. Six and a half million acres of northern Maine are, to this day, served by 5,000 miles of roads, all of them private. The Brown Company, a logging concern, is more important to the daily life of several townships than is any agent of the state government. Robert Hallowell Gardiner still occupies one of the few continuous squirearchies in the United States, in the town of Gardiner, on Gardiner lands that have been in the family since the mid-eighteenth century and were parts of the Kennebec purchase, thirty miles square. (These Gardiners are not to be confused with the Gardiners of Gardiners Island, New York, though the latter have held their isolated manor even longer.)

Despite our democratic preference to think of this region as owing its charm to the reign of independent yeomen, there is no denying the fact that some of its large landowners have bestowed upon it a benign tradition of conservation practices and public service. The remarkable legacy of the Gardiners is just one example. It is the strange outcome of Maine's reliance upon lumber as a cash crop that some of its proprietors have taken a very long view of their interests and responsibilities. Three-quarters of the "old-growth" timber in all northern New England was recently transferred to a conservancy in the block around Seven Ponds, north of Mount Katahdin, by the heirs of David Pingree, who acquired this domain in 1820. The Seven Ponds reserve is one of the two largest surviving tracts of unspoiled America north of the Smokies (the other is Ramsey's Draft, in Virginia); both are considerably larger than any similar tract in the Adirondacks.

Much of what now looks "wild" in northern New England is merely abandoned, indelibly affected by the farming and grazing that were done in the eighteenth and nineteenth centuries. Even before the arrival of Europeans, the Native Americans had already altered the landscape by purposeful burning and by agriculture. But in Vermont there are thirteen acres of large, old-growth pines in the Fisher-Scott Memorial, north of the village of Arlington, and sixteen acres of climax sugar maples and beech in the Gifford Woods State Park, east of Rutland. Not far away, in the Tinker Brook Natural Area south of West Bridgewater, there are forty-five acres of hemlock and red spruce. Even with the addition of the Battell Stand in Middlebury and more remote stands of timber, such as the Lord's Hill Tract in Marshfield, the diminutive size of these remnants makes the point: We have left very little of the terrain unaffected by our ambitions.

In the countryside, life goes on much as it did in the past. Along the coast, the fishermen and subsistence farmers remain as suspicious of strangers as the Abenaki had been. It is to continuities like this that I wish to draw attention: The extent of northern New England's ancient landholdings, its perpetual clearing of land for planting and grazing, and, despite the felling of white pines so tall that their first branches were higher than the rooftops of a Manchester textile mill, the intractability of the fundamental North Country to any human intervention.

The moose go on searching for succulent stems of arrowroot, the mosquitoes seek the nourishment of blood, the eagles ride the currents sent upward by the sun's earnest effort to thaw Katahdin, and the wolves, it is said, are coming back.

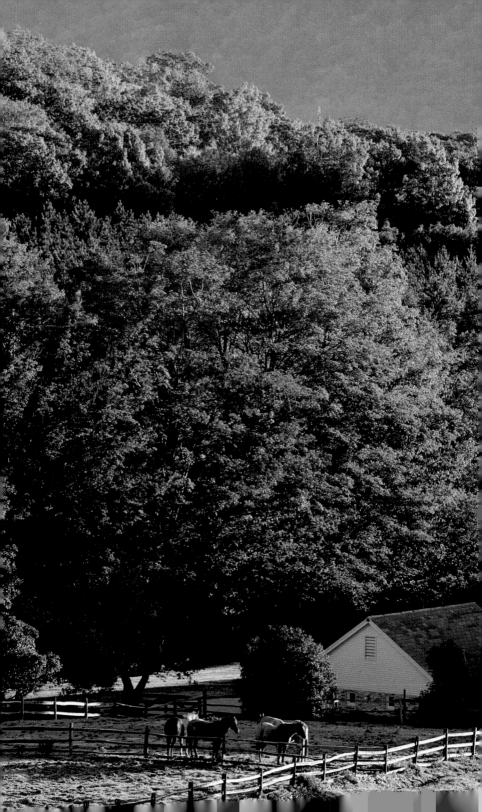

WESTERN VERMONT

In its pre-colonial days, Vermont was the hunting ground of Iroquois and Algonquin Indians who traveled the small waterways—the Winooski, Lamoille, and Missisquoi rivers and Otter Creek—to and from the territory's long western lake. Samuel de Champlain gave his name to that lake in 1609, when he sailed down from Canada, trading with the Algonquin along the way. The explorer's countrymen would attempt Vermont's first settlement on Lake Champlain in 1666 at Isle la Motte.

Shared by New York and Canada, Lake Champlain stretches for over a hundred miles within Vermont (its total length is 120 miles). The lake developed as an important artery for France's colonial commerce in furs and was a vital waterway during the Revolution. Britain's plan to send an invasion force down the lake to the Hudson Valley and split the rebellion was delayed for a year by Benedict Arnold's little fleet at Valcour Bay. During the War of 1812 another small American force, under Thomas Macdonough, won an important American victory on the lake. Later in the century Burlington grew into a rich port city as timber harvests were shipped south on flatboats and steam-powered sidewheelers.

The early French settlement at Isle la Motte failed to survive; it was the English, in 1724, who succeeded in establishing the state's first permanent European settlement at Fort Dummer, near the site of present-day Brattleboro. In 1764 Governor Benning Wentworth of New Hampshire, liberally interpreting his colony's royal charter, began granting towns west of the Connecticut River. The region between the Connecticut and Lake Champlain became known as the New Hampshire Grants. New York also had a claim to this area and began granting towns as well.

When the king decreed in 1770 that New York's claim was the valid one, settlers who had acquired land from New Hampshire found themselves thrown off their land or forced to buy it again from New York proprietors. Anger boiled into action, as Ethan and Ira Allen, Seth Warner, and other leaders organized the Green Mountain Boys, a vigilante group that resisted by force any effort of a New Yorker to evict a Vermonter. Settlers from New York were beaten and their houses burned; New York sheriffs were prevented from serving eviction papers and driven off.

The Green Mountain Boys launched the first offensive of the Revolution, taking Fort Ticonderoga from the British in May 1775. The only Revolutionary battle in Vermont was a rear guard action at Hubbardton in which the Americans stopped the British from

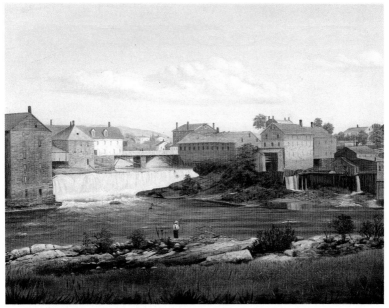

A view of Middlebury Falls, ca. 1865, attributed to James Hope (detail).

pursuing an American column retreating from Fort Ticonderoga. Although the 1777 Battle of Bennington is named for a Vermont town, the actual fighting in that engagement took place in New York. A Hessian raiding party, detached from General John Burgoyne's Hudson Valley invasion force, was on its way to seize supplies at Bennington when it was stopped by John Stark at Walloomsac in New York.

After the war, Vermont announced itself an independent republic. Still concerned about the possibility that New York's land claims would be held valid, Vermont held out the threat that it would join Canada instead of the United States. In 1781 Ethan Allen wrote a firm letter to Congress: "I am as resolutely determined to defend the independence of Vermont as Congress [is] that of the United States, and rather than fail will retire with the hardy Green Mountain Boys into the desolate caverns of the mountains and wage war with human nature at large." The dispute was settled in 1791, when Vermont was admitted as the fourteenth state. Its constitution prohibited slavery and guaranteed suffrage to males whether they owned property or not. The authors of Vermont's constitution also mandated free public education.

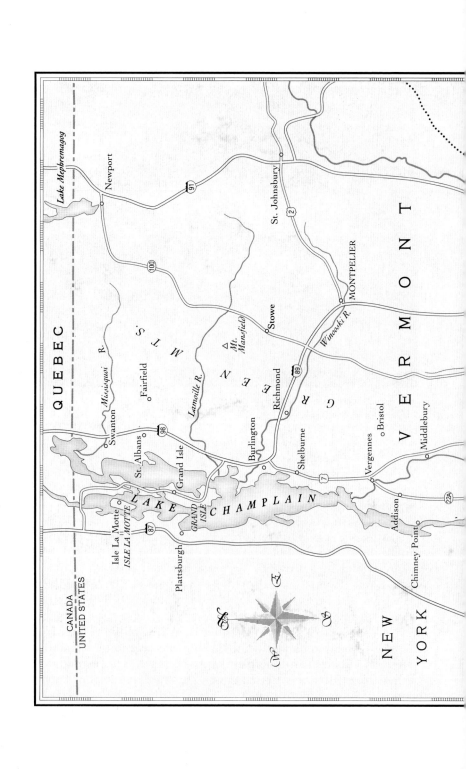

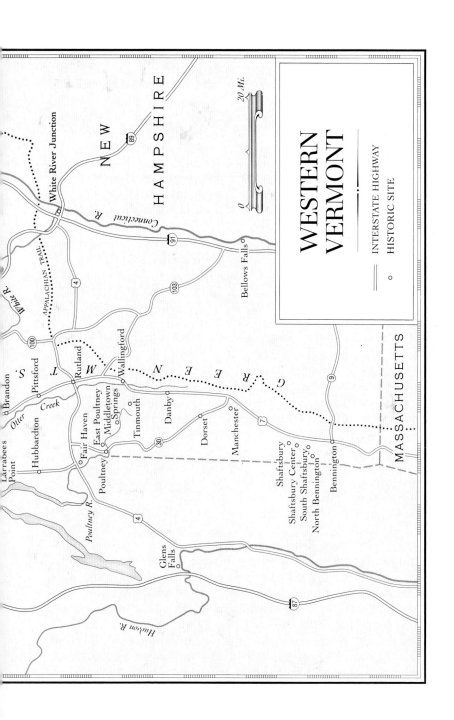

WESTERN VERMONT

— INTERSTATE HIGHWAY

∘ HISTORIC SITE

20 Mi.

NEW HAMPSHIRE

White River Junction

Connecticut R.

APPALACHIAN TRAIL

Bellows Falls

WEST · VERMONT · GREEN

Rutland

Wallingford

Tinmouth

Danby

Middletown Springs

East Poultney

Fair Haven

Poultney

Poultney R.

Dorset

Manchester

Shaftsbury

Shaftsbury Center

South Shaftsbury

North Bennington

Bennington

MASSACHUSETTS

Larrabees Point

Hubbardton

Brandon

Pittsford

Otter Creek

White R.

Glens Falls

Hudson R.

After 1791 the state's population surged. French Canadians settled on Lake Champlain and along the northern border. Scottish immigrants came to work the new state's rock quarries, as did Welsh, Italian, and Spanish settlers. Though Vermont lacked the natural water resources of its neighboring states, there were a sufficient number of rivers and streams to power some mills, and young manufacturing towns attracted other New Englanders as well as Polish and Scandinavian immigrants. The Irish came to build canals in the 1820s and railroads in the 1840s and 1850s.

Sheep and cattle raising dominated Vermont agriculture and led to the establishment of woolen mills and creameries throughout the state. Abundant maple trees made Vermont the sugar and syrup capital of the country. Native manufacturing often was small-scale and specialized—ranging from farm tools and fishing rods to papermaking and book publishing. Noah Webster's 1828 dictionary was among the state's early publishing enterprises.

The quiet countryside of Vermont has long attracted artists and writers—Rudyard Kipling, Emily Dickinson, Daniel Chester French, Sinclair Lewis, Pearl Buck, and Norman Rockwell among them. Anna Mary Robertson, the painter known as Grandma Moses, kept a summer studio outside Bennington. Vermont has also attracted sportsmen and vacationers—the state's year-round resort industry has thrived since the mid-nineteenth century. City people still come for the cool lakes and mountain air, foliage, and snowy slopes.

Vermont's towns, farms, and small cities reflect the modesty and thrift of their builders. Executed in clapboard and native stone, the buildings seem as sturdy and pure as the state character. Exuberant, highly decorated architecture is rare in this state—even the Greek Revival, often a showy style, is subdued here. More than any individual structures, entire villages make the strongest architectural impression in Vermont (and indeed, many are designated historic districts), the white steeple of a white church within a white picket fence identifying the scene as quintessential pre-industrial New England. The term "continuous architecture" describes the rural compound of farmhouse, barn, sheds, and other buildings, all connected to one another. The design made life easier in a cold climate, allowing the farm family to rise each morning, milk cows, gather eggs, and perform other chores without having to step into the sub-freezing outdoors. It also kept the family unto itself, out of view. Such compounds are no longer built (chiefly because of sanitation), but many from the last century may be seen along Vermont's country roads. Also identified with the state are covered bridges, which still charm and confound visitors. Why build a roof over a bridge? The best explanation seems to be the simplest one— to protect the bridge structure itself from the weight and damp of the snow.

Rocky and mountainous, with thin soil and lacking a network of powerful rivers, Vermont never spawned major farming or industrial centers, and over the years it has lost people to the more populous, industrialized states to the west and south. Vermont remains the most rural of the United States, with the fewest number of people residing in cities, and its population is the smallest east of the Mississippi River. But it still exemplifies Yankee independence. For the most part, Vermonters are of Anglo-Saxon descent, grassroots conservatives who continue to hold town meetings the first Tuesday of every March.

This chapter begins in the southwestern corner of the state at Bennington (the first New Hampshire Grant town chartered by Governor Benning Wentworth), then proceeds north to the Lake Champlain area.

BENNINGTON

Built on the banks of the Walloomsac River, Bennington encompasses both the Old Town—established in the 1760s—and the nineteenth-century industrial district of textile and paper mills. The town is set off by hills to the north and east. It was on these slopes that Ethan Allen organized his Green Mountain Boys in 1770. Seth Warner, who was elected commander of that group, had his home in Bennington.

Bennington's earliest citizens, a group of families from Massachusetts, settled along a rise of land that now defines the **Old Bennington Historic District,** site of a concentration of Federal and Greek Revival houses along Monument Avenue, all private. This district went into a decline beginning in the 1820s, when the area that is now downtown Bennington started its industrial boom, but revived later in the century as a fashionable residential enclave. Some of the houses were remodeled in the late 1800s and early 1900s, and new houses, in the Colonial Revival style, were built into the 1930s. A plaque on the avenue marks the site of the **Catamount Tavern,** a gathering place for the Green Mountain Boys.

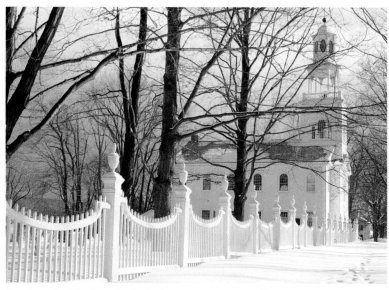

Bennington's Old First Church, built in 1805, has been officially designated "Vermont's Colonial Shrine." The poet Robert Frost is buried here, in the state's oldest graveyard.

Also on Monument Avenue is the handsome, white clapboard **Old First Church,** officially designated as "Vermont's Colonial Shrine." Built in 1805, it was designed by Lavius Fillmore, who followed a popular building handbook, Asher Benjamin's *The Country Builder's Assistant.* Fillmore made his own adaptations to the basic Federal scheme, adding a belfry to the steeple, and enormous Palladian windows above the front entrance and behind the high pulpit. In 1937 the church underwent restoration and Robert Frost was among the project's patrons; the poet and his family are buried behind the church, in the oldest graveyard in the state.

Located across the street from the church, the **Walloomsac Inn** (Monument Avenue and West Road, private) was built in 1766 by Elijah Dewey, the son of Bennington's first minister and later a veteran of the Battle of Bennington. British and Hessian prisoners taken at the battle were brought here for their meals.

Bennington Battle Monument

At the northern end of the historic district a 306-foot-high dolomite obelisk commemorates a 1777 Revolutionary War battle that occurred two miles away in New York. It was there that General

John Stark, reinforced by Seth Warner and the Green Mountain Boys, defeated two British columns advancing toward an American storehouse which was then located on the monument grounds. The New Hampshire and Vermont militia defended the supply depot in one of the significant battles of the Revolution. The battle denied General John Burgoyne crucial supplies, and contributed to the subsequent American victory at Saratoga. In 1891, the state of Vermont erected the monument near the old arsenal. An elevator takes visitors to an observation gallery 200 feet up the shaft.

LOCATION: Monument Circle. HOURS: April through October: 9–5 Daily. FEE: Yes. TELEPHONE: 802–447–0550.

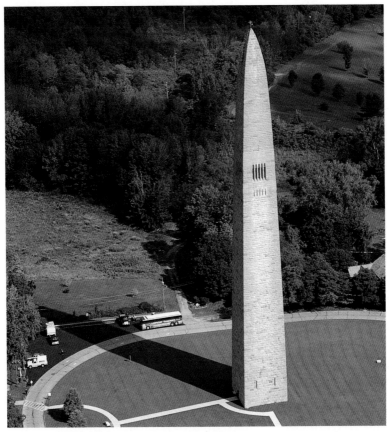

The Bennington Battle Monument, erected in 1891, commemorates the historic defeat of the British by Vermont's Green Mountain Boys on August 16, 1777.

East of Monument Avenue, along the Walloomsac River, is Bennington's **nineteenth-century milling and manufacturing district.** Set up along both sides of the river were paper mills, gristmills, and brick and pottery factories. Two notable buildings are the 1865 **Big Mill** (Benmont Avenue, along the river), a brick structure in the Italianate style with a lofty bell tower, and the Romanesque Revival **Bennington and Rutland Railroad Station** (River Street), built of marble in 1898. The downtown historic district along Main, North, and South streets is a busy mingling of Victorian commercial architecture, including the **Putnam Block** at South and Main and the 1870 **Pennysaver Building** (107–111 South Street).

Bennington Museum

This museum, specializing in the region's art and history, displays the most complete collection of Bennington pottery in existence, as well as a collection of pressed glass, blown glass, and some items by the Tiffany studio. Its exhibits of local military items include the flag flown at the 1777 Battle of Bennington, believed to be the oldest surviving Stars and Stripes. The painting collections encompass works by Erastus Salisbury Field, a 1798 *View of Bennington* by Ralph Earl (one of the oldest landscape paintings in the country), and many works by Anna Mary Robertson ("Grandma") Moses. A collection of Moses memorabilia is displayed in the schoolhouse she attended, which was moved here from its original site in Eagle Bridge, New York, in 1972.

LOCATION: West Main Street. HOURS: March through December: 9–5 Daily; January through February: 9–5 Saturday–Sunday. FEE: Yes. TELEPHONE: 802–447–1571.

A few miles northeast is **North Bennington,** where woodworking and furniture making were local specialties. Paran Creek powered the community's mills, few of which survive. Early mill-workers' housing, however, stands along Sage Street. Rail lines to Massachusetts and New York converged at the **North Bennington Depot,** a small brick train station and former headquarters of the Bennington and Rutland Railroad.

Park-McCullough House

This Second Empire–style, thirty-five-room mansion was begun in 1863 and completed in 1865 by Trenor Park, who made his initial fortune managing California gold mines. The house has important

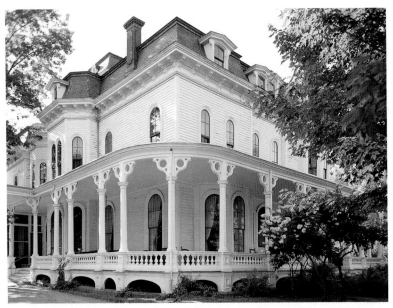

Two of Vermont's governors, Hiland Hall and John G. McCullough, lived in North Bennington's Park-McCullough House, one of the country's earliest Second Empire style residences.

collections of nineteenth-century furnishings, decorative arts, and fine arts. It was home to two Vermont governors, Hiland Hall (Trenor Park's father-in-law) and John G. McCullough (his son-in-law). The house's archival collection includes the papers of Park and McCullough, as well as rare photographs by the renowned photographer of the American West, Carlton Watkins.

LOCATION: Park and West streets. HOURS: June through October: 10–4 Daily. FEE: Yes. TELEPHONE: 802–442–5441.

THE SHAFTSBURYS

Strung together by Route 7A, "the Shaftsburys"—**South Shaftsbury, Shaftsbury Center, Shaftsbury**—were settled by newcomers from Connecticut and Rhode Island in the 1760s.

Some of the Shaftsburys' earliest settlers (founders of Vermont's first Baptist congregation, in 1768) are buried in the eighteenth-century graveyard next to the **Center Shaftsbury Baptist Church** (Route 7A). The church, a Greek Revival structure built in 1846, houses the **Shaftsbury Historical Society Museum** (802–442–4580). Exhibits include church artifacts, hand tools, wedding dresses, locally made spinning wheels, historic flags, and tools used by the Eagle Square Manufacturing Company, which forged the first steel carpenter's tools. The **Peter Matteson Tavern,** a restored farmhouse and tavern operated by the Bennington Museum (East Road in Shaftsbury, 802–447–1571), is furnished with many pieces from the late 1780s period of its construction. The **Munro-Hawkins House** (Route 7A, 802–447–2286) is a fine two-story Georgian structure, built in 1808 by a successful wheat farmer, Joshua Munro, who exported wheat to France during the Napoleonic Wars. The house has been converted to an inn.

In 1920, the poet Robert Frost bought the oldest house in South Shaftsbury, the 1769 **Homer Noble Farm** (Route 7A, private), with twenty-two-inch thick stone walls. Just off the highway, the house did not afford sufficient privacy and Frost moved.

MANCHESTER

Manchester has been one of New England's prime resort towns since the middle of the nineteenth century. Along **Main Street,** which preserves its old marble sidewalks, are private houses and resort buildings once visited by Mrs. Ulysses S. Grant, Theodore Roosevelt, and William Howard Taft. Mrs. Abraham Lincoln stayed at the **Equinox Hotel** (Route 7A, Manchester Village, 802–362–4700), one of the great resorts of the day; it is still operating.

Hildene

Hildene was the summer home of Robert Todd Lincoln, the only one of Abraham Lincoln's four children to survive to adulthood. The twenty-four-room house was completed in 1904, when Robert was president of the Pullman Company; he died there in 1926. Today it is maintained as a house museum, with many original furnishings, including a 1908 Aeolian pipe organ, with 1,000 pipes and a player attachment. A narrow cabinet in the office contains a few of Abraham Lincoln's personal items, including a stovepipe hat.

The 400-acre estate includes a carriage barn (now the visitor center) and a magnificent formal garden in the shape of a Gothic window, designed by Robert's daughter, Jesse.

LOCATION: Route 7A South. HOURS: Mid-May through October: 9–4:30 Daily. FEE: Yes. TELEPHONE: 802–362–1788.

OPPOSITE: *Hildene, now a house museum, was built in 1904 by Robert Todd Lincoln, the son of Abraham Lincoln.* OVERLEAF: *Dorset is the site of America's first marble quarry.*

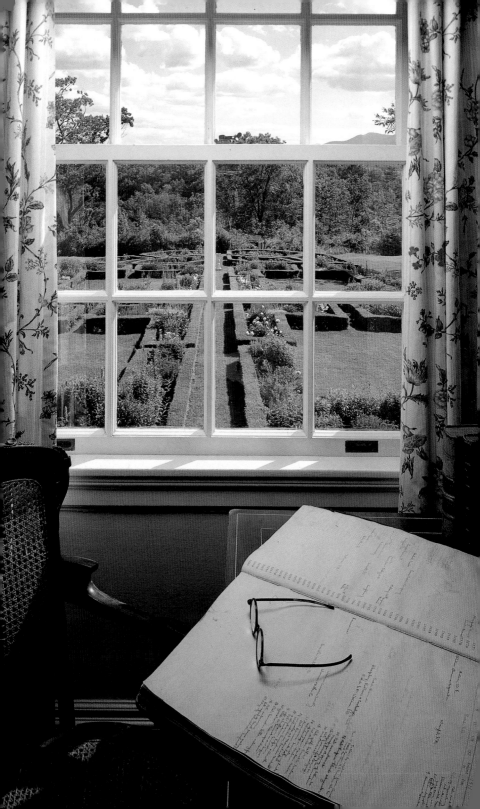

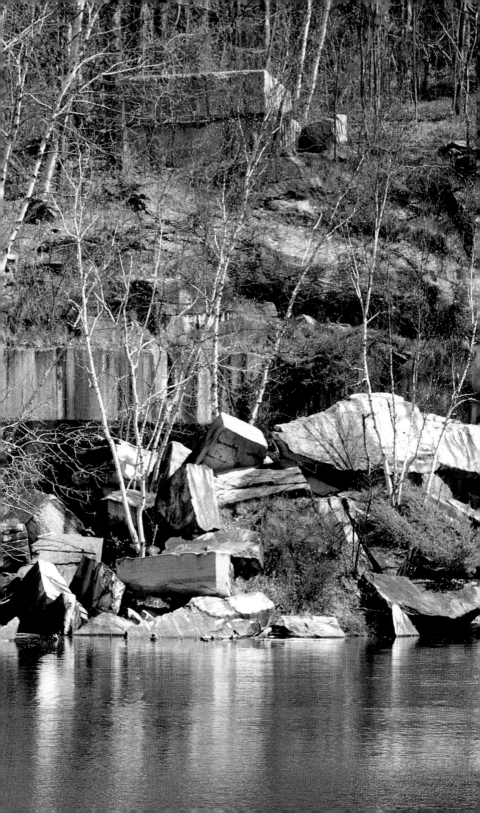

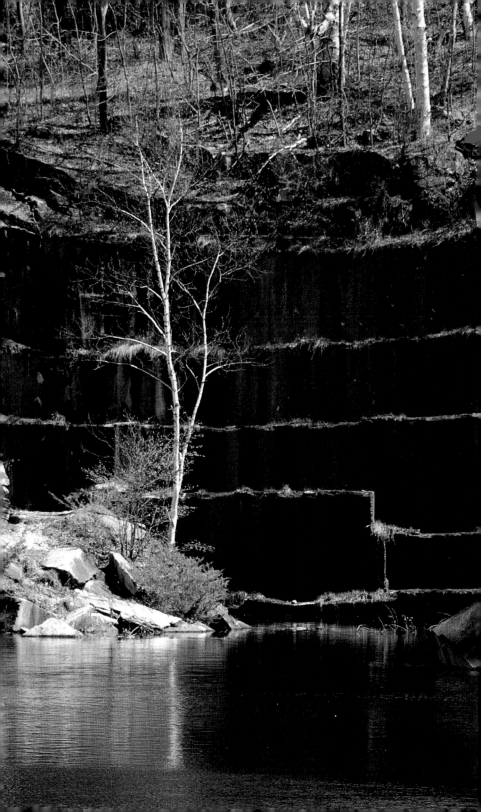

DORSET

Dorset is the site of the first (1785) marble quarry in the United States. In 1776 Vermont's leaders, including Thomas Chittenden, Seth Warner, and Ira Allen, convened at a tavern here and proclaimed the "Free and Independent State of Vermont." The town's eighteenth-century landmarks include the **Memorial Library** (Route 30, 802–867–5774), housed in a 1790 tavern, and the **United Church of Dorset and East Rupert** (Church Street, 802–867–2260), constructed of local marble. The **Kent Neighborhood Historic District** (surrounding the intersections of Dorset West Road, Lane Road, and Nichols Hill Road) contains clapboard homes from the eighteenth and early-nineteenth centuries.

DANBY

This village was settled largely by Quakers in the 1760s, and grew into a prosperous town in the nineteenth century as men opened quarries and harvested forests, and sent the stone and lumber south on the Rutland Railroad. Silas Griffith, one of Vermont's first millionaires, made his fortune cutting the Danby forests. The writer Pearl S. Buck moved to Danby toward the end of her life; by the time she died in 1973 she had restored several houses on the village's historic Main Street.

A manufacturing specialty developed north of Danby in the town of **Wallingford.** Hand garden tools (rakes, forks, spades) were produced at the **Old Stone Shop** (South Main Street), built in 1848, and other small factories. West of Wallingford, across Otter Creek, is **Tinmouth.** One of Vermont's first iron forges was started here in 1781. Later enterprises included sawmills, gristmills, tanneries, and creameries. Chartered in 1761, the town has a number of imposing Federal houses within its compact **historic district.**

MIDDLETOWN SPRINGS

This isolated mountain community came to life a century after it was founded in 1784 with the discovery of a spring. In the late-nineteenth century, people came to take the waters and relax in the Victorian "Springhouse," a replica of which has been built off Burdock Avenue by the **Middletown Springs Historical Society.**

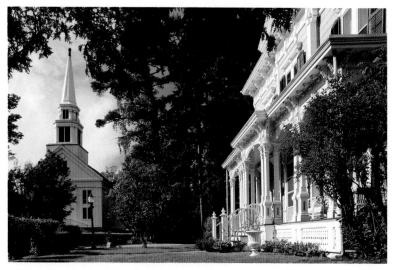

Middletown Springs was founded in 1784 and became a fashionable spa and resort in the 1860s. One elegant place to stop was the Middletown Springs Inn, at right.

The society maintains a small **museum** (802–235–2322) on the town green that displays artifacts of local history. Fine Federal and Greek Revival houses surround the green on three sides.

POULTNEY AND EAST POULTNEY

Until the 1860s the village of East Poultney was the commercial center of the immediate area. The region's chief town is now Poultney, farther to the west. East Poultney was settled in the early 1770s by people from Connecticut, led by Heber Allen of the famed Allen family. They were driven from their new homes in 1777 by Burgoyne's troops during the British march from Canada to the Hudson Valley. The settlers later returned, establishing a string of busy mills and shops along the Poultney River up to Middletown Springs. These businesses, and the bridges that crossed the river, were wiped out by a flood in 1811, an event from which East Poultney never quite recovered.

The Poultney River plain is rich in slate. Federal and Greek Revival houses on East Poultney's **green** are roofed with the native slate—green, purple, or mottled. The handsome **United Baptist Church** (802–287–5577), with a Palladian window and clock tower, dominates the green. Built in 1805 from designs in Asher Benjamin's guide, *The Country Builder's Assistant,* it has been recently restored. The **Eagle Tavern** (on the green, 802–287–9498), a 1785 stagecoach inn, has put up many boarders, including the famous newspaperman Horace Greeley, founder of the *New York Tribune.* Greeley apprenticed at a local newspaper, the *Northern Spectator,* from 1826 to 1830. George Jones, one of the founders of the *New York Times,* was born in this town. Local history collections are at the **Poultney Historical Society Museum** (off Route 30, 802–287–4042). In the 1840s and 1850s Welsh quarry workers settled in the area to mine the slate deposits. The rise of the slate industry and the coming of the railroad led to the development of the town.

FAIR HAVEN

This town was another center of the slate industry in the nineteenth century, and like Poultney, attracted Welsh quarrymen. The town's early history was dominated by an Irish immigrant, Matthew Lyon, who arrived in 1783 and started sawmills, paper mills, an ironworks, and a printing press. Lyon also published the town's newspaper, and built its meetinghouse and school. He went on to become one of Vermont's best-known politicians, a controversial foe of President John Quincy Adams and the Federalists. In 1801 Congressman Lyon cast the tie-breaking presidential vote for Thomas Jefferson against Aaron Burr. Before the Civil War Fair Haven's houses were stops on the Underground Railroad, by which runaway slaves escaped to Canada.

RUTLAND

Vermont's "Marble City," Rutland is spread out in the Otter Creek valley, with the Green Mountains to the east and the Taconic range to the west. By the 1770s settlers, mostly from Connecticut, were farming in the town, which had been chartered by Governor Benning Wentworth in 1761. During the Revolution they built Fort Rutland, which burned in 1777. It was replaced the following year by Fort Ranger in Center Rutland.

The town boomed as a center of commerce and manufacturing after 1849 when the Rutland Railroad connected it to Boston. After the Civil War a returning veteran, Redfield Proctor, turned the town's sleepy marble business into one of the nation's biggest. Proctor's Vermont Marble Company employed thousands, many of them new immigrants from Ireland, Italy, Poland, and Sweden.

With its other attractions—milling and lumber industries, a lively retail trade, mountain resorts—Rutland tripled its population by 1880. The people built a handsome city, with some of the finest structures of that era in the **Rutland Courthouse District,** along Main, Center, and Washington streets. Two of the most notable and monumental are the **Rutland Free Library** (Court Street), designed by Ammi B. Young to house the post office and federal court, and the 1871 **county courthouse** (83 Center Street). The **Gryphon Building, opera house,** and other brick business blocks line **Merchants Row.** The former Rutland Bank at 101 Center Street was built in 1825. In 1989 the **Rutland Historical Society** opens its new museum in an 1850, Italianate-style building (formerly a firehouse) on Center Street. The 1892 Queen Anne–style house of marble magnate George Chaffee is now the **Chaffee Art Center** (16 South Main Street, 802–775–0356).

PROCTOR

The **Vermont Marble Exhibit** (61 Main Street, 802–459–3311), housed in the still-operating Vermont Marble Company, displays locally quarried marble and shows the process by which the raw material is turned into the carved and polished finished product.

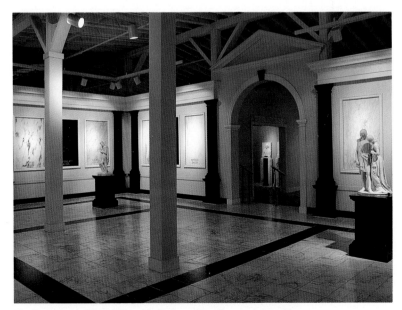

The Vermont Marble Exhibit, with displays of locally quarried marble.

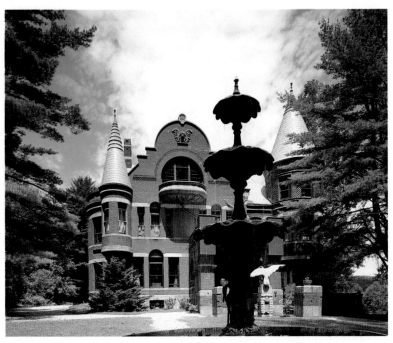

Wilson Castle, Proctor. OPPOSITE: *The grand stairwell of Wilson Castle.*

Wilson Castle

Wilson Castle, an eclectic blend of European styles surrounded by a 115-acre estate, has a facade of brick and marble, and, as befits its name, boasts a turret, parapet, and balcony, as well as nineteen proscenium arches. The thirty-two rooms, spread over three floors, feature French, German, Italian, and English antiques, as well as rugs, scrolls, and statues from the Far East. Particularly notable are the grand stairwell, with its mahogany panelling and frescoed ceilings, and the frescoed and gold stencilled walls and ceilings of the art gallery. Tiffany chandeliers hang in both the library and dining salon, and there are 84 stained-glass windows scattered throughout the Wilson home. Though it lacks a moat, the estate is suitably grand, with barns and stables, a carriage house, and an aviary stocked with peacocks, the bird traditionally owned by royalty.

LOCATION: West Proctor Road. HOURS: Mid-May through October: 8–6 Daily. FEE: Yes. TELEPHONE: 802–773–3284.

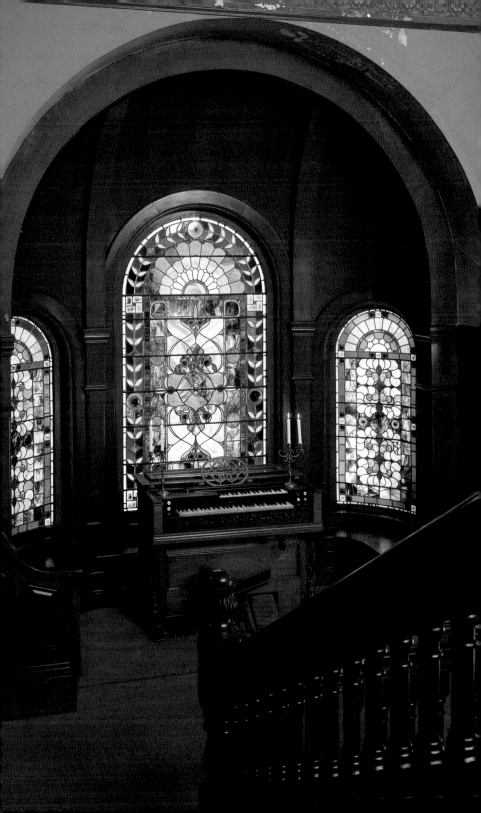

PITTSFORD

Saw and grist mills operated along two brooks that run through Pittsford, and the town was noted for its iron foundries. Nineteenth-century churches, commercial buildings, and houses surround the town's triangular green. Pittsford has three covered bridges, all built in the 1840s: the **Cooley,** the **Gorham,** and the **Hammond.** The **New England Maple Museum** (Route 7, 802–483–9414) has exhibits on the history of Vermont sugaring, beginning from the time of the Indians.

HUBBARDTON BATTLEFIELD

The only battle of the Revolutionary War fought on Vermont soil took place here on July 7, 1777. British and Hessian troops, commanded respectively by General Simon Fraser and General Baron Friedrich von Riedesel, were pursuing the American forces that were evacuating Fort Ticonderoga. The American rear guard, about 1,200 men commanded by Seth Warner of the Green Mountain Boys and two other officers from Massachusetts and New Hampshire, was waiting at Hubbardton with orders to delay the British advance as long as possible and then scatter. The British reached the American position just before dawn. In the sharp two-hour fight that ensued, the New Englanders were holding their own against highly trained, select British units, until the Hessians arrived. The Americans then scattered into the woods. Both sides suffered heavy losses; but the Americans achieved their purpose of stopping the British pursuit of the main American column.

The battle has been a controversial one: Warner was accused of tarrying at Hubbardton in defiance of his orders and of failing to post guards, thus allowing the British to surprise the camp. Recent scholarship, however, tends to vindicate Warner. There is evidence that he was in fact following orders when he made his stand here, that he did post guards, and was prepared for the British attack. The **Hubbardton Battlefield Monument,** a spire of solid Vermont marble, commemorates the battle and marks the burial spot of Colonel Ebenezer Francis, who led the Massachusetts detail and lost his life in the battle.

LOCATION: Seven miles north of Route 4, Hubbardton. HOURS: Late May through mid-October: 9:30–5:30 Wednesday–Sunday. FEE: None. TELEPHONE: 802–828–3226.

BRANDON

Northeast over the mountains is Brandon, birthplace of Stephen A. Douglas (1813), who later became the Democratic senator from Illinois and foe of Abraham Lincoln. In the senatorial campaign of 1858, the occasion for the famed Lincoln–Douglas debates, Douglas was the victor. In 1860, as the first Vermont native to be nominated for president, he lost to Lincoln. The village is sited on the Neshobe River, which powered its marble-cutting mills. Ironworks also were active in the area—ruins of the 1810 **Forestdale Iron Furnace** are preserved nearby (Route 73 and Furnace Road, 802–828–3226). Adding to the local industry were factories producing stoves and scales.

MOUNT INDEPENDENCE

After the Americans captured Fort Ticonderoga in 1775 they fortified this point on Lake Champlain, opposite Ticonderoga, and connected the two with a floating bridge. When Burgoyne recaptured Ticonderoga in 1777 the bridge served as the American garrison's escape route. Today the site contains the ruins of fortifications and gun batteries.

LOCATION: West of Route 22A, in Orwell. HOURS: June through mid-October: 9:30–5:30 Wednesday–Sunday. FEE: None. TELEPHONE: 802–828–3226.

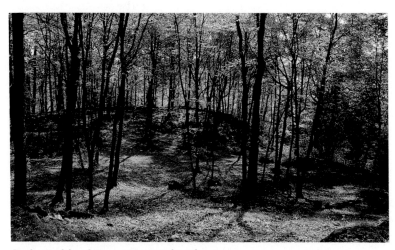

Bunkers and foundations at Mount Independence.

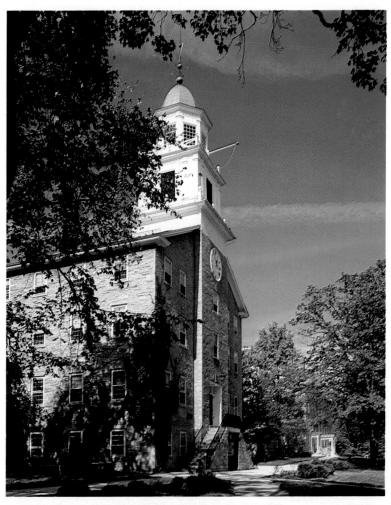

The stately Old Chapel at Middlebury College is one of several early campus buildings constructed of local limestone.

LARRABEE'S POINT

Once a busy landing place for commercial traffic on Lake Champlain, this town became a trading center for quarried stone, lumber products, furniture, and textiles. Local black marble was a profitable export. The place was named for John Larrabee, who in 1823 built a **warehouse,** still standing on the lake's edge. Within the town's historic district are the **ferry dock** (for Ticonderoga traffic) and a few lakeside **cottages** dating from Larrabee's late-nineteenth-century resort days. Larrabee's Point lost its commercial thrust in the mid-nineteenth century when the northeastern network of railroads began to move merchandise more efficiently than had the waterways. The 108-foot **Shoreham Covered Railroad Bridge** was built by the Rutland Railroad in 1897.

Further up the Lake Champlain shoreline is the green promontory of **Chimney Point,** named for the ruins of an early French settlement on this strategic site. Indians had settled here before the French; in fact, this area has been settled for over 12,000 years. According to popular belief, Samuel de Champlain stood at this point in 1609 when he gave his name to the lake. The French raised their stone fortress in 1690. Nearly a century later, local ferry operator Benjamin Paine refashioned it as the **Chimney Point Tavern** (Route 17, 802–828–3226). Its taproom, visited by soldiers on both sides of the Revolution, is open to the public; a museum is scheduled to open in the summer of 1989.

MIDDLEBURY

Northeast toward Vermont's interior is Middlebury, lying on Otter Creek. Middlebury was chartered in 1761, though its early European settlers were unable to sustain their incursion into Indian lands; another settlement was begun twenty years later. The town sits on a deep bedrock of marble, quarried since 1803. Two important industrial innovations have come from Middlebury: the sand-and-water process of sawing marble, and the welding of cast steel. Falls on Otter Creek powered textile mills, and wool processing grew into Middlebury's major industry. Another important local enterprise was the manufacture of doors and window sashes.

In 1800 **Middlebury College** (College Street, 802–388–3711) was chartered. Among the campus's historic buildings (many made of local limestone) are **Mead Memorial Chapel, Hepburn Hall, Starr Hall, Starr Library,** and the college's oldest structure, the 1815 **Painter Hall.** The **Emma Willard House National Historic Landmark,** site of the Middlebury Female Seminary established in 1814, is now the admissions office for Middlebury College.

The village historic district, along Otter Creek, contains many eighteenth- and nineteenth-century structures. Among them are the **Battell Block** (Merchants Row and Main Street), the **Beckwith Block** (Main Street), and the **Congregational Church** (Main and

North Pleasant streets, 802–388–7634), completed in 1809 to designs by Lavius Fillmore. The Ionic columns inside are of solid wood, each made from a single tree.

Sheldon Museum

Located in an 1829 Federal-style house, the Sheldon Museum features everyday objects from the nineteenth century displayed in period settings. Permanent exhibits include furniture by Vermont artisans, fine and decorative arts, farming and carpentry tools, household utensils, and toys; these are supplemented by special exhibits. The house, built by local marble merchant Elias Judd, is a three-story brick mansion. Its Ionic columns, sills and lintels, and six fireplaces are made of black marble quarried in Shoreham.

LOCATION: 1 Park Street. HOURS: June through October: 10–5 Monday–Saturday; November through May: 1–4 Wednesday and Friday. FEE: Yes. TELEPHONE: 802–388–2117.

John Strong Mansion

This elegant brick mansion, built in the 1790s, stands near the site of Strong's first home, a frame house burned by the British in 1777. Shutters, door hinges, and iron-walled fireplaces all reflect fine craftsmanship. One of the bricks, on display in the mansion, bears the engraved signature of the bricklayer. The house has four "hidey holes," each large enough to hold several people. Although it is said that Strong built the hiding places as refuge from possible Indian raids, it is possible that he was also worried about bear attacks—a group of bears had come into his first house looking for food, sending his wife and children to a loft for safety. The mansion contains furnishings from the 1800s and some original Strong family pieces; among these are a 1749 tall clock and a ca. 1790 painted fireboard with a beautifully stenciled border.

LOCATION: Route 22A. HOURS: Mid-May through mid-October: 10–5 Friday–Monday. FEE: Yes. TELEPHONE: 802–759–2309.

BRISTOL

Situated near the New Haven River on a plateau at the base of Hogback Mountain is the village of Bristol. In the late-nineteenth century, sawmills along the New Haven produced furniture and caskets, and local cabinetmakers won national renown for their fine work. The Bartlett Plow Manufactory produced equipment for the farmers of the Midwest. The chief architectural sites here are commercial blocks, clustered near the green. The **town hall**—part Queen Anne, part Romanesque Revival—and a **gristmill** also are within the downtown historic district.

VERGENNES

The territorial disputes between New Hampshire and New York were briefly focused here in 1773 when the Green Mountain Boys burned a settlement of Scotsmen established at the behest of a New Yorker. Vergennes was incorporated as a city in 1788 and named for the Comte de Vergennes, the French minister of foreign affairs whose support of America during the Revolution was crucial. It is the nation's smallest city, being only one mile square. What it lacked in size Vergennes made up in energy—by the early 1800s it was a bustling place of iron forges, rolling mills, and sawmills. During the War of 1812, Commodore Thomas Macdonough selected Vergennes as the 1813–1814 winter quarters for his small Lake Champlain fleet. The town's forges produced 177 tons of shot for him and, working with incredible speed, local carpenters built a flotilla for Macdonough, including the twenty-six-gun corvette *Saratoga,* the twenty-gun brig *Eagle,* and ten small gunboats propelled by oars. With these vessels Macdonough defeated the British at Plattsburgh on September 11, 1814—an important victory that thwarted British plans to prolong the war. A **monument** to Macdonough stands in the town green.

Nearby buildings, most of them constructed between 1825 and 1900, reflect Vergennes's industrial prosperity; chief among them are the **Ryan commercial block,** the **Stevens House Hotel,** and **Victorian houses,** all on Main Street; the elegant 1911 **Bixby Memorial Library** stands nearby. **Mill buildings** are preserved below Otter Creek Falls.

FERRISBURG

The Underground Railroad ran through western Vermont, but its operations in this region were less clandestine than those farther south. Perhaps because of a prominent Quaker community, the general sentiment in the region was largely abolitionist. Rowland Thomas Robinson, a Quaker and founder of the Vermont Anti-Slavery Society, used his house as a stop on the Underground

Railroad; escaped slaves worked for wages on his farm and ate with the family. Rowland Evans Robinson, his son, was a nineteenth-century writer and illustrator who chronicled the dialect and folkways of the region in a series of enormously popular stories and essays. His wife, Anna Stevens Robinson, was a portrait painter, and their two daughters were also artists. The 1786 late Federal-early Greek Revival farmhouse where four generations of Robinsons lived is now the **Rokeby Museum** (Route 7, 802–877–3406), furnished entirely with family pieces ranging from the 1780s to the 1890s, including many portraits, landscapes, and genre scenes by this family of artists. Across the road from the museum is a working farm (private) with a round barn, one of only twenty left in the state.

BASIN HARBOR

The history of Lake Champlain and the surrounding region is examined in the **Basin Harbor Museum** (Basin Harbor Road, 802–475–2317) which features historical exhibits and an exact replica of an eighteenth-century *bateau,* based on a wreck found in the lake. The museum supports ongoing underwater research in Lake Champlain, including the exploration of **Arnold's Bay,** about five miles north of Panton, where Benedict Arnold ran five of his ships aground on October 13, 1776, after the battle of Valcour Bay, New York. Arnold—whose treason was to come four years later—delayed a British invasion along Lake Champlain by constructing a small fleet and deploying it brilliantly. The onset of winter prevented the British from continuing their invasion until 1777. After his successful delaying action at Valcour Bay, Arnold beached his vessels north of Panton and set them afire to keep them from British hands. Parts of one ship still lie at the bottom of the lake.

RICHMOND

In 1813 the people of Richmond, a quiet dairy-farming community, built a multidenominational church that looked like no other in the state, but harkened back to the round churches of early Christianity and of early French Protestantism. The **Old Round Church** (off Route 2) actually is sixteen-sided and is topped by an octagonal belfry. It has not been used as a church since 1879 but serves a variety of public functions.

OPPOSITE: *Richmond's striking Old Round Church—which actually has sixteen sides—was constructed in 1813 to serve five denominations.*

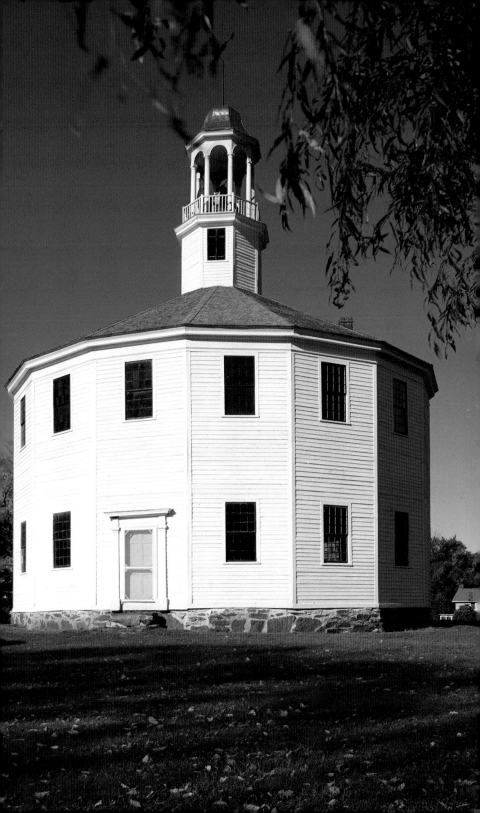

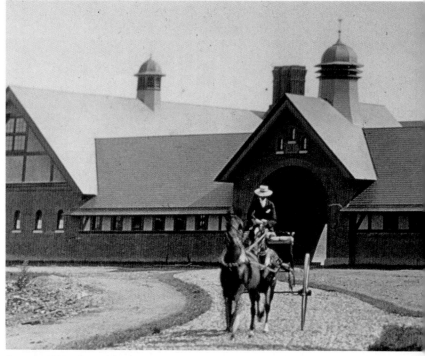

An early 1900s photo of the Queen Anne Revival Coach Barn at Shelburne Farms, on the

SHELBURNE FARMS

In the late-nineteenth century the dairy country below Burlington attracted railroad magnate William Seward Webb, who had married Lila Vanderbilt. The Webbs built a 110-room English cottage–style manor house on 4,000 acres. Frederick Law Olmsted advised the Webbs on the landscaping of the grounds. The estate is smaller now—1,000 acres—and is open to the public; the visitor center is located in the ca. 1890 **Gate House,** a cottage-style shingle building once occupied by the Webbs's gatekeeper. **Shelburne House,** the 1889 main house, has been restored with original furnishings and is operated as an inn. The formal gardens, overlooking Lake Champlain, are also being restored to their original design. The five-story **Farm Barn,** which surrounds a central courtyard, currently houses a bread bakery, furniture shop, and offices; restoration is scheduled to begin in the summer of 1989, and a museum with interpretive exhibits on conservation and agricultural history

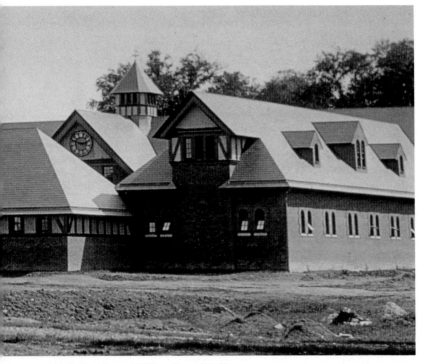

estate of railroad mogul William Seward Webb.

will be added. Also notable is the brick Queen Anne Revival **Coach Barn,** now an education center. The complex also includes a working dairy housed in modern buildings.

LOCATION: Off Route 7, eight miles south of Burlington. HOURS: June through mid-October: 9–5 Daily. FEE: Yes. TELEPHONE: 802–985-3222.

SHELBURNE MUSEUM

The Shelburne Museum houses one of the finest collections of American folk art in the world. It is a complex of thirty-seven buildings, many of them historic structures moved to the museum from other sites in New England. Some of the buildings, which include seven houses, a one-room schoolhouse, a general store, and a railroad station, are furnished in period style; others simply display the immense art and Americana collection of Electra Havemeyer Webb, who, together with her husband, J. Watson Webb

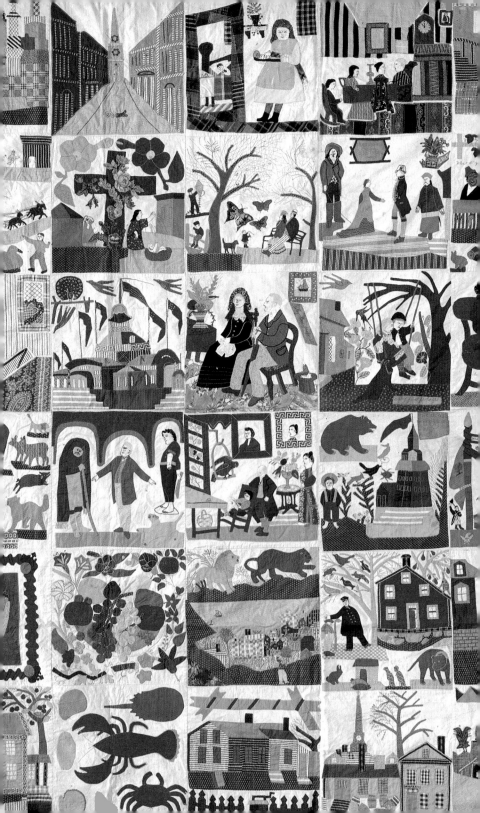

(son of the Webbs of Shelburne Farms), founded the museum in 1947. One of the first structures was a huge horseshoe-shaped barn (constructed from pieces of eleven older barns and two gristmills) built to house the Webb family's collection of carriages and sleighs. Also on the site are a jail, a blacksmith shop, a covered bridge, and the SS *Ticonderoga*. The magnificent collection of quilts, coverlets, and other textiles is housed in the Hat and Fragrance Unit; weathervanes, cigar-store Indians, and other folk art objects are on display in the Stagecoach Inn; and the Colchester Reef Lighthouse is now a gallery of maritime art and ship figureheads. Two modern buildings hold fine collections of paintings and antique furniture.

LOCATION: Route 7, south of Shelburne. HOURS: Mid-May through mid-October: 9–5 Daily. FEE: Yes. TELEPHONE: 802–985–3346.

BURLINGTON

Settled in the early 1770s, Burlington was nearly abandoned during the Revolution, when most of its inhabitants went off to the fighting. But the pioneers returned, to resume building the town on a triple-tiered slope above Lake Champlain. The general plan is still evident, with wharves and warehouses on the shoreline, a business district on the second tier, and residences taking in the whole scene from the top.

Many enterprises went into making Burlington Vermont's largest city. Ira Allen established a shipyard on the Winooski River in 1772. A few years later, he dammed the river and put in sawmills. In 1791, the Vermont legislature called for the establishment of a state university. Accordingly, the University of Vermont was founded here, adding academic affairs to the local business activity. Entrepreneur Gideon King was one of the first to realize the commercial implications of Lake Champlain traffic to and from Canada, and one of the men joining him in exploiting it was John Jacob Astor, the New York fur merchant. Furs and lumber came down from the north woods to markets south and west of Burlington.

Steamboats and the railroads quickened the pace of trade. The *Vermont*, launched in 1809 from Burlington, was the second commercial steamboat in the country, coming two years after Robert

OPPOSITE: *This appliquéd album quilt, from the extensive textile collection of the Shelburne Museum, was made in 1876 to celebrate the nation's centennial by a member of the Burdick-Childs family.*

Fulton made history on the Hudson River with his *Clermont*. Passenger crossings were a popular diversion, and in 1823 when the Champlain Canal opened a path to the Hudson and the sea, Burlington saw the arrival of first-class passenger steamers. The railroad came at mid-century, with the Rutland and Central Vermont lines. The first ran to Boston via Rutland, the second by way of White River Junction.

By 1880, the city had a magnificent courthouse and grand residences (still standing) on fashionable Main, Pearl, and Willard streets. From the city's nineteenth-century boom period are private residences and commercial buildings along Battery Street, Court House Square, South Willard Street, South Union Street, and on the university green.

The square steeple tower of Burlington's 1816 **Unitarian Church** (Church and Pearl streets, 802–862–5630) is topped by a double octagonal spire. The interior gallery is supported by Doric columns. Also on Church Street are the Romanesque **Masonic Temple,** built in 1898 (now converted to offices), and the **Richardson Building,** an 1895 department store and rooming house built in a chateau style.

One of the city's most handsome lakefront houses belonged to railroad executive and county judge Timothy Follett. Known as **Follett House** (63 College Street), the 1840 Greek Revival residence designed by Ammi B. Young now is used for offices. Several of the day's prosperous merchants built their houses on Pearl Street. Still private residences today, they include the **Buell House** at number 303, **Deming House** at number 308, and **Loomis House** at number 342. The **Moore-Woodbury House** (416 Pearl Street), with two late-nineteenth-century elaborations to the 1815 original, once belonged to Urban Woodbury, Burlington mayor and Vermont governor from 1894 to 1896. It is now an apartment house.

University of Vermont

The University of Vermont was founded in 1791 by an act of the state legislature, which endowed the school with a grant of some 29,000 acres of land in parcels all over the state. (Since 1777 the government had been setting aside land for a college in each new town that was chartered—all of these lands were turned over to the new university.) On a smaller but no less important scale, Ira Allen gave the university fifty acres in Burlington for its campus. A statue

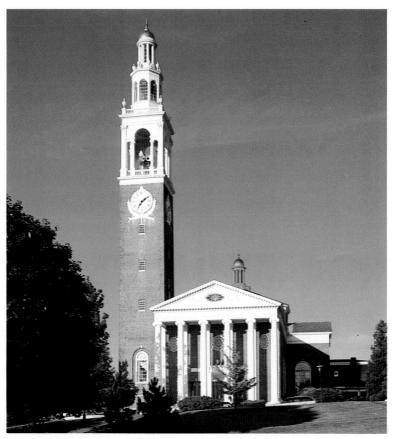

The University of Vermont, in Burlington, is graced with buildings designed by several of America's most distinguished architects. McKim, Mead & White's Chapel was built on the college green in 1927.

of Allen stands on the college's **green,** and the **chapel** (1927) is named for him. Designed by the firm of McKim, Mead & White, the chapel rises above the northeast side of the green.

Adjacent to the chapel is the Romanesque **Billings Building,** designed by Henry Hobson Richardson. Originally the library, it was completed in 1885. Richardson called it "the best thing I have yet done." Next door is the Gothic-style **Williams Science Hall.**

Grassmount, the five-bay brick residence of Vermont governor (1823–1826) Cornelius P. Van Ness, at 411 Main Street, is now the university's alumni office. A fraternity occupies the 1891

Queen Anne **Edward Wells House,** at 61 Summit Street. The original owner hired local woodworker Albert M. Whittekind to execute intricate carving, inside and out.

LOCATION: Route 2. TELEPHONE: 802–656–3480.

The redoubtable Revolutionary War hero and founding father of the state, Ethan Allen, is said to be buried at **Greenmount Cemetery** (Colchester Avenue) under a forty-two-foot-tall column, topped by a statue of Allen. He is depicted at the moment of his great triumph, the surrender of the British garrison at Fort Ticonderoga. He died in 1789.

East of Burlington, on the Browns River in **Jericho,** is the 1856 **Old Red Mill** (Route 15, 802–899–3225). Shut down at the turn of the century, the flour mill is now a museum, with its water-driven machinery on view.

STOWE

Originally a logging and farming community, Stowe has been primarily a resort since the mid-1800s, when city-bound New Englanders began to flock here for winter sports and mountain air. The resort is sited between Mount Mansfield (at 4,393 feet the highest peak in Vermont) and Hogback Mountain. Handsome commercial and public buildings reflect its prosperity. Among the most notable within the compact historic district are the **Green Mountain Inn, Community Church, Carlson Building,** and the **Akeley Memorial Building,** housing the **Stowe Historical Society Museum,** all on Main Street.

The **Fisher Covered Railroad Bridge** spans the Lamoille River east of **Morrisville.** The 1908 wooden bridge has been strengthened with steel beams. Its long clerestory is a chimney for locomotive smoke. **Grand Isle,** in the northern reach of Lake Champlain, is connected to the mainland of Vermont by ferry and highway. The abundant wildlife was hunted and fished by Indians, then by settlers of English descent in the late-eighteenth century. Until it was discovered a century later as a summer resort, Grand Isle was a small but thriving lake and apple-orchard community.

One of the oldest surviving log cabins in the United States, built in 1783, is on Route 2 just north of the town of Grand Isle.

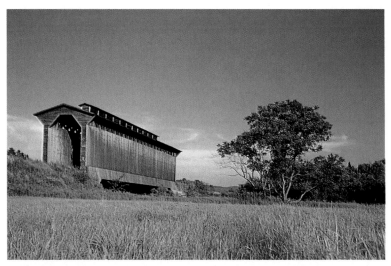

The last covered railroad bridge still in regular use in Vermont, the Fisher Covered Railroad Bridge was reinforced with heavy steel beams in 1968 to allow the preservation of the historic wooden structure.

Made of cedar logs, the twenty-by-twenty-five-foot cabin has a half-story loft and a large fireplace at one end. It is called **Hyde Log Cabin** (802–372–8830) after its builder, Jedediah Hyde, Jr., a veteran of the Revolution.

ISLE LA MOTTE

Closer to Quebec than to the Vermont mainland, Isle la Motte is the site of Vermont's first (though not permanent) French settlement. In 1666 Captain de la Motte led 300 men, Jesuits among them, to this small island near the top of the Champlain. To ward off a counterattack from the Mohawk Indians, the French raised Fort Sainte-Anne; the first Catholic mass in the state was celebrated here. Today, the site is marked by **St. Anne's Shrine** (off Route 129, 802–928–3362), which consists of an open-air chapel, a marble statue of Saint Anne, and several small outdoor shrines. A granite statue of Samuel de Champlain marks the spot where he is believed to have landed in 1609. Relics of the island's history are also on display.

The island's rich deposits of black marble were quarried in the late 1800s—the stone was used in the construction of New York's Brooklyn Bridge and Rockefeller Center.

ST. ALBANS

Situated close to Canada, St. Albans, settled just after the Revolution, has been the scene of many illegal escapades and political maneuvers of the type that often beset border towns. When Jefferson's embargo on trade with Britain was in effect from 1807 to the War of 1812, smugglers did a brisk business here, plying various kinds of contraband into and out of Canada. Three Federal officers were killed by gunmen protecting a smuggling craft. In 1837 when French Canadians were plotting a revolt against Britain, St. Albans was one of their rallying places. The most spectacular border incident took place during the Civil War in 1864, when twenty-two Confederate agents (part of a well-organized Confederate terrorist group operating out of Canada) simultaneously robbed all the banks in town, making off with some $200,000. Brought to trial in Canada, the raiders were acquitted on the grounds that their raid was an act of war and not a criminal offense. In 1866 members of an Irish political group, the Fenians, planned to use St. Albans as a jumping-off point for a raid on Canada, but were thwarted by the arrival of federal troops.

The railroads arrived in 1850, and St. Albans became not only an important railroad center but headquarters of the Central Vermont Railroad. Dairy farming, lime processing, and the manufacture of animal feed, maple sugar, and sugar-making equipment added to the economy. The wealth of the town is apparent in monumental public buildings on **Taylor Park,** the **Central Vermont Railroad Headquarters** (Kingman Street), and the large private houses on Main Street.

Occupying an 1861 nine-room school, the **Franklin County Museum** (Church and Bishop streets, 802–527–7933) contains a variety of exhibits depicting aspects of Vermont history: memorabilia of the Central Vermont Railway, winter sports equipment, an Indian canoe, a country doctor's office, and articles relating to the Confederate raid of 1864.

CHESTER A. ARTHUR HISTORIC SITE

Chester A. Arthur was born in 1829. In 1848, after graduating from Union College in New York State, he returned to Vermont to teach at the North Pownall Academy. Two years later, he moved to New York City to pursue a career in law and, later, the civil service. In 1871, President Ulysses S. Grant named him customs collector of the Port Authority of New York. The abuses of the Grant administration had resulted in widespread corruption within the civil service, however, and when the next president, Rutherford B. Hayes, undertook to reform the system, Arthur's appointment was rescinded. When the Republicans nominated James A. Garfield (who had also taught at North Pownall Academy) to run for president in 1880, Arthur was chosen as his running mate to appease an anti-reform faction. A few months after he was elected, Garfield was assassinated and Arthur became president. Against all expectations, he continued the reforms initiated by Hayes and supported the Pendleton Act of 1883, which established the Civil Service Commission. Although Arthur was passed over for nomination in 1884, historians credit him with restoring a measure of dignity to the presidency.

This thirty-five-acre park features a replica of the simple clapboard house where Arthur lived as a child. The building was reconstructed using a photograph of the original; it houses interpretive exhibits about Arthur, his family, and Fairfield County. Also on the site is the ca. 1830 brick church, where Arthur's father preached.

LOCATION: Off Route 36, Fairfield. HOURS: By appointment. FEE: None. TELEPHONE: 802–828–3226.

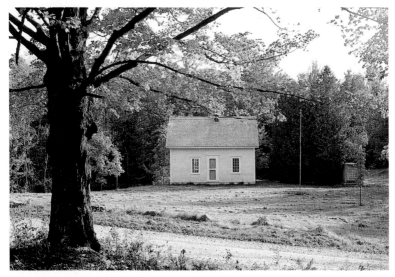

This modest clapboard house replicates the birthplace of Chester A. Arthur, who became the twenty-first president of the United States when James A. Garfield was assassinated in 1881.

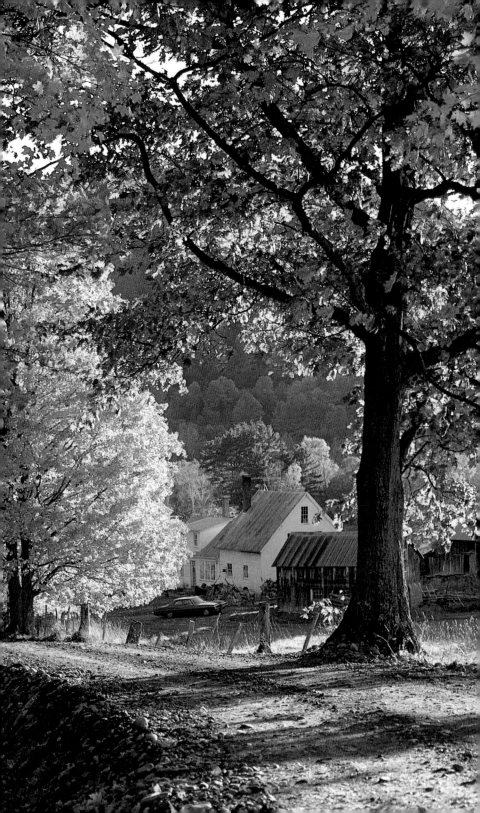

EASTERN VERMONT

OPPOSITE: Autumn in South Woodstock.

To the east and west of the Green Mountains that form Vermont's great backbone, the land falls away to the flat valleys of Lake Champlain and the Connecticut River. The river was the most important corridor of settlement and commerce in the eighteenth century. Like their neighbors on the eastern side of the river, the towns were founded by people from Connecticut and Massachusetts. Puritan and relatively sophisticated, they looked with some horror on the rough-and-tumble settlements on the western side of the Green Mountains, the domain of the "awful infidel," Ethan Allen, and his rowdy cohorts. During and after the Revolution, towns on both sides of the Connecticut considered joining together to form their own state. The plan was promoted by the founder of New Hampshire's Dartmouth College, Eleazor Wheelock. Alarmed that the new republic of Vermont might lose its eastern flank, the Allen brothers decided to hold the 1777 constitutional convention at an eastern locale, in Windsor. Although the Allens and their Green Mountain Boys were not active in eastern Vermont, one town, Irasburg, was named after Ira Allen in recognition of his role in the founding of the state.

In the nineteenth century the Green Mountains yielded a harvest of stone. Granite was quarried in Bethel, Mount Ascutney, Derby, and Woodbury; soapstone in Springfield; and slate in Fair Haven. Northeastern Vermont is still a place apart—known as the Northeast Kingdom, a name first applied to the region in the 1930s. Isolated and still largely undeveloped, this mountainous, forested territory is partly owned by paper companies. Many of the towns are unincorporated.

This chapter begins in the Northeast Kingdom at the Canadian border and descends south to St. Johnsbury, Montpelier, Barre, and then along the Connecticut River to Brattleboro.

NORTHEASTERN VERMONT

North of the Green Mountains are eighteenth-century settlements that would develop into lumber towns in the nineteenth century— **Troy, Irasburg, Coventry**—tied to the south by railroads. One of the more isolated of these was **Brownington.** Virtually the entire village is a historic district. Notable within it is the **Old Stone House Museum** (802–754–2022), a four-story school built of granite blocks in the 1830s by the Reverend Alexander Twilight, one of

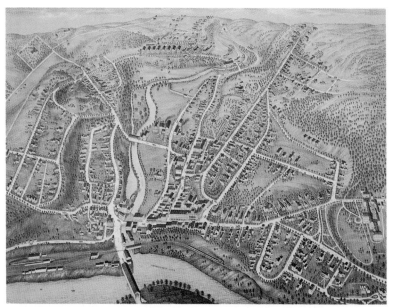

An 1876 lithograph depicting Brattleboro, along the Connecticut River (detail)

America's first black college graduates. The museum displays tools, furniture, and household items, and is operated by the Orleans County Historical Society.

Above Brownington is Lake Memphremagog—"Beautiful Waters" to the Indians who crossed it in birch canoes. **Newport,** the border city on the western bank, grew into a thriving lumber town, railroad center, and a resort favored by Americans and Canadians. Recalling the town's late-nineteenth-century heyday are the **Goodrich Memorial Library** (802–334–7902), and the old **Federal Office Building** (now a state office complex), both on Main Street. A 1905 railroad car is part of the permanent exhibits of industrial machinery and equipment at the **Old Colony Maple Sugar Factory** on Bluff Road outside of Newport (802–334–6516).

Across the lake, the international border line runs along the maple-shaded streets of **Derby Line** straight through the **Haskell Free Library and Opera House** (Caswell Avenue, 819–876–2471), donated to the communities of Derby Line and Rock Island, Quebec, just after 1900 by patron Martha Stewart Haskell.

Eastward, the border dips into valleys, climbs hills, and levels out on large plains, almost always in view of water—northern

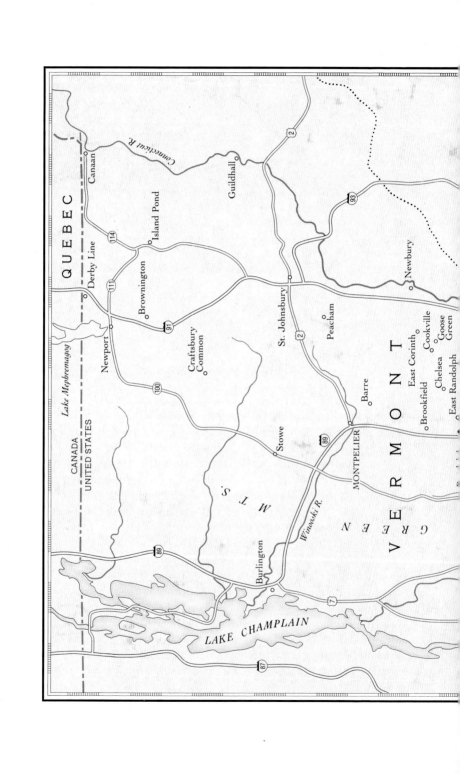

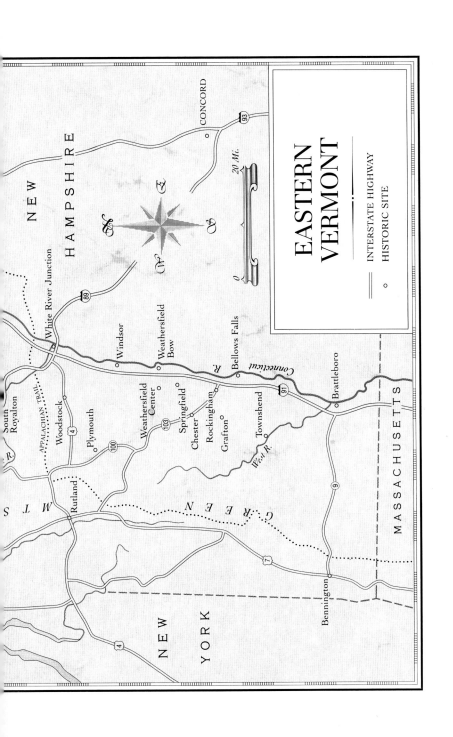

EASTERN
VERMONT

— INTERSTATE HIGHWAY
○ HISTORIC SITE

NEW HAMPSHIRE

CONCORD

93

White River Junction

89

Windsor

Weathersfield
Bow

Bellows Falls

Connecticut R.

91

Brattleboro

South
Royalton

APPALACHIAN TRAIL

Woodstock

4

Plymouth

100

Weathersfield
Center

103

Springfield

Chester

Rockingham

Grafton

Townshend

West R.

G R E E N

Rutland

M T S

9

NEW
YORK

7

MASSACHUSETTS

Bennington

4

20 Mi.

0

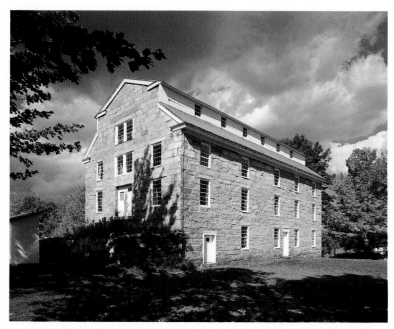

*Headmaster Alexander Twilight built the 1836 Old Stone House as a dormitory for Browning-
ton Academy after the school's trustees refused to do so; local legend has it that he quarried the
granite himself. Twilight was without doubt a remarkable man, serving as the headmaster of
the school for twenty-one years and in the Vermont state legislature for two. Middlebury College
claims him as the first black college graduate in the United States.*

Vermont is rich in streams, ponds, and small lakes. The highest
elevations of Vermont's "Northeast Kingdom" look west to the
Adirondacks, south to the Green Mountains, and east to the Connecticut River and the White Mountains of New Hampshire. Before the railroads **Canaan** was a stage stop on the river valley route
from Franklin, New Hampshire, to Montreal. **Ward Library** (Park
Street, 802–266–8676), the 1846 house of abolitionist Fernando C.
Jacobs, was known for years as Jacob's [sic] Stand, being the northernmost hideout on the Underground Railroad.

The midpoint between Montreal and Portland, Maine, **Island
Pond** became one of Vermont's vital economic links when the
Grand Canadian Trunk Railway first came to this forest town in
1853. The 1903 **depot** is made of native timber and granite, as are
other commercial buildings within the small historic district.

Guildhall is the oldest community in northeastern Vermont,
settled in 1764. Early houses and public buildings, including the

Greek Revival **Essex County Court House** and **Guild Hall,** a portion of which dates from 1795, surround the small green, which leads to the Connecticut River.

CRAFTSBURY COMMON

This classic hilltop village is named after Revolutionary Colonel Ebenezer Crafts, who founded Craftsbury proper in 1788 (Crafts' son Samuel was governor of Vermont from 1828 to 1831). Eighteenth-century gravestones dot the iron-fenced **cemetery** at the west end of the village. The **United Church of Craftsbury, Craftsbury Academy,** and the **Craftsbury Public Library** face the large green common, surrounded by a white wooden fence.

ST. JOHNSBURY

A quiet farming village settled by Rhode Islanders in 1786, St. Johnsbury landed on New England's industrial map in 1823 when two brothers, Thaddeus and Erastus Fairbanks, established a small iron foundry here. Thaddeus was an inventor and won his first patent for a cast-iron plow. The family soon specialized in the manufacture of scales, from the smallest (for measuring doses of medicine) to the largest platform (which could hold railroad cars).

Maple sugaring also enlivened the local economy. Exhibits at the **Maple Grove Maple Museum** (East of town on Route 2, 802–748–5141) illustrate the process and history of indigenous maple sugaring. By 1850 three railroads served the town, including the 1883 **Canadian-Pacific Depot** (Depot Square, 802–748–4401).

On and near Main Street are St. Johnsbury's most important buildings, many of them built by the Fairbanks family. Among them are the **Fairbanks Block,** distinguished by fancy brickwork and **Brantview,** a Queen Anne house at the foot of Main Street designed by Lambert Packard, a Vermont architect, for William P. Fairbanks in 1883. **St. John the Evangelist** and **North Congregational** churches, both Packard creations, contrast sharply with the Neoclassical **South Congregational Church** farther down Main Street at number 11. The **Fairbanks Museum and Planetarium** (Main and Prospect streets, 802–748–2372), founded by industrialist Franklin Fairbanks in 1889, occupies a towered, Romanesque building of red sandstone, also the work of Lambert Packard. The **Caldedonia County Courthouse,** at 27 Main Street, faces a monument to Vermont's Civil War soldiers.

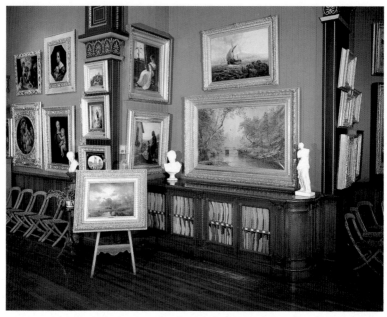

*The St. Johnsbury Athenaeum, one of many local benefactions of the Fairbanks family,
incorporates a library and a gallery containing a significant collection of American paintings.*

St. Johnsbury Athenaeum

The town's library and art museum are housed in another Fairbanks legacy, the Athenaeum. The library, built in 1871, still contains many of the original books. Wooden spiral staircases lead
from the main floor to graceful balconies, and the main reading
room has retained its original gas chandeliers (now converted to
electricity). The gallery, which was added in 1873, houses an excellent collection of Hudson River School paintings as well as copies of
old master paintings commissioned by Horace Fairbanks. The
centerpiece of the collection is Albert Bierstadt's *Domes of the Yosem-
ite;* the 116-by-180-inch painting takes up the entire back wall of
the gallery and is lit from above by a skylight. The building may
actually have been designed to accommodate the painting.

LOCATION: 30 Main Street. HOURS: June through August: 9:30–8
Monday and Wednesday, 9:30–5 Tuesday, Thursday, Friday, 9:30–2
Saturday. September through May: 9:30–8 Monday and Wednesday,
9:30–5 Tuesday, Thursday–Saturday. FEE: None. TELEPHONE: 802–
748–8291.

Below St. Johnsbury is the town of **Peacham**. With its apple orchards and stately white houses, it is among the most picturesque towns in a state famous for them. The white clapboard **Congregational Church** was built in 1806.

MONTPELIER

The name of Vermont's capital was apparently the whim of Francophile Jacob Davis, a veteran of the Revolutionary War who led a band of settlers to this Green Mountain gap in 1788. Davis and his fellow pioneers cleared land along the Onion River, cutting paths that became State and Court streets. Seat of Vermont's government since 1805, the city is dominated by the capitol's gleaming gold dome.

Vermont State House and State Complex

The present statehouse was designed by Thomas Silloway and built in 1857 to replace the capitol designed by Ammi B. Young in 1833. Young's capitol was destroyed by fire; however, Silloway incorporated the Doric portico, which is derived from the ancient Greek temple of Theseus. The exterior is of Vermont granite. Interior details are rich, particularly the molded plaster ceilings in the Governor's Office, Representatives' Hall, and Senate Chamber, and the black marble on the lobby floor, quarried from Isle la Motte. Fine granite from Millstone Hill in nearby Barre also was used in the state house.

LOCATION: 115 State Street. HOURS: 8–4 Monday–Friday. FEE: None. TELEPHONE: 802–828–2228.

The capitol is the centerpiece of a complex that includes the **Supreme Court Building** and the **Pavilion Building** (109 State Street), now a state office building. The Pavilion is a 1970 copy of its 1876 predecessor, which, as a hotel, was the center of the city's social and political life. The first floor of the building is given over to the Vermont Historical Society's **Vermont Museum** (802–828–2291), in which permanent and rotating exhibits illustrate Vermont's way of life from prehistory to the present day. Montpelier's

OVERLEAF: *The Vermont State House was built in 1857, incorporating the portico of an 1833 capitol that had burned down. Atop the golden dome is a statue of Ceres, the Roman goddess of agriculture.*

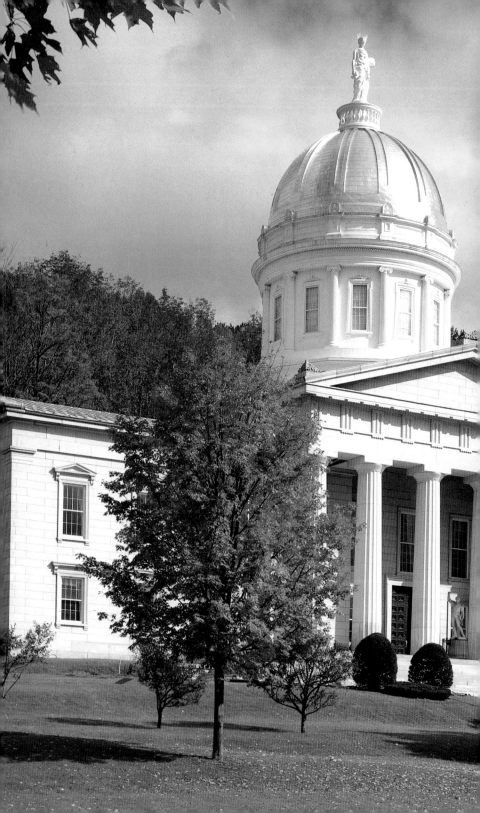

residential and commercial districts contain many attractive Victorian buildings, including **city hall,** the Gothic, all-granite **Christ's Church, Washington County Court House,** and the **Blanchard and Walton commercial blocks.**

BARRE

Since the early 1800s more than 100 quarrying companies have harvested Barre's granite and marble deposits. The business was local for many years, but in 1875, when the Central Vermont Railroad connected the town to southern markets, Barre's economy boomed—and the population more than tripled in the following decade. Scotsmen, Scandinavians, and Italians arrived, already skilled in stonecutting. Barre became as rambunctious as a logging town, with no shortage of pubs and saloons to serve the male working population.

In construction and detail, buildings in downtown Barre reflect extravagant use of the native stone, to particularly graceful effect in the 1899 **Barre City Hall,** which contains the local opera house, and the 1924 **Soldier and Sailors Memorial** in City Park. The 1899 **Robert Burns monument,** in front of the Spaulding School, is also carved from local granite. The abbeylike **Episcopal Church** and **Aldrich Public Library** (housing the **Barre Museum**) are on the park. The museum (6 Washington Street, 802–476–7550) has permanent exhibits on the history of the town and the granite industry, as well as rotating exhibits on various subjects. Barre's **Rock of Ages Company** (Main Street in Graniteville, just outside Barre, 802–476–3115) still harvests a twenty-acre quarry, and its massive operations are open to the public. Many of Barre's stoneworkers are buried in **Hope Cemetery** (Upper Merchant Street), their headstones and monuments a testament to the skills of the local craftsmen.

NEWBURY

On the **town common** stands the **Jacob Bayley Monument,** honoring one of the men who founded the town in the 1760s and who played a significant role in the development of this region of the state. A vocal Patriot, Bayley was nearly arrested by the British while plowing his fields, but a friend warned him of the approaching patrol and he escaped. Across the common from the monument are the **Methodist Church** and a marker for the Newbury

Seminary, which operated from 1834 to 1868. It was the first Methodist theological school in the country. The town's **Congregational Church,** with its white siding, tall spire, and portico, was built in 1856, replacing an earlier one that had burned. The congregation, organized in 1764, was the second in Vermont. A half-mile north of the church is **Oxbow Cemetery,** with many markers dating to the 1700s.

To the west, where the terrain turns mountainous and streams run a little faster, is **Brookfield,** a former milltown (the power came from nearby Sunset Lake) with a manufacturing specialty—pitchforks, in this case. Brookfield's library was established in 1791. What may look like the earliest houses in the village were actually built as taverns. Sunset Lake boasts an unusual "pontoon" bridge, a floating platform buoyed by wooden barrels. The **Historical Society of Brookfield** (Ridge Road, Brookfield Center) occupies an 1835 house and displays pitchforks along with other farm tools, boot dryers, and a washing machine patented in 1861—all made in Brookfield—and local furniture and clothing.

RANDOLPH

The railroad came to Randolph in 1848 to take the village's produce and manufactured products to market. The resulting nineteenth-century development of downtown Randolph is apparent in the Italianate **Central Vermont Railway Depot,** the Second Empire **DuBois and Gay commercial block,** other commercial buildings in the Italianate and Queen Anne styles, and the Gothic Revival **United Church of Randolph. Chandler Music Hall** was built in the early 1900s and is still used for the performing arts. The **Randolph Historical Museum,** located on the second floor of the Village Building (Salisbury Street, 802-728-5398), preserves the town's drugstore and soda fountain, in operation from 1893 to 1958, as well as tools, signs, and other items from the area.

STRAFFORD

East of Randolph is the small village of Strafford. The **town hall** was built on the town green in 1799, the year the farming and dairy community was founded in the Ompompamoosuc River valley.

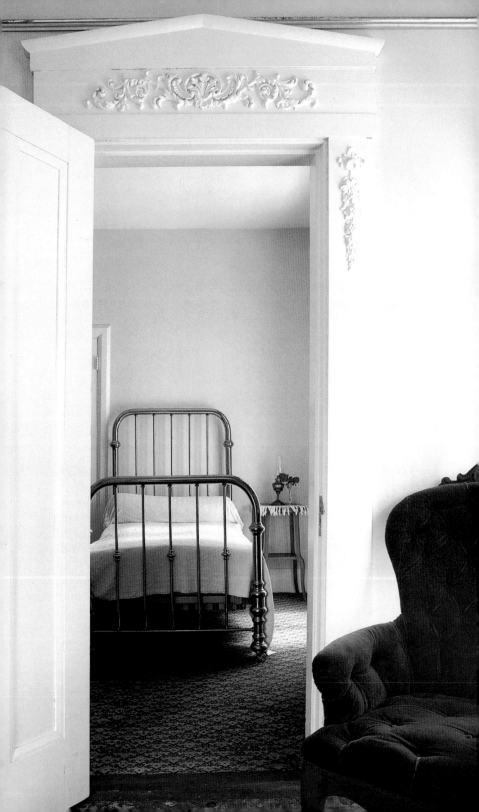

Justin Morrill Homestead

This two-story Gothic Revival house was built by Justin Morrill, who served in both the House of Representatives and the Senate. The son of a blacksmith, Morrill was forced to leave school at age 15 and work as a store clerk. He soon had a store of his own and was so successful that he was able to retire at age 38, to lead the life of a country gentleman. He was elected to the House in 1854 and the Senate in 1866, where he sponsored the Land-Grant College Acts of 1862 and 1890.

Morrill began building his house in 1848, the year he retired; it was completed in 1851. The seventeen-room frame house is painted pink to imitate sandstone, and is embellished with elaborate carved details. Family antiques, paintings, murals, and decorative objects are on display.

LOCATION: Strafford Village. HOURS: June through mid-October: 9:30–5:30 Wednesday–Sunday. FEE: Yes. TELEPHONE: 802–828–3226.

SOUTH ROYALTON

South Royalton grew as a freight depot when the Vermont Central came through in 1848. Around Village Park, houses were built in the popular revival styles of the Victorian period—late Greek Revival, Queen Anne, and Italianate. Those styles also are seen in the 1886 **Railroad Station and Baggage House** and the two-story brick **commercial block,** built in 1887. The centerpiece of the park is an ornate bandstand dating from the 1880s; the park also contains a granite arch that stands as a memorial to Hannah Handy, who rescued nine children from British-led Indian raids in 1780.

The Mormon prophet Joseph Smith was born on a farm in the hills east of Royalton in 1805, and spent his first decade there. His family moved across the border into New York in 1816, during a period of evangelistic revivals. As a young man, Smith had the visions that led him to establish the Church of Jesus Christ of Latter-Day Saints. The monolithic **Joseph Smith Monument** (Dairy Hill Road, 802–763–7742) of Barre granite marks the Smith property and a chapel, museum, and visitor center stand on the site of the family farmhouse.

OPPOSITE: *The Justin Morrill Homestead, built in the 1840s by the Vermont congressman and senator who sponsored the Land Grant College Acts, is furnished with many original Morrill family pieces.*

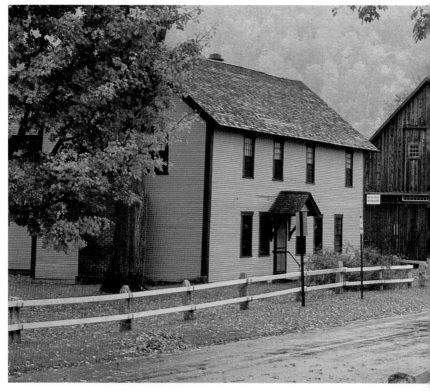

President Calvin Coolidge was born in this modest dwelling on July 4, 1872. After many

PLYMOUTH NOTCH

This village, administered by the state of Vermont, is best known for the **Coolidge Birthplace,** a modest five-room frame house attached to the village's general store. The thirtieth president was born in the downstairs bedroom on July 4, 1872. When he was 4 years old, the family moved to a larger house, now known as the **Coolidge Homestead.** It is here that Coolidge assumed the country's highest office. Colonel John Coolidge administered the presidential oath to his son on August 3, 1923, at 2:47 AM—President Warren G. Harding had died a few hours before.

The Coolidge family had lived in the shadow of the Green Mountains for generations. Coolidge attended Plymouth's school, and stones from that first structure went into the foundation of the present **One-Room Schoolhouse.** Schoolteacher Carrie Brown,

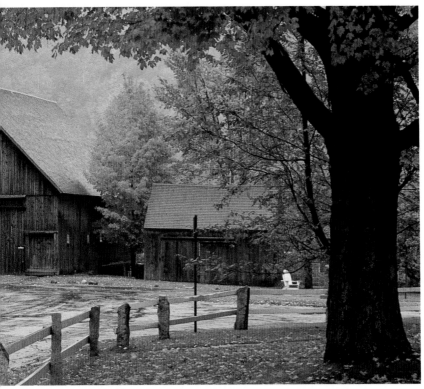

alterations, the Coolidge Birthplace was restored to its 1872 appearance in 1968.

who greatly influenced the young Calvin, married his widower father in 1891. Coolidge began his political career in Massachusetts, where he became mayor of Northampton after attending Amherst College; in 1919 he was elected governor of that state. In 1920, he and Harding defeated James Cox in the presidential election. Coolidge was home visiting Plymouth when he became president—no other president has been sworn into office at his ancestral home. Plymouth Notch includes the Coolidge compound of houses and barns and its surrounding village, touched only by preservationists and restorers since the late-nineteenth century. Six generations of Coolidges, including the president, his father, mother, and stepmother, are buried in **Plymouth Cemetery**.

LOCATION: Off Route 100A. HOURS: June through mid-October: 9:30–5 Daily. FEE: Yes. TELEPHONE: 802–828–3226.

WOODSTOCK

Settled in 1765, Woodstock is situated between hills on the Otta-quechee River. Almost from the beginning, the town seemed rar-efied—from Massachusetts and Connecticut came professionals, scholars, and superior craftsmen. Around the oval **green** were the shops of hatters, tailors, silversmiths, jewelers, cabinetmakers, and weavers. Literate Woodstock had bookbinders and publishers and, by the 1850s, five weekly newspapers. Musical instruments were made here—flutes, pianos, and violins. Four bells cast by Paul Revere survive in Woodstock; three of these still ring from local steeples while the fourth is displayed at the **Congregational Church** on Elm Street. From 1827 to 1856, Woodstock boasted the state's premier medical school.

Virtually all structures in the village date to the nineteenth century, from the houses and public buildings on the green (still dominated by the octagonal tower of the 1855 **Windsor County Courthouse**) to the rows of stone business buildings north of it. The **Woodstock Historical Society** occupies the 1807 **Dana House** (26 Elm Street, 802–457–1822). Built for merchant Charles Dana in 1807, the house remained in the family until 1943. It displays furniture, silverware, and china dating from the periods of the Dana family's occupancy. Nearby is the ca. 1806 **First Congrega-tional Church** (Elm Street at Pleasant).

Vermont congressman, linguist, lawyer, conservationist, ar-chaeologist, and diplomat, George P. Marsh grew up in Wood-stock, in an 1807 brick and frame Federal house (54 Elm Street, private). When Robert Mills's original design for the Washington Monument in the national capital was put aside, Marsh recom-mended the monument be an obelisk and, from his diplomatic post in Rome, sent the engineers accurate measurements of an ancient example. On the town green is the 1804 **Ottaquechee D.A.R. House,** which displays toys and railroad memorabilia.

At the edge of the village, the **Billings Farm and Museum** (Route 12 and River Road, 802–457–3555) is a working farm that demonstrates nineteenth-century agricultural methods.

WINDSOR

Popularly known as the birthplace of Vermont, Windsor is the home of the **Old Constitution House** (Route 5, 802–828–3226), the eighteenth-century tavern where representatives met in 1777

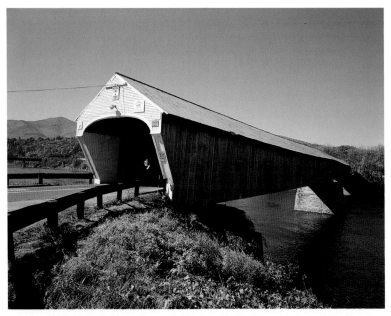

The Windsor-Cornish Covered Bridge, the longest in the United States, connects Vermont and New Hampshire.

to adopt Vermont's first constitution. The convention was a dramatic one, seven days in duration; on July 8, the day of adjournment, the delegates received news of the costly American rearguard action at Hubbardton. The first legislature met in Windsor in March 1778, and remained independent until 1791, when Vermont became the fourteenth state.

The Georgian-style wooden building no longer stands on its original site, having been moved twice to accommodate downtown expansion. The interior is currently (1988) being renovated; a major interpretive exhibit, with mounted displays and period rooms, will be installed. One artifact that will remain is the tavern table on which, according to tradition, the constitution of the Vermont Republic was written.

The manufacture of firearms became an important local industry in the mid-nineteenth century, and this, in turn, led to important developments in standardization and mass production. In 1846 a local firm built an armory and machine shop to produce rifles with interchangeable parts—a new technology at the time. The company's exhibit at the Crystal Palace Industrial Exhibition in London in 1851 led to widespread interest in the system, and soon the Windsor factory was exporting machine tools and finished products to England. The building—a three-story structure made, ironically, of handmade bricks—now houses the **American Precision Museum** (South Main Street, 802–674–5781), which traces the history of manufacturing by displaying various products, such as rifles, typewriters, engines, and even an automobile, together with the tools used to make them.

Alexander Parris designed the classic **St. Paul's Episcopal Church** (State and Court streets, 802–674–2926) on a monumental scale; the two-story brick church, built in 1822, has round-arched windows that conceal the actual interior height, and the gabled roof is topped by a dome-capped, tiered bell tower. The 1798 Federal-style **Old South Congregational Church** (Main Street, 802–674–5087) is attributed to Asher Benjamin. Windsor's Italianate **U.S. Post Office** (Main Street, 802–674–5822), designed by Ammi Burnham Young in 1857, is the oldest active post office–courthouse in the country.

The houses of Windsor encompass a wide range of architectural styles, from the simple Federal-style **Skinner House** (Main Street, private) built in 1820, to the gingerbread-rich **McIndoe House** (Court Street, private), an 1849 Gothic Revival cottage noted for the elaborate decorative elements and details that seem to animate its exterior. The ca. 1785 **Nathaniel Leonard House** (Main Street), a Federal-style wood-frame house with a gabled roof and a Palladian window, was partially destroyed by fire in 1881 and restored in 1919; it is now used as a Masonic lodge.

Merino sheep, prized for their thick white fleece, were introduced into Vermont south of Windsor at **Weathersfield Bow,** named for its location at a crook in the Connecticut River. William Jarvis, U.S. consul to Portugal during the first decade of the nineteenth century, returned to his native Vermont in 1811 with a large flock of the sheep (acquired at distress prices during the Peninsular War). The ensuing wool production added substantially to the state's economy.

West of the river is **Weathersfield Center.** Its Federal-style **meetinghouse** was built in 1821 to replace an earlier one that had

OPPOSITE: *The Federal-style Weathersfield Meetinghouse, built in 1821, was remodeled forty years later to accommodate both church and state. The first floor was used for town meetings and the second by the Congregational Church.*

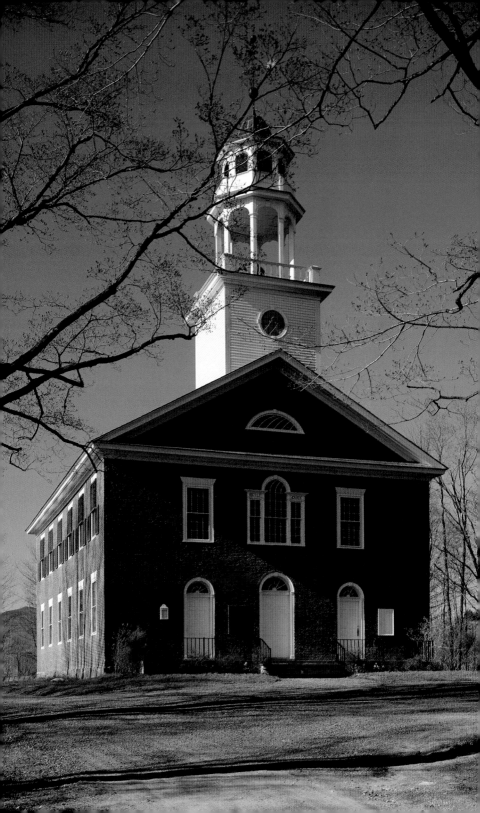

been destroyed by fire. The two-story building served public and religious functions—town meetings on the ground floor, Congregational services on the second. In 1985 the building was gutted by fire but has been meticulously restored. The first pastor of the church lived nearby in the **Reverend Dan Foster House** (802–263–5239), which now houses the historical society's museum. It was built during the Revolution and expanded in 1787, 1825, and 1888.

SPRINGFIELD

The early industrialization of Springfield has been credited to Isaac Fisher, who came from New Hampshire in 1808 and bought frontage along the Black River for mills and foundries. Although no longer water driven, some of the mills still operate on the Black River, along with more recent machine tool companies.

In the 1750s, Abenaki Indians shared the valley with English and French settlers; together they harvested the forest, fished, and worked a generally good soil. Further settlements grew up along the Springfield section of the **Crown Point Military Road,** blazed across Vermont in 1759 to connect the Connecticut River to Lake Champlain.

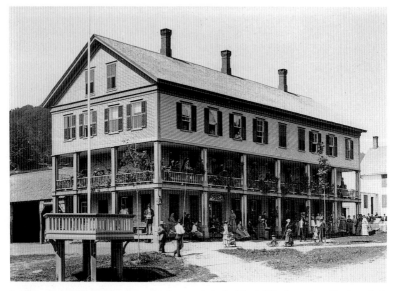

A photo of the Old Tavern Inn, Grafton, as it looked in 1885, from the collection of the Grafton Historical Society.

In 1790 those first settlers built **Eureka Schoolhouse** (east of Springfield on Route 11, 802–828–3226), one of Vermont's few surviving eighteenth-century public buildings, and the state's oldest one-room schoolhouse. Adjacent to it is the **Baltimore Covered Bridge,** built over Great Brook in 1870, tying Springfield to the smaller town of Baltimore.

Springfield's second generation built a sawmill on the falls, then gristmills, cotton mills, and a foundry. By the late-nineteenth century a third of the town's population came from Eastern Europe.

CHESTER VILLAGE

This town suffered religious factionalism early in its life, in 1785, with Congregationalists isolating themselves in the north end of town (now known as **Stone Village**), and the Baptists taking over the south. The buildings in the Stone Village area—which consists of a single street—are, indeed, of stone. The work probably was executed by Scottish stonemasons in the early nineteenth century.

Many fine buildings are in the **Chester Village Historic District,** particularly the Italianate **Fullerton House** (now converted to an inn) on the common.

GRAFTON

This virtually unspoiled nineteenth-century village boasts two steepled churches—the 1833 **Brick Meeting House** and the nearby **Baptist Church** (both on Main Street), notable for its Sandwich glass chandeliers. In 1790 the first of six dams was built along Saxtons River; by 1824 the dams furnished power to more than a dozen mills. A large woolen mill was built in 1831 to process the wool yielded by Grafton's 10,000 merino sheep.

From 1825 to 1900 one of the country's largest soapstone quarries brought much prosperity to Grafton, as did the manufacture of carriages, sleighs, butter churns, fine fishing rods, and violins. Logging, dairying, and the production of cheese and maple syrup were also important industries here.

The **Grafton Historical Society Museum** (Main Street, 802–843–2388) displays a fine collection of local artifacts and more than 500 old photographs. The **Old Tavern Inn** (Main Street) was built in 1801. The Grafton cornet band has played on the green every summer Sunday evening since 1867.

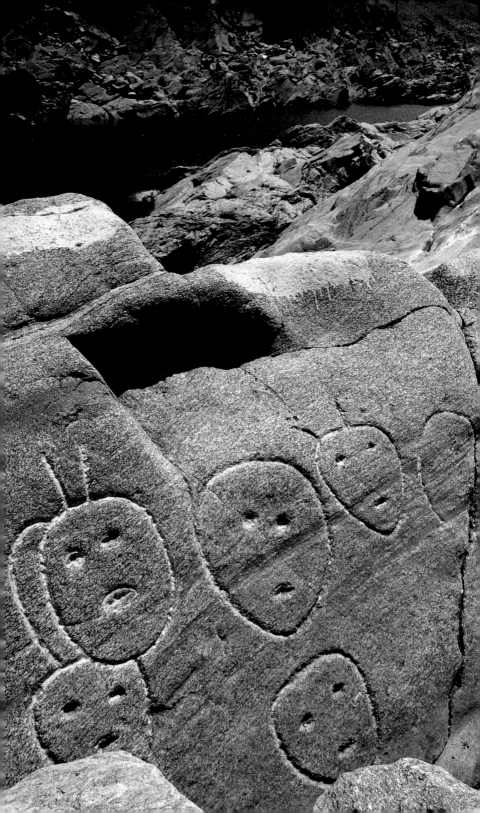

BELLOWS FALLS

A variety of Native American groups knew the area of Bellows Falls before its settlement in the 1780s and left stone carvings on the rock walls of the falls of the Connecticut River. When the light is right, the **petroglyphs** are visible downriver from the **Vilas Bridge.** In order to develop commercially the river had to be made navigable, and in 1792 settlers began construction of a canal. Completed in 1802, the canal was one of the first in the nation. For a half century, barges, rafts, and then steamers made their way to and from the town's mills and other businesses. When the railroad came to Bellows Falls in 1875, the canal became less important for transportation but more important for hydroelectric power. It was enlarged in the 1870s and again in the late 1920s to its current width of 125 feet. The power station built in 1928 is still in use.

The 1831 **Adams Old Stone Grist Mill** (Mill Street, 802–463–3706) preserves its original machinery. The mill was water powered until 1926, when it was electrified; it ceased operations in 1956. The building also houses exhibits on the region's history and locally made churns and creamery equipment.

A small rag-paper mill that went up in 1802 marked the beginning of a major industry—seventy years later, the state's first pulp mills were in operation and Bellows Falls was home of the International Paper Company. A landmark of industrial Bellows Falls is the 1925 crenellated clock tower on the town hall.

The town gained a famous resident in 1867 when local businessman Edward H. Green married financier Henrietta Howland Robinson. Born in New Bedford, Massachusetts, in 1835, "Hetty" inherited the family fortune made in the China trade, and increased her holdings tremendously as a crackerjack operator on Wall Street. (It has been said that she learned about finance as a youngster when she read the business pages aloud to her grandfather.) She had a reputation as a miser—detractors called her "The Witch of Wall Street."

Hetty Green's desk is in the **Rockingham Free Public Library** (65 Westminster Street, 802–463–4270), as well as Indian artifacts, antique dolls and a dollhouse, locally made farm machinery, and other articles relating to local history.

OPPOSITE: *With a certain slant of light, mysterious Indian petroglyphs are visible on the rocky banks of the Connecticut River below the Vilas Bridge in Bellows Falls.*

North of Bellows Falls in the small village of **Rockingham** is a hilltop **meetinghouse** (off Route 103) built in 1787. South and west, on Route 30 in **Townshend,** is the longest wooden highway span within Vermont, the **Scott Covered Bridge,** spanning the West River. The original section was built by Vermont engineer Harrison Chamberlain in 1870 and is 166 feet long. As the bank eroded, the bridge was lengthened; it is now 276 feet long. Between 1894 and 1910, Chamberlain's colleague, James Otis Follett, became known for his arched stone bridges, four of which are near Townshend, off Route 30.

BRATTLEBORO

The land on which modern Brattleboro stands was bought at auction in 1718 at a price of approximately one farthing an acre by a group of Massachusetts notables that included the lieutenant governor, William Dummer, and financier William Brattle. Although the town was later named for him, Brattle never was to see it. In 1724 a blockhouse, called Fort Dummer, was built on the bank of the Connecticut River and became the first permanent British settlement in what is now Vermont.

Various industries have thrived here: cotton weaving, woolen milling, bottling, printing, and the manufacture of paper, organs, and wood products. In 1845 D. Robert Wesselhoeft established a hydropathic center here, treating a variety of illnesses with Brattleboro mineral water. Downtown Brattleboro reflects the range of nineteenth-century architectural styles and the scale of building associated with industrial prosperity.

Among the local historical exhibits in the **Brattleboro Museum and Art Center** housed in the 1915 **Union Railroad Station** (Main and Vernon streets, 802–257–0124), are organs made by Jacob Estey, whose 1855 company became the country's largest manufacturer of pipe organs. Seven of the Estey factory buildings stand on Birge Street. The collections in the **Brooks Memorial Library** (224 Main Street, 802–254–5290) include nineteenth-century Vermont arts and crafts, paintings, and furniture.

Brattleboro cultivated artistic and literary talent. Rudyard Kipling built a house (private) in nearby **Dummerston,** where he lived from 1892 to 1896 and wrote *The Jungle Book* and *Captains Courageous.* Accomplished natives included Richard Morris Hunt, the society architect who designed some of the most opulent mansions

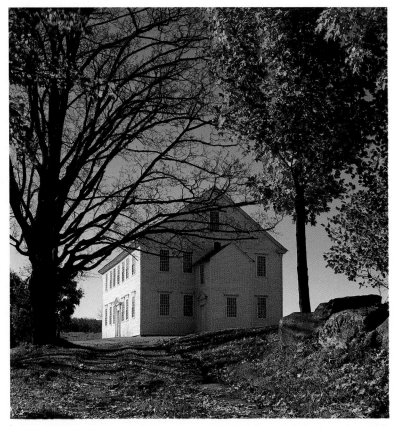

The severe 1781 Rockingham meetinghouse, north of Bellows Falls, is the earliest public building that survives in nearly original condition in Vermont.

of the Gilded Age, and his brother, William Morris Hunt, a noted portrait painter. (The brothers sometimes shared clients, one designing their palatial houses, the other painting their portraits.)

Another Brattleboro-born architect, William Rutherford Mead, joined in partnership with Charles McKim and Stanford White in 1879 to create the famous firm of McKim, Mead & White. Mead's older brother, Larken G. Mead, Jr., was a sculptor who designed the figures on Abraham Lincoln's tomb in Springfield, Illinois, a statue of Ethan Allen for the Vermont state capitol, another statue of Allen for the national Capitol, and the tomb monument for the robber baron Jim Fisk, who is buried in Brattleboro.

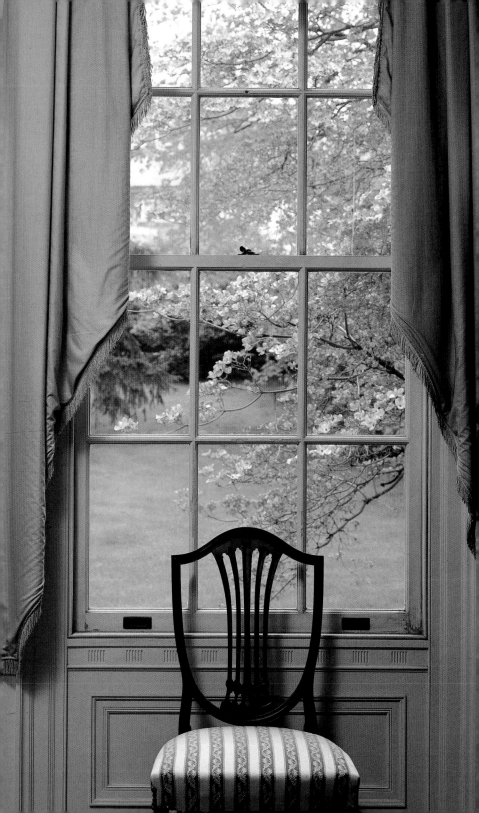

PORTSMOUTH
AND
SOUTHEASTERN
NEW
HAMPSHIRE

OPPOSITE: *Of all the houses in Portsmouth in the late eighteenth century, George Washington claimed that Colonel John Langdon's ". . . may be esteemed the first."*

"Air pure and salubrious; the country pleasant, having some high hills; the rivers well stored with fish . . . meadows full of timber-trees"—thus did an explorer glowingly describe the land that would become New Hampshire. The pure air apparently did prove salubrious to the settlers, often said to be pugnacious and the toughest of New England. New Hampshire is known as the Granite State not just for the plentiful bedrock, but for the character of its people, who, early on, survived more than their share of disillusion as they discovered the harsh truth behind the optimistic promises of sea captains and entrepreneurs.

The European settlement of New Hampshire began at the mouth of the Piscataqua River, which had been explored, on separate occasions, by Martin Pring (in 1603), Samuel de Champlain (1605), and Captain John Smith (1614). All found the spot suitable for settlement—Pring noted its "goodly groves and woods and sundry sorts of beasts." The first settlers were not seekers of religious or social freedom, but colonists dispatched from England by merchants to establish a profitable trade in furs and fish. In 1620 Sir Ferdinando Gorges persuaded royal officials to create a Council of New England that would control the territory between the fortieth and forty-eighth parallels. The Council granted patents to many commercial ventures, notably three run by Gorges, by David Thomson, and by Sir John Mason. In 1623 Thomson himself led a small group of about a dozen settlers to Odiorne's Point on the Piscataqua, only to find that he had vastly overestimated the ease of life in New England. A man who visited Odiorne's Point in 1624 wrote a sarcastic letter back to England: "I will not tell you that you may smell the corn fields before you see the land, neither must men think that corn doth grow naturally (or on trees), nor will the deer come when they are called or stand still and look on a man until he shoots him . . . which is no truer than that the fowles will present themselves to you with spits through them." Thomson left after four years for Boston, where he died.

New Hampshire owes its name to another of its early would-be developers, John Mason, who obtained a patent to the land between the Merrimack and the Piscataqua Rivers in 1629. He never laid eyes on it, but named the region after his home county of Hampshire. (The boundaries of his patent more or less define New Hampshire's present eighteen-mile-long coastline.) Mason and Gorges founded the Laconia Company to establish settlements along the Piscataqua and trade with the Indians for furs. When no

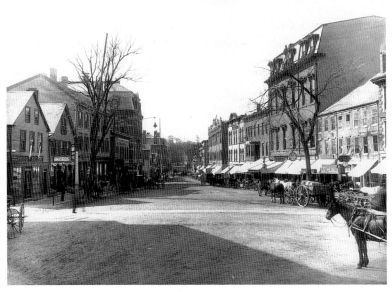

An early photograph of Congress Street, Portsmouth, between 1890 and 1895. Once a residential area, the street succumbed to commercial interests after the Civil War.

profits ensued the merchants ordered the settlers to switch to fishing; but the colony still struggled. Just as the colonists were hoping for a fresh infusion of cash, Mason died, and the Laconia Company was subsequently dissolved. Some of the Piscataqua settlers dispersed to Maine and Massachusetts, but a group at Strawbery Banke, the future Portsmouth, hung on and thrived.

The Piscataqua settlers built squared-log cabins, simple meeting houses that doubled as town hall and church, and mills to saw wood and grind grain. The lumbermen among them harvested the forests and sold valuable white pine timber to carpenters and shipbuilders in the coastal towns. Shippers exported the timber, and fur pelts, in an increasingly profitable trade with Britain and the West Indies.

Until 1675 there were only four towns in New Hampshire—Portsmouth, Dover, Exeter, and Hampton. In 1641 Massachusetts Bay Colony asserted its control over them. In 1679 New Hampshire was split off as a separate colony; briefly came under Massachusetts rule again; and was permanently separated in 1692. However, both colonies were ruled by a single governor until 1741.

New Hampshire's growth was slow in the seventeenth and early eighteenth centuries, hindered in large part by the resistance of the Indians to white encroachment. Incited by the French, Abenaki and Pennacook Indians killed many settlers along the Cocheco River in 1689 and at Salmon Falls and Exeter the following year. In the 1690s Portsmouth and Dover were repeatedly raided. This stage of the fighting ended with a treaty in 1713, but the fighting was renewed in "Governor Dummer's War" of the 1720s. Intent upon driving the Indians out once and for all, the provincial government offered high bounties to Indian hunters who could present a scalp. The grim policy worked: by 1730 there were few natives left in the Piscataqua and lower Merrimack regions to contest white settlement.

Around that time an important new group of settlers arrived. Several hundred Scotch-Irish Presbyterians, originally invited to settle in Massachusetts, opted for southern New Hampshire when they found that the Puritans expected them to convert to Congregationalism. They settled along the Merrimack Valley, founded the town of Londonderry, and prospered from the home manufacture of very high-quality linen. In the mid-1700s prosperity was spreading across the colony. Agriculture flourished, and was given an additional boost by the French and Indian War, when New Hampshire farms profited from sales to the British army. Meanwhile, Portsmouth merchants carried on a lucrative business in lumber and, particularly, in selling pine masts.

New Hampshire's highly disputed border with Massachusetts was finalized in 1741, but a further ambiguity remained to the west. Governor Benning Wentworth granted lands on the western side of the Connecticut River—territory, known as the New Hampshire Grants, that is now Vermont. By 1764 Wentworth had granted 131 towns across the river, only to have New York assert its claim to the region and begin granting towns. The confusion of claims and grants was not sorted out until Vermont was admitted as a state in 1783.

No Revolutionary War battles were fought in New Hampshire, but the colony provided two of the Revolution's important military leaders, John Stark and John Sullivan. The latter was one of the commanders in a pre-Revolutionary raid on Fort William and Mary, outside Portsmouth, in which the Americans, without firing a shot, made off with a large amount of supplies. In the war itself Sullivan commanded forces at battles in Pennsylvania and Rhode

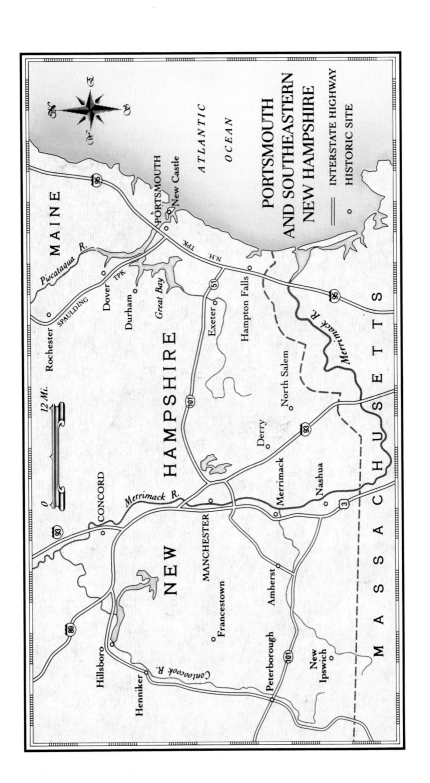

PORTSMOUTH
AND SOUTHEASTERN
NEW HAMPSHIRE

—— INTERSTATE HIGHWAY
○ HISTORIC SITE

MAINE

ATLANTIC

OCEAN

PORTSMOUTH
New Castle

Piscataqua R.

SPAULDING

Rochester

Dover TPK

Durham

Great Bay

N.H. TPK

Exeter

Hampton Falls

Merrimack R.

North Salem

NEW HAMPSHIRE

12 Mi.

0

CONCORD

Merrimack R.

Derry

Merrimack

Nashua

MASSACHUSETTS

MANCHESTER

Francestown

Amherst

Peterborough

New
Ipswich

Contoocook R.

Henniker

Hillsboro

Island, and conducted a controversial "search-and-destroy" campaign against the Iroquois in New York. Stark, whom the military historian John Elting described as a combination of "New England cantankerousness with Scots-Irish contentiousness," played a large role in the Battle of Bunker Hill in Boston. In that contest the British succeeded in ousting the Americans from their fortification, but at a terrible cost. Having ordered his men to march to Bunker Hill at a regular pace despite a heavy British bombardment, Stark was urged by one of his officers to quicken the pace. In response, as the officer later recalled, "With a look peculiar to himself, he fixed his eyes on me and observed with great composure—'Dearborn, one fresh man in action is worth ten fatigued.'" Stark is also remembered for a remark to his men before the Battle of Bennington in New York: "There, my boys, are your enemies—We'll beat them before night, or Molly Stark will be a widow."

New Hampshire's role in the ratification of the Constitution was the decisive one. It was the ninth state to vote its approval, providing the two-thirds majority needed for ratification. At the birth of the republic New Hampshire was itself a house divided—the old colonial towns along the coast and just inland were isolated from the settlements on the Merrimack and the Connecticut, and from the northern frontier. In addition, the Portsmouth merchants were distrusted by the farmers of the interior. Sectional tensions and jealousies were such that the state could not decide on the location of its capital until 1806.

One of the country's most important political figures of the nineteenth century, Daniel Webster, was born in New Hampshire in 1782. After attending Phillips Exeter Academy and Dartmouth College, Webster began a law practice first in Boscawen, then in Portsmouth. As counsel to many corporations, he became rich. He represented Massachusetts in the U.S. House and Senate, and served as Secretary of State under presidents Harrison, Tyler, and Fillmore. A lifelong defender of the Union, and a superlative speaker, he became a Northern hero. In his January 1850 debates with Senator Hayne of South Carolina he attacked the states' rights theory with the memorable phrase, "Liberty and Union, now and forever, one and inseparable." However, his willingness to compromise on the slavery issue was not popular in New England.

The state remained largely agricultural in the first half of the 1800s, but by the mid 1800s thousands of farmers were abandoning their rocky fields for richer lands in the West. In the 1860s the state's population actually began to shrink. After the Civil War, industry surged as agriculture declined markedly (in the middle decades of the century the acreage under cultivation fell by 20 percent). Mills produced miles of woolen and cotton goods every day, and shoe factories operated in overdrive. The old colonial towns of Dover and Exeter, as well as newer settlements such as Keene and Nashua, grew into small mill cities.

The behemoth of New Hampshire industry was Manchester, site of the massive Amoskeag Manufacturing Company operations, which produced mainly cotton cloth but also machinery, locomotives, fire engines, and other items. As were Lowell and Lawrence farther down the Merrimack River in Massachusetts, Manchester was completely a company town, owned by Bostonians. Virtually all aspects of life in the town were determined by the company's planners. A strike in 1922, followed by several years of declining profits, led to the closing of the huge Amoskeag mills. New Hampshire's other mills were also closing, faced with competition from the South. Agriculture also continued its decline in the early decades of the twentieth century: by the 1930s only a little over ten percent of the populace was involved in farming. The economic decline began to reverse itself, however, in the 1960s, with a boom in recreation and manufacturing.

New Hampshire's historic heritage is reflected in well-planned towns and the formal designs of their churches, government buildings, and private houses—New Hampshire's early Colonial and Federal architecture ranks with the finest in New England. And its old mill buildings, in such towns as Salmon Falls, Dover, and Newmarket, often made of native brick that ranged from salmon to dark red in color, are landmarks as important to New Hampshire's past as the celebrated frame houses and spired churches.

This chapter covers the southeastern portion of New Hampshire, focussing on the original colonial settlements and on the manufacturing centers along the Merrimack. It begins in Portsmouth, and traces a loop through Nashua and Manchester, detouring briefly to the west, and ending with Concord.

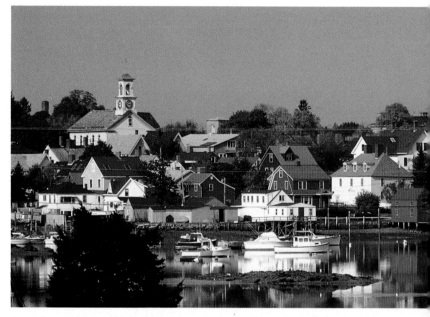

Located at the mouth of the Piscataqua River, on the Atlantic coast, Portsmouth became a

PORTSMOUTH

Located at the mouth of the Piscataqua River, one of the finest natural harbors on the east coast, Portsmouth was preeminent in the economic and political affairs of colonial New Hampshire. The first settlements, funded by English merchants and led by John Mason and Sir Ferdinando Gorges, were established in the 1620s and 1630s. The company's high hopes for making a quick profit from the sale of furs and fish were not realized. Mason wrote, "I have disbursed a great deal of money in the plantation, and never received one penny." After Mason's death in 1635 the company ceased to support its operations on the Piscataqua; some settlers returned to England, some dispersed to other points on the New England coast, but others decided to continue.

In its early years Portsmouth was a refuge for religious dissenters and common criminals from Puritan Massachusetts, whose authorities complained that the settlement attracted "desperately wicked" characters and welcomed "all such lewd persons as fled from us to them." John Winthrop accused one colonial leader of living "very wickedly in whoredom, drunkenness and quarelling."

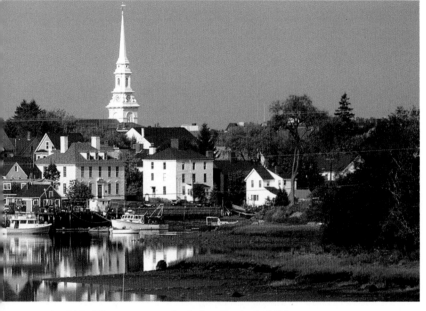

major shipbuilding center soon after its founding in the 1620s.

Able-bodied workers, regardless of religious beliefs or criminal pasts, were always in demand on the Piscataqua, a busy scene of shipbuilding from the 1630s into the nineteenth century. The profusion of timber in the forests that ran right to the sea enabled shipwrights to produce trading vessels far cheaper than European shipyards. By the early 1700s British shipyards were feeling a marked decline in their business, leading their shipwrights to emigrate to the colonies, including Portsmouth. Timber was also shipped to the British colonies in the West Indies, along with agricultural products. But among the most important of Portsmouth's commodities were masts for the Royal Navy. The nearby forests produced straight, tall pines — 3 to 6 feet in diameter and up to 200 feet in height — ideally suited for masts. As these behemoths took five to ten centuries to reach that height and girth, they were not a readily renewable resource and had to be harvested with care. Royal officials scoured the woods, placing the king's mark on mast trees and imposing heavy fines on anyone who felled one without authorization. Profits from the sale of masts, ships, fish, furs, and other goods created a wealthy trading class in Portsmouth.

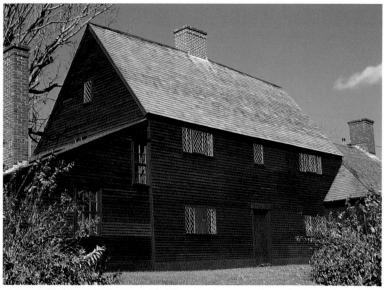

The seventeenth-century Richard Jackson House.

A tight little aristocracy of loyalists revolved around the royal governor. John Adams referred to "the pomps and vanities and ceremonies of that little world, Portsmouth." But the middle class of tradesmen and artisans, as well as the laboring class were firmly in support of independence. Although the Revolution destroyed Portsmouth's trade with England and the West Indies, business subsequently revived, and the town enjoyed several decades of prosperity. Portsmouth declined as fortunes were being made from manufacturing along the rivers of the interior.

Despite an 1813 fire that destroyed many of the oldest buildings, Portsmouth preserves handsome vestiges of its eighteenth- and early-nineteenth-century heyday.

Richard Jackson House

The state's oldest residence surviving in its original form, the Richard Jackson House is a weathered saltbox named for the shipwright who built it ca. 1664. His descendants lived here for nearly three centuries, adding a lean-to on one side and a wrap-around addition on the other. The central, oldest portion of the house is immediately recognizable by its seventeenth-century windows, which have been reconstructed and fitted with leaded glass.

The old-style windows are much smaller than those in the additions. The house, a study property of the Society for the Preservation of New England Antiquities, is not furnished.

LOCATION: Northwest Street. HOURS: By appointment. FEE: Yes. TELEPHONE: 617–227–3956.

Wentworth-Coolidge Mansion

This house was the seaside home of the first royal governor, Benning Wentworth (his term was from 1741 to 1766), who wrote "The place of my residence is within a mile of . . . the harbor . . . and no vessel can come into port without coming into my sight, which . . . has contributed in great measure to the chastity of the port." The governor's brother, Mark, carried on a brisk business in masts, selling them to all comers "at his own price." One large parlor was used as the council chamber for the provincial government. The fireplace in that room is flanked by a sculptured pair of comely women with half-bare breasts. Some original Wentworth pieces are in the house: a punch bowl (invitations to the house always mentioned a toast to the king's health), some Chinese export porcelain, and a late-eighteenth-century spinet. The wallpaper in the parlor and a bed chamber is original, a 1740s pattern put up in the 1750s;

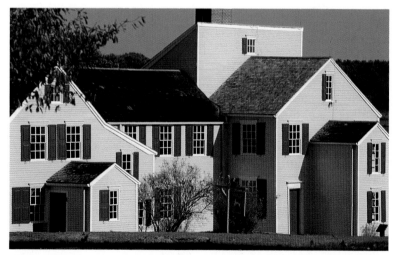

The Wentworth-Coolidge Mansion, home of New Hampshire's first royal governor, Benning Wentworth, in the 1750s. It is one of the few colonial governors' residences to survive unchanged.

the old colors, gold and crimson, of the costly flocked damask paper have faded. The lilacs on the grounds were the first in the country—brought by the governor from England.

In 1885 the house was purchased by J. Templeman Coolidge (no relation to the president), whose father-in-law, the eminent historian Francis Parkman, came to the house in the summer to write. One room has been furnished to the period of the 1880s. The exterior colors—dark mustard and dark green—were chosen in the nineteenth century.

LOCATION: Little Harbor Road. HOURS: Memorial Day through mid-June: 10–5 Saturday–Sunday; mid-June through August: 10–5 Daily. FEE: Yes. TELEPHONE: 603–436–6607.

MacPheadris-Warner House

Portsmouth's oldest brick residence, this three-story, fourteen-room house was built ca. 1716 by John Drew for Captain Archibald MacPheadris, who married into the Wentworth family. The bulk of the house—the red brick walls are eighteen inches thick—is lightened by the doorway and windows, perfectly ordered in the Georgian style. The roof has been remodeled; it was once two parallel gables, in an M shape.

The house's remarkable feature is the painted murals in its stair hall. Dating to about 1720, they may be the oldest such paintings in the country still in their original setting. The subject matter of the murals is puzzling in its variety: They depict a British soldier on horseback; two Mohawk Indians (these portraits were apparently not made from life but were copied from engravings made in England when four Mohawks visited the queen); the biblical episode of Abraham's intended sacrifice of his son Isaac, interrupted by the appearance of an angel; and an allegorical scene of hawks attacking a chicken. The murals, covered with wallpaper, were discovered in 1852 and restored several times, most recently in 1988. A ceiling mural may be hidden under a coat of paint.

The house preserves some original family furnishings, such as a set of six chairs made about 1810, books from the 1740s, a coverlet of the 1760s, and a silk dress given to Sarah Warner by the wife of John Wentworth, the royal governor.

LOCATION: 150 Daniel Street. HOURS: June through mid-October: 10–4:30 Tuesday–Saturday. FEE: Yes. TELEPHONE: 603–436–5909.

Moffatt-Ladd House

This three-story Georgian residence, topped by a captain's walk, was built in 1763 by John Moffatt and occupied by the same family until 1913. Because two inventories were made of the objects in the house, in 1768 and 1786, this is one of the best-documented Colonial residences in the state. It is furnished with eighteenth- and early-nineteenth-century items, many of them original to the house, such as silver, jewelry, clothing (including wedding dresses), family portraits (one by Gilbert Stuart), and eight samplers. A set of Chinese Chippendale chairs, bench, and settee on display was purchased by the Moffatts at an auction of the belongings of Governor John Wentworth. The carving on the staircase is especially fine. The garden at the rear of the house retains its nineteenth-century arrangement, with arbors and beehives. Also on the grounds are a coach house and counting house (the family was in the shipping business), displaying shipping artifacts, a telescope, and an early wall safe.

LOCATION: 154 Market Street. HOURS: Mid-June through mid-October: 10–4 Monday–Saturday, 2–5 Sunday. FEE: Yes. TELEPHONE: 603–436–8221.

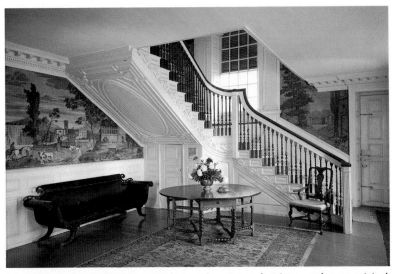

The 1763 Moffatt-Ladd House contains an elegant carved staircase and many original furnishings.

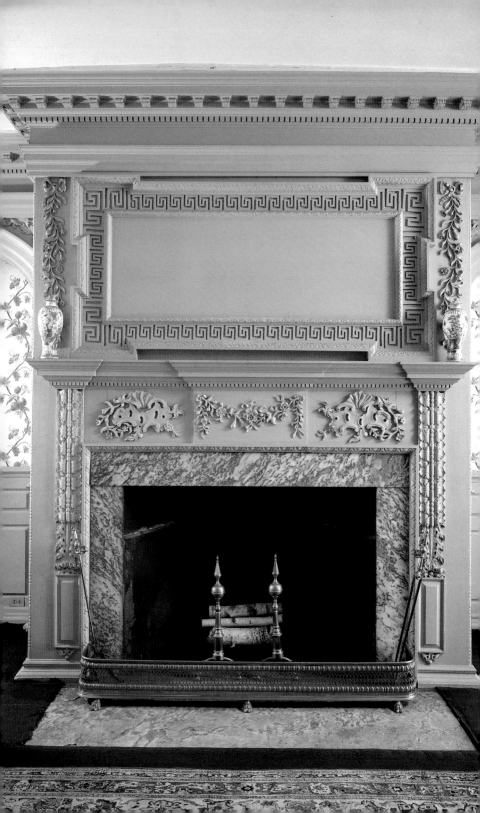

Governor John Langdon House

John Langdon was one of the most prominent New Hampshire men of his day. He served as president of the state, as its governor, and as a U.S. senator. He made his fortune during the Revolution in shipbuilding and privateering, thanks in part to his position as the government's agent for procuring new ships and for distributing the goods captured by privateers. It is often noted that he financed several military campaigns out of his own pocket—but he was always careful about getting repaid. In 1783 work began on this grand residence.

The house was admired by George Washington, an astute judge of architecture and the status it implied, who was a guest here in 1789. In his diary he wrote that among Portsmouth's houses, "Col. Langdon's may be esteemed the first." Langdon's house clearly was a statesman's, from the monumental exterior enhanced by gardens to the exquisitely carved interior woodwork. The drawing room fireplace is a particularly fine example of late-eighteenth-century woodworking. Langdon descendants have furnished the house with antiques of the period; it is now a property of the Society for the Preservation of New England Antiquities.

LOCATION: Off Route 95. HOURS: June through mid-October: 12–5 Wednesday–Sunday. FEE: Yes. TELEPHONE: 617–227–3956.

John Paul Jones House

While his ship *America* was being readied in October and November 1782, John Paul Jones stayed in the commodious house of Sarah Purcell, who was operating it as an inn after the death of her husband. The master carpenter who built it in 1758 may have been the mulatto Hopestill March, renowned in the Portsmouth area for his fine gambrel-roofed houses. The house and its exhibits are the property of the Portsmouth Historical Society.

LOCATION: 43 Middle Street. HOURS: July through August: 10–4:15 Monday–Saturday, 1–4:15 Sunday. FEE: Yes. TELEPHONE: 603–436–8420.

OPPOSITE: *Exquisitely carved interior woodwork graces the Governor John Langdon House, built in 1784 by the wealthy Portsmouth merchant and statesman.*

Rundlet-May House

A farm boy named James Rundlet moved from Exeter to Portsmouth in the 1790s and amassed a comfortable fortune as a merchant. To proclaim his success in this town of aristocratic airs, he built an elegant three-story house with extensive gardens on an artificial terrace eight feet above the level of Middle Street. Located in a then-unfashionable, indeed, almost empty, part of town, the house stirred envy and disdain in the hearts of some townspeople, who predicted that the Rundlets would fall as fast as they had risen. But the house remained in the family for four generations until it was given to the Society for the Preservation of New England Antiquities. Rundlet's careful accounts show that he imported wallpaper from England but preferred locally made furniture, resulting in the house's fine collection of Portsmouth's Federal furniture.

LOCATION: 364 Middle Street. HOURS: June through mid-October: 12–5 Wednesday–Sunday. FEE: Yes. TELEPHONE: 617–227–3956.

The **Wentworth-Gardner House** (140 Mechanic Street, 603–436–4406) is another of Portsmouth's fine Georgian residences, built by Elizabeth Wentworth as a wedding present for her son, Thomas. It has eleven fireplaces and is celebrated for its hand-painted wallpapers and graceful carvings—woodworkers are said to have labored on cornices and pilasters the entire year of 1760. The pineapple within the entrance pediment is a symbol of welcome.

Portsmouth's 1804 **Athenaeum** (9 Market Square, 603–431–2538), housed in a fine Federal building, contains collections of books, early manuscripts, and other historical documents; portraits of important local figures (two painted by Samuel F. B. Morse); Indian artifacts; ships' models; and curiosities from around the world brought home by seamen.

The **Portsmouth Public Library** (8 Islington Street, 603–431–2007) was built as a private boys' school, the Portsmouth Academy, in 1809. Once thought to be the work of Charles Bulfinch, the building was designed by James Nutter, who also did the interior of St. John's Church. The brick structure has housed the library since the 1890s.

The brick **St. John's Church** (101 Chapel Street), built in 1807, stands on the site of its 1732 predecessor, Queen's Chapel. Portsmouth's first church, also Anglican, was built a century earlier at the southwest corner of Court and Pleasant streets. After the Revolution, Queen's Chapel was rechristened St. John's; it was de-

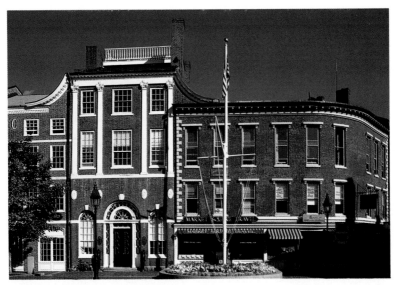

The 1804 Portsmouth Athenaeum contains a variety of curiosities brought home by seafaring adventurers and traders.

stroyed by fire on Christmas Eve 1806. Surviving the blaze are the altar, now known as the Credence Table, in the chancel; the baptismal font; and the box pews in the south gallery. The church's Brattle organ, imported to Massachusetts from England before 1708, is the oldest operating pipe organ in the United States. Plaques on some pews commemorate former parishioners such as Daniel Webster. On display is a rare 1717 Vinegar Bible, so named for a misprint of "vineyard." Royal Governor Benning Wentworth is buried in the churchyard.

The 1826 **South Church** (292 State Street) was designed and constructed by Jonathan Folsom, a local contractor, church builder, and stonemason. Built in massive proportions with two-foot-thick granite walls and in Greek Revival style, this building is one of the first in New England to utilize a truss roof and hung ceiling.

Strawbery Banke

Settled in 1630, this ten-acre site was established as a plantation compound by the English. Originally named for the abundance of wild berries growing along the shores of the Piscataqua River, the settlement was renamed Portsmouth in 1653 and became a thriving waterfront neighborhood during the seventeenth and eighteenth

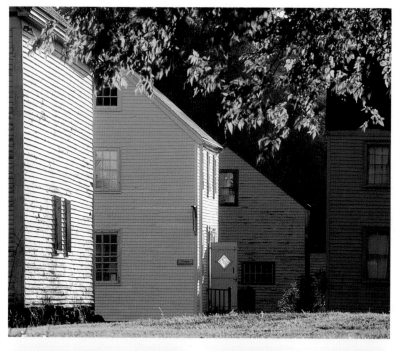

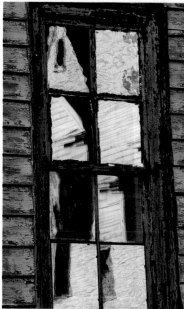

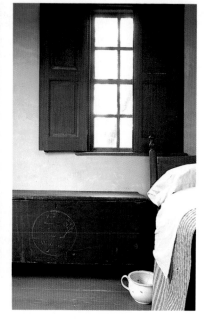

centuries. Rescued from many years of neglect, the area is now an outdoor history museum, with ongoing archaeological excavations. Collections include ceramics and other decorative objects, household furnishings and implements, artifacts from the settlement's earliest period, and books and other scholarly materials relating to the history of the compound. Functioning crafts shops include a cooper at the **Dinsmore Shop,** a weaver at **Shapley-Cotton House,** potters at **Cotton Tenant House,** a cabinetmaker at **Peacock House,** and boat builders at the **Boat Shop.** An exhibition on early tools and craftmanship is in the **Lowd House.** Seventeenth-century construction techniques are on view in **Sherburne House.**

There are forty-two historic houses from the 1600s to the 1900s, most of which stand on their original foundations. Seven are furnished to illustrate different time periods in Strawbery Banke's history: the 1850s **Goodwin Mansion,** home of Governor Ichabod Goodwin; **Chase House** (1790–1830); **Wheelwright House** (1780s); **Walsh House** (spanning 1790–1830); **Pitt Tavern** (ca. 1800); the **Thomas Bailey Aldrich House,** a 1908 restoration of a mid-nineteenth-century home; and the **Drisco House,** in which domestic life in the 1790s is contrasted with that of the 1950s. Gardens include the vegetable and herb beds of the 1695 **Sherburne House.** The elaborate **Victorian Garden** of the Goodwin Mansion, the special domain of Mrs. Sarah Parker Rice Goodwin, is planted today according to her detailed 1862 diaries and sketches.

LOCATION: Marcy Street. HOURS: May through October: 10–5 Daily. FEE: Yes. TELEPHONE: 603–433–1100.

The most historically significant commercial buildings in Portsmouth are the wood-frame and brick warehouses along the waterfront. While outfitting the *Ranger,* John Paul Jones used the **Sheafe Warehouse** (Mechanic Street at Prescott Park). The warehouse, framed and shingled about 1705, is now a museum of folk art, featuring wooden sculptures of wildlife and boats and a replica of a gundalow, a flat-bottomed boat used to transport cargo on the river during the nineteenth century.

NEW CASTLE

New Castle, off the coast on Great Island, was first settled in 1623 and received its royal charter in 1693. An early provincial capital, the town was scattered with simple fishermen's cottages as well as

OPPOSITE: *Strawbery Banke, a ten-acre outdoor history museum commemorating Portsmouth's long history, re-creates the appearance of a colonial settlement.*

the elegant houses of the Frost, Pepperrell, and Jaffrey families. English loyalists realized the island's strategic importance early on and built a redoubt on a rocky point there in 1632. A timber blockhouse was added in 1666; in 1692, cannon and military stores were brought in from England and a breastwork erected to protect them. The fort was named Fort William and Mary in 1694, in honor of the king and queen, and was the scene of one of the first overt acts leading to the Revolution: On December 13, 1774, Paul Revere brought the message from Boston that the British were on their way with reinforcements; the following day, the Portsmouth colonials (led by Major John Langdon) raided the fort and removed approximately five tons of gunpowder from the magazines. The next day, Major John Sullivan led them in a second raid. Some of the guns and powder taken from the fort were sent on to Patriots at Bunker Hill. New Hampshire gave the facility to the United States government in 1791; the fort was renamed **Fort Constitution** five years later. The site consists of the ruins of the seventeenth-century walls and later constructions.

A very different attraction in New Castle is **Wentworth-by-the-Sea** (Wentworth Road, private), a resort hotel built at the height of the Victorian era. Since 1874, its verandas and mansard towers have looked out to the **Isles of Shoals.** Four of the nine isles belong to New Hampshire, five to Maine. Dotted with weathered cottages, stone churches, fishing shacks, and inns, the rocky little islands were strategically important to colonists, pirates, and fishermen.

Toward the coast from Exeter, **Hampton** and **Hampton Falls** (incorporated separately in 1726) preserve many eighteenth- and nineteenth-century houses along and off Route 1. At the center of Hampton Falls is the **First Congregational Society Unitarian Church**, built in 1843 in the form of a small Greek temple.

EXETER

Exeter lies on the Squamscott River at the southeastern point of an irregular box shape it forms with Dover, Portsmouth, and Hampton. Together the towns share New Hampshire's richest Revolutionary history. Like Dover, Exeter is inland, but only just, and its access to the sea bestows a coastal air. It was founded in 1638 by Reverend John Wheelwright, who was expelled from Boston by the

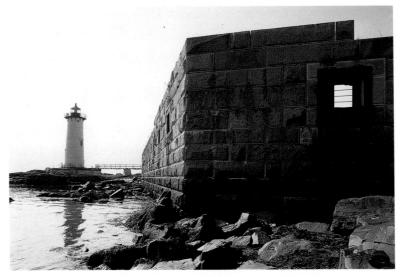

Fort Constitution, originally named Fort William and Mary, the site of one of the first overt acts leading to the Revolution.

Massachusetts General Court for "contempt and sedition." His "sedition" had been to publicly disagree with the Puritan church on a theological matter. Wheelwright and some followers secured a large tract of land here (thirty miles square) from the Squamscott Indians and established an independent government. In 1643, when the majority of the townspeople decided to seek annexation by Massachusetts, Wheelwright left for Maine.

As the town grew in the eighteenth century, prospering from fishing and lumbering, it retained its independent spirit. Like many coastal towns, Exeter profited from the sale of masts—legally to the Royal Navy and illegally to every other shipbuilder. When royal agents visited Exeter in 1734 to reassert the official monopoly on the colony's masts, the townspeople burned the ship. As the Revolution neared, it was common to see British officials burned in effigy on the Exeter green. In 1775, New Hampshire moved its capital from loyalist Portsmouth to more patriotic Exeter. In 1776 the Provincial Congress adopted the first independent state constitution, making New Hampshire the first of the thirteen colonies. Throughout the Revolution, the state's Legislative Assembly met at the **Exeter Town House,** its site marked at Court and Front streets. The current **Town Hall** (Front Street) dates from 1855.

Gilman Garrison House

For decades after its construction in the 1650s or 1660s, this fortified refuge was a garrison, built by John Gilman near his sawmill. The door of the house was protected by a portcullis, metal bars that could be dropped in front of the door to bar entrance. The house was constructed of massive logs, some of which show the marks of Gilman's sawmill. One of the first-floor rooms was a fort within a fort—its ceiling is as thick as its walls—so that if attackers managed to break into the house the defenders would have a fall-back. Peter Gilman, grandson of John Gilman, was a brigadier general in the New Hampshire militia in the expedition against Crown Point in 1745. He made additions to the house in 1725 and again in the 1770s. His remodeling, in a more formal Georgian style, is in sharp contrast to the old portions of the house. The house, one of the oldest in New Hampshire, is a property of the Society for the Preservation of New England Antiquities.

LOCATION: 12 Water Street. HOURS: June through mid-October: 12–5 Tuesday, Thursday, Saturday, Sunday. FEE: Yes. TELEPHONE: 617–227–3956.

Cincinnati Hall

Also known as the **Ladd-Gilman House,** the 1721 building is owned by the New Hampshire chapter of the Society of the Cincinnati, a group composed of descendants of Revolutionary officers. The house, the state treasury from 1775 to 1782, displays an important collection of historical papers, including documents signed by Washington, Lafayette, and John Hancock. Memorabilia of the Gilman family and of others who served in the Revolution with them are also exhibited. Colonel Nicholas Gilman, Sr., was the treasurer and receiver general of the state in 1775. Captain Nicholas Gilman, Jr., held a high post on George Washington's staff and participated in many major campaigns of the war. The room used as the treasury during the Revolution is restored.

LOCATION: 1 Governor's Lane. HOURS: May through October: 12–5 Tuesday, 12–5 Sunday. FEE: Yes. TELEPHONE: 603–772–2622.

As trade and commerce quickened after the Revolution, **Front Street** became Exeter's fashionable address. A number of fine Federal houses survive along that tree-shaded street. Among them are the 1809 **George Sullivan's House** (4 Front Street), now converted to apartments and offices; the 1826 **Gardner House** (12 Front Street, private); and the 1815 **Perry-Dudley House** (14 Front Street, now offices). The Federal style gives way to the Greek Revival at number 81, the **Otis-Gorham House,** built in 1820 as a residence with office attached. Also on Front Street is Exeter's 1798 **Congregational Church** at number 21 and the 1831 **Granite Bank.** At **65 High Street,** where it was moved from beside the Town Hall, is an exceptionally handsome early-nineteenth-century house (private) designed by Ebenezer Clifford.

An important part of Exeter's post-Revolutionary development was **Phillips Exeter Academy,** founded in 1781 by John Phillips. Having joined his brother in endowing an academy in his hometown of Andover, Massachusetts, Phillips determined to do the same for his adopted Exeter. The college preparatory school's campus, composed of more than 100 buildings, lies on both sides of Front Street. All except one of the academy's buildings date to the late nineteenth or early twentieth century. The academy's ornate English Gothic church was built in 1897.

NORTH SALEM
America's Stonehenge

Once known as Mystery Hill, this thirty-acre archaeological site — dated to about 1000 B.C., it is among the oldest man-made complexes in North America — has confounded scholars and delighted other visitors. The stone slabs, chambers, tunnels, and wells seem to have been arranged as a great outdoor astronomical facility, used to observe stars and chart the seasons. Or it may have been used for other rituals: One slab, weighing nearly five tons and standing on stone legs, is known as the Sacrificial Table, etched with channels that might have conveyed blood into stone receptacles. Many guesses have been made about its builders, obviously strong, clever, and numerous: ancient Greeks or Phoenicians, medieval explorers, North American Indian tribes, aliens from another planet. In the nineteenth century, the stones may have been put to practical purposes — according to local legend, a cobbler who lived nearby used chambers in an elaborate liquor-distilling operation and to shelter runaway slaves.

OVERLEAF: *Most of the buildings at Phillips Exeter Academy date from the late nineteenth and early twentieth centuries.*

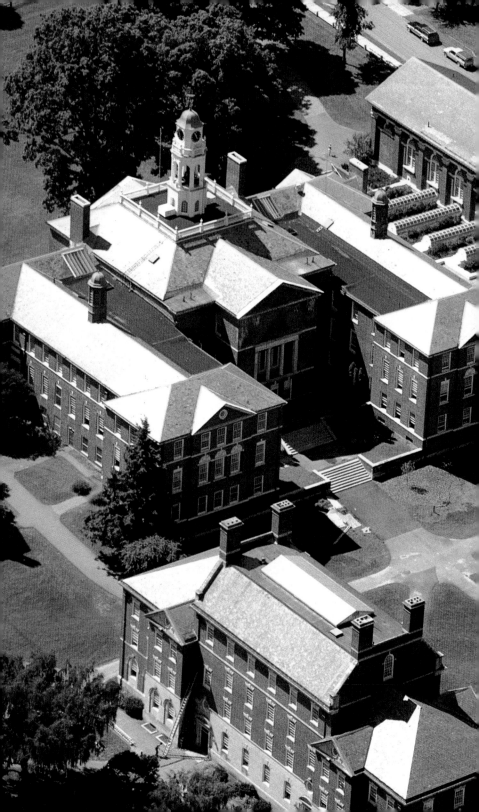

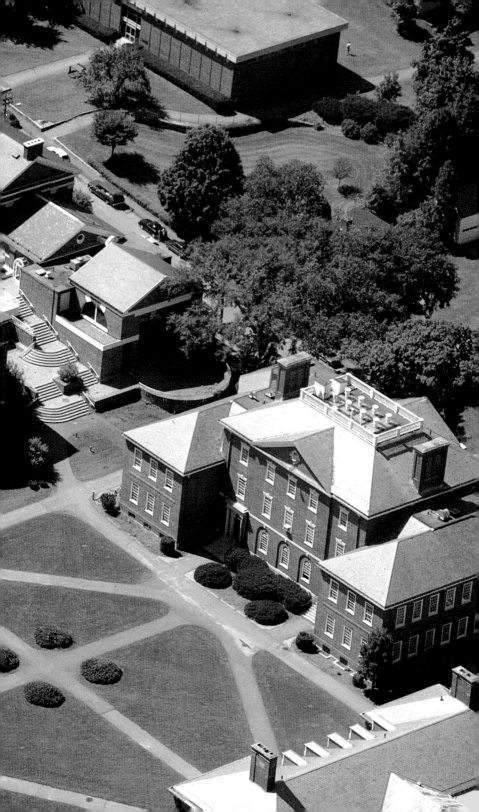

DERRY

Scotch-Irish families settled here, east of Beaver Brook, in the early 1700s. They cultivated potatoes, and their linen making was the first of Derry's manufacturing enterprises (later came shoes, woolens, and hats). Derry's **Pinkerton Academy** (Route 93), named for the Scotch-Irish family that founded it in 1814, remains a premier educational institution. The original wood-frame **Old Academy** was the school's sole building until 1887, when officials built a high-towered Romanesque companion next to it. Pinkerton's most famous alumnus is Admiral Alan B. Shepard, Jr. (class of 1940), the first American in space. Pinkerton's best-known teacher, on faculty in the early 1900s, was the poet Robert Frost. Born in California in 1874 to New Englanders, Frost moved back East with his family when he was 10 years old to live at the place, south of Derry, preserved as the **Robert Frost Farm** (off Route 28, 603–432–3091). "Stopping by Woods on a Snowy Evening" is one of the works Frost set in the Derry countryside.

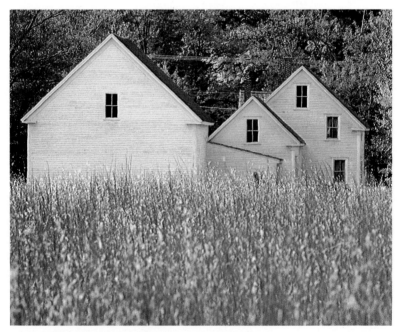

Home to Robert Frost from 1900 to 1911, this farm in Derry allowed the young poet the "time and seclusion" to develop his poetic voice.

MANCHESTER

The history of New Hampshire's largest city is interwoven with the textile industry on the Merrimack River. But long before the falls turned industrial wheels, Manchester was a gathering place for Algonquian Indians, who trapped and fished here. Early in the 1700s, Archibald Stark, the father of Revolutionary War general John Stark, bought land in Londonderry. Here his famous son, a Rogers' Ranger in the French and Indian War, was born in 1728, in the northwest section of Londonderry called Derryfield. A memorial to the hero stands in **Stark Park** on North River Road. Derryfield became Manchester in 1846.

After the Revolution a growing milling industry began to attract thousands of immigrants—French-Canadian, Greek, Polish, Italian, Turkish, and English. The **Amoskeag Manufacturing Company** grew out of a small mill built on Amoskeag Falls in 1805 by New Ipswich's Benjamin Prichard. It attracted investors in Boston and New York, who incorporated a new company in 1831. The red-brick mill buildings, put up between 1838 and 1910, stretch for a mile along the east bank of the Merrimack River in downtown Manchester. The grimness of the long brick walls is relieved somewhat by granite trim and by ornamented stair towers.

In the nineteenth century the Amoskeag company owned nearly all of the land in the city and in 1838 drew up a master plan for development. It built housing for its workers, gave land for churches and cultural centers, and regulated private development. In addition to its weekly output of 4 million yards of cloth, the company produced its own machinery, bricks, locomotives, fire engines, and, during the Civil War, muskets. By the beginning of the twentieth century, Amoskeag claimed to be the largest textile mill in the world, employing 17,000 people. But not even the great Amoskeag company was immune to the various factors that led to the demise of New England textile milling—a drop in demand for cotton with the coming of rayon in the 1920s, labor disputes, and competition from southern mills. In 1936, more than a century after it had opened, the Amoskeag Manufacturing Company filed for bankruptcy. But other manufacturing developed, some of it in heavy machinery, putting people back to work and the mill buildings back in use. Information on tours of the Amoskeag Mills is available at the **Manchester Historic Association** (129 Amherst Street, 603–622–7531).

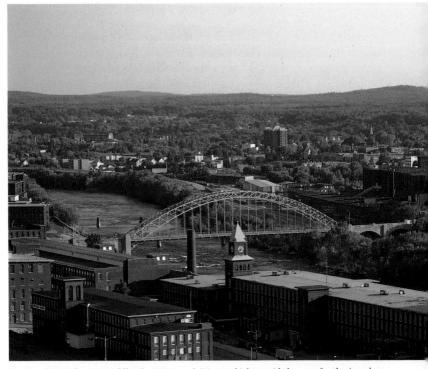

The city of Manchester straddles the Merrimack River, which provided power for the Amoskeag

Manchester's nineteenth-century prosperity is reflected in several impressive buildings, including its **City Hall,** an 1845 Gothic Revival edifice (Elm and Market streets); the towered, Romanesque **Webster Street Fire Station,** built in 1887 on Webster at Chestnut Street; and the 1874 **Ash Street School,** whose pair of mansard-roofed towers give it a storybook air (Ash at Bridge Street). **Grace Episcopal Church** (106 Lowell Street), designed in 1860 by Richard Upjohn, and the **Alpheus Gay House,** the 1870 villa of one of the city's prominent men (Myrtle and Beech), are also of note.

MERRIMACK

The Merrimack River meets the Souhegan below Manchester, and Merrimack, compared with its northern neighbor, developed modestly as a mill town. It was the hometown of Matthew Thornton, born in 1714, when Merrimack was known as Dunstable. Thornton, Revolutionary soldier and signer of the Declaration of Indepen-

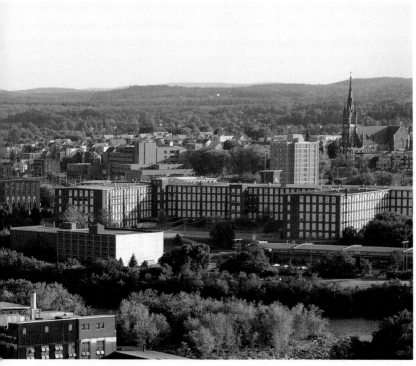

Mills, in the foreground.

dence, presided over the Provincial Congress in 1775. His grave **memorial** is across from the **Thornton homestead** (private) on Daniel Webster Highway in the Thornton's Ferry district.

NASHUA

A fur-trading post turned mill town, Nashua lies on the hilly western bank of the Merrimack. The Nashua River, which runs through the city, drove gristmills as early as 1700 and textile mills in the 1820s. The **Nashua Manufacturing Company,** a Romanesque complex of brick and stone, extends along the aptly named Water and Factory streets. Through the nineteenth century, Nashua developed other manufacturing industries, and the diversity of its international population matched that of Manchester.

Fine Victorian residences, all privately owned, may be seen on Concord Street: the **Shattuck-Tolles House** at number 65 and the **Elijah Shaw House** at number 85, both built in 1890; the 1879

Dana King House at number 47; the **Samuel Dearborn House** at number 6, built in 1886; and the **F. D. Cook House,** built in the Shingle style in 1889. The villa-style, 1856 **George Stark House,** at Concord and Manchester streets, now contains offices. Its wooden construction softens the Italianate styling, usually executed in stone. The white clapboard **Abbot-Spalding House** (5 Abbot Street, 603–883–0015), finished with red brick ends, was built by lawyer Daniel Abbot in 1804; it is owned by the Nashua Historical Society. Among the city's public buildings are the Romanesque **First Church,** erected in 1893 on Library Hill, and the **John H. Hunt Memorial Building,** built as the Main Street library in 1902. The **First Unitarian-Congregationalist Society** church, with a portico overlooking Concord and Grove streets, may be the work of architect Asher Benjamin, who in 1825 had been commissioned by the Nashua Manufacturing Company to lay out new city streets.

Heading northwest from Nashua, travelers dip into one green valley after another, white church steeples visible from one village to the next in **Hollis, Milford, Wilton,** and **Greenfield.**

Northeast from New Ipswich, Route 101 leads through a long valley that grew in population through the eighteenth century with the increasing stagecoach traffic on the Boston Post Road. In **Amherst,** near the Bedford border, is the **Birthplace of Horace Greeley,** a small one-story frame house (just off Route 101 on Horace Greeley Road, private). Greeley, the legendary newspaperman who founded the New York *Tribune* in 1841, was born here in 1811 and brought up on the Puritan simplicity and discipline he considered the great heritage of his home state. As a newspaperman he was a foe of slavery and an advocate of granting free land in the West to farmers and to new colleges. His name is forever linked with the phrase "Go West, young man, and grow up with the country," which appeared in his July 13, 1865, editorial in the *Tribune.* (Greeley had actually found those words in an 1851 editorial in an Indiana paper—he freely acknowledged his borrowing.) Greeley went on to become a congressman and presidential candidate. He ran against Grant in 1872 on the ticket of the newly formed Liberal Republican Party and garnered 2,800,000 votes, more than 40 percent.

OPPOSITE: *Nashua's 1893 First Church, a substantial example of the Romanesque style.*

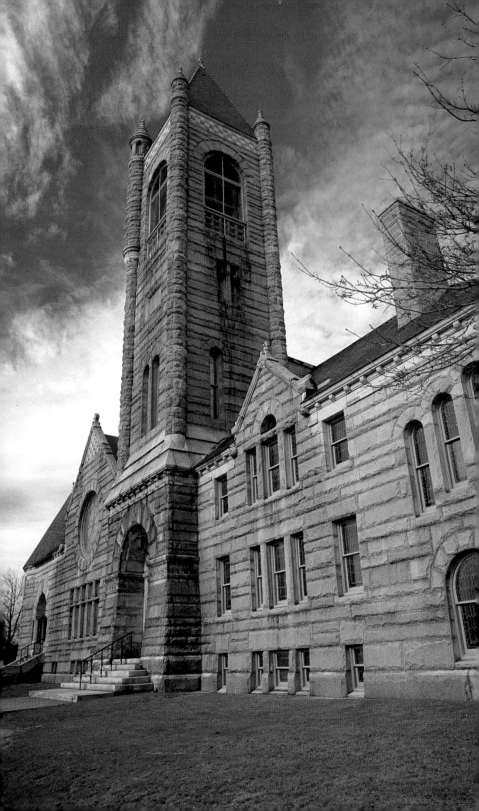

NEW IPSWICH

A group of settlers arrived here from Ipswich, Massachusetts, in 1738; by the end of the eighteenth century, the town had a population of about 1,000. Most of them were farmers, but factories turned out potash, linseed oil, glass, and other products. In 1803 a cotton mill, probably the first in the state, was built here; Benjamin Prichard, a carpenter who helped with its construction, later started the great textile factory on Amoskeag Falls in Manchester. In 1810, Peter Wilder brought in another local industry with his chair and stool factory. The 1875 **Columbian Mill** rises above the Souhegan, on a site of two earlier mills; the cotton-processing complex includes a picker house and storage facility.

Barrett House

One of New Ipswich's leading industrialists, Charles Barrett, gave his son this great hilltop estate as a wedding present. The property includes a three-story main house, a summer house, and extensive grounds. It is now administered by the Society for the Preservation of New England Antiquities. The facade of the three-story, Federal-style main house, built in 1800, features four pilasters and a handsome doorway topped by a pediment. Inside are many of the original furnishings given to the young Barretts by the bride's father, including portraits and musical instruments.

LOCATION: Main Street. HOURS: June through mid-October: 12–5 Thursday–Sunday. FEE: Yes. TELEPHONE: 617–227–3956.

FRANCESTOWN

Named for the wife of Governor John Wentworth, last royal governor of New Hampshire, Francestown was incorporated in 1752. The first and only industry to speak of was soapstone quarrying; an enormous deposit of the mineral was discovered by accident in 1794. Francestown soapstone was used in the manufacture of sinks, hearths, mantels, and water pipes. On the common, next to the **Old Meeting House,** is a **memorial** to Levi Woodbury (1789–1851), a Francestown native who served as state legislator, judge, governor, U.S. senator, treasury and naval secretary, and Supreme Court justice. Woodbury's **birthplace** (private), across the street, is in the Federal style, with pilastered doorways and elaborate stencilwork; among the eighteen rooms is a ballroom.

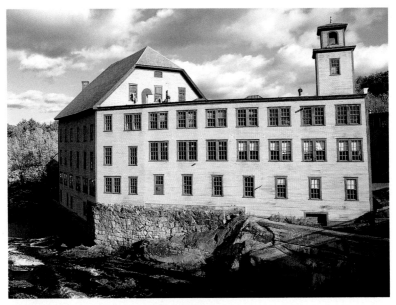

The nineteenth-century Contoocook Mills, Hillsboro.

HILLSBORO

This town, known primarily as the boyhood home of President Franklin Pierce, also has an industrial past. The **Contoocook Mills** (Bridge Street), begun in 1828 on the riverbank near the center of town, operated grist- and sawmills and cotton and wool manufacturing through the nineteenth century. The library and community center occupy the **Governor John B. Smith House** (School and Myrtle streets), a local landmark since its construction in 1892. Architectural details are intricate, from the molded chimney and irregular windows to the wooden carvings inside the house.

The Franklin Pierce Homestead

General Benjamin Pierce, Revolutionary War hero and twice governor of New Hampshire, finished his family's large, two-story Federal house below Hillsboro in 1804, just six weeks after the birth of his son on November 23. The general's son Franklin—the seventh of eight children—would become the fourteenth president of the United States and the only New Hampshire man to occupy the White House.

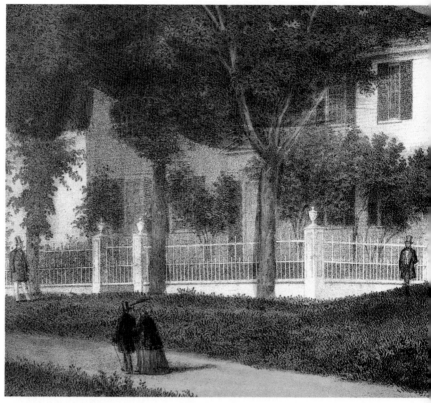

A Currier and Ives lithograph of the Franklin Pierce Homestead.

After studying law at Bowdoin College in Brunswick, Maine, Franklin returned to New Hampshire to join the ranks of the state's other political leaders—Daniel Webster, Isaac Hill, Levi Woodbury, Horace Greeley, and Salmon P. Chase, many of whom would visit the Hillsboro house. He won his first election at the age of 25, serving in the state legislature when his father was governor. At the outbreak of the Mexican War he enlisted in the state militia as a private, later being appointed colonel, and then general, by President Polk. He met Jefferson Davis at that time and formed a lifelong friendship with the future president of the Confederacy. The politics of the two were compatible—Pierce, in the rough political parlance of the day, was a "doughface," a northern man of southern principles. In 1852 a divided Democratic Party nominated him for president; his campaign biography was written by his

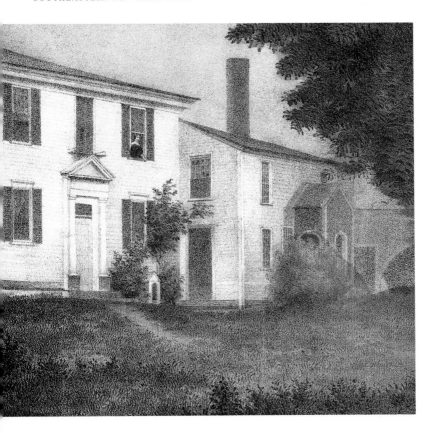

old friend from Bowdoin, Nathaniel Hawthorne. Pierce won, but his was not a popular presidency—one of his critics said that he managed to further divide not only North and South but also industry and agriculture, town and country. In 1854, as president, he signed the Kansas-Nebraska Act, which opened the territories north and west of Missouri to slavery.

The Pierce home, restored to the period of the late 1830s, is typical of Federal houses in this section of New Hampshire, only grander, with a ballroom, French scenic wallpaper depicting the Bay of Naples, and particularly handsome pedimented doorways.

LOCATION: Near the junction of routes 9 and 31 in Hillsboro. HOURS: June, September, October: 10–4 Friday–Saturday, 1–4 Sunday; July through August: 10–4 Saturday, 1–4 Sunday. FEE: Yes. TELEPHONE: 603–478–3165.

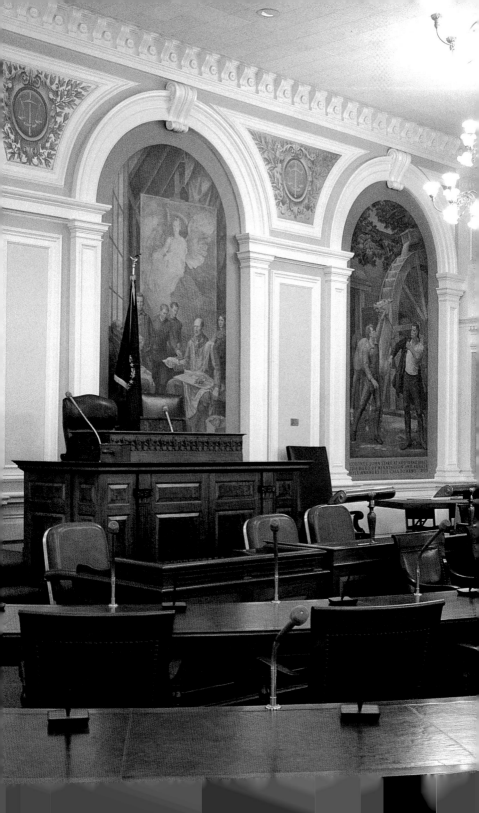

HENNIKER

The charming pirate tale of "Ocean-Born" Mary is told in this landlocked village. According to the story, Mary was born at sea to a couple emigrating from Ireland in 1720. Pirates captured their ship, then took kindly to the young parents and their baby girl. The pirate captain promised safe passage if they would name the child after his deceased wife, Mary. He gave the couple a bolt of brocaded silk, asking that the girl wear it on her wedding day. Years later, "Ocean-Born" Mary, who grew up in Londonderry, did indeed have her wedding gown made of the pirate captain's silk. She and her husband, James Wallace, moved to Henniker, where she died at the age of 94. She is buried in the cemetery behind the town hall.

CONCORD

First settled around 1733, Concord was originally named Rumford. The colonies of New Hampshire and Massachusetts had both issued grants to settlers in this place. This confusion of sovereignty wended its way through colonial and English courts until the king decided in 1741 that New Hampshire owned the town. Perhaps to symbolize that the dispute had been settled amicably, the town was renamed Concord.

State House

After the Revolution the state legislature met at various times in eight different towns, delaying designating a permanent capital because any choice would inevitably annoy one region of the state or another. In 1806, at last, Governor Langdon urged the legislature to settle at Concord. State records were transported to the town in 1808, but there was as yet no capitol, something of an embarrassment—in 1814 a committee pointed out to the legislature that New Hampshire was the only state that did not have a capitol building. The lack was soon remedied. The people of Concord donated land and granite, which was transported to a state prison where convicts worked it into blocks; the cut stone was then hauled to the building site in oxcarts. Despite the undoubted reluctance of the forced labor that produced the raw material, the

OPPOSITE: *The New Hampshire legislature still meets in its original chambers in the 1819 State House in Concord.*

foundations were pronounced to be "a specimen of workmanship, not deficient in beauty, and in strength not exceeded by any work of the kind" in the nation.

The original structure, completed in 1819, was a simple and dignified Federal design with a central pavilion flanked by wings and topped with a tower. It was enlarged and remodeled by the Boston architect Gridley J. F. Bryant in the 1860s. He added a third story and the mansard roof, as well as the two-story portico to the front, and replaced the tower with an octagonal, domed cupola, transforming the Federal building into a more stylish expression of the Second Empire mode. A 1910 addition by architects Peabody and Stearns doubled the amount of space in the building; this addition houses the executive chambers and legislative offices. After its early era of wandering the state, the legislature has exhibited a marked reluctance to change its quarters: It has met in the same room since 1819, a record unparalleled in the nation.

LOCATION: Main Street. HOURS: 8–4:30 Monday–Friday. FEE: None. TELEPHONE: 603–271–2154.

The **New Hampshire Historical Society Museum and Library** (30 Park Street, 603–225–3381) occupies a Neoclassical building of white granite, the gift of businessman and philanthropist Edward Tuck. On permanent display are a Concord coach and other examples of local craftsmanship. The museum frequently hosts traveling historical exhibits. One of the most famous artifacts of the Old West—the stagecoach—was a Concord product. Concord Coaches were manufactured by Abbot, Downing & Company at a factory (now demolished) on South Main Street, its spot marked by a plaque. They were a common sight in the American West and were exported to Mexico, South America, South Africa, and Australia. Pulled by four or six horses, a Concord Coach could carry nine passengers inside, with a few more on the roof. Traveling around the clock, a coach could cover about 100 miles in a day.

The state's **Legislative Office Building** (North State Street), built by the federal government in 1889 to house the federal court and the post office, is an impressive and picturesque example of the Romanesque Revival style. One of Concord's oldest (ca. 1735) houses is the **Rev. Timothy Walker House** (276 North Main Street, private); Walker was Concord's first minister. Immediately north of it is the **Joseph B. Walker Cottage** (private), based on a pattern-book design by one of the prominent advocates of the Gothic

Revival, Andrew Jackson Downing.

Mary Baker Eddy, founder of Christian Science, lived for a time on Concord's Pleasant Street. She was born just south of Concord, in **Bow**, in 1821. The **First Church of Christ, Scientist** (North State and School streets) was her 1903 gift to Concord.

Franklin Pierce bought the 1838 **Pierce Manse** (14 Pennacook Street) when he came to Concord to practice law in 1842. He and his family lived there for six years. The two-story clapboard house has been restored to that period and contains many Pierce family furnishings, including Pierce's writing table, his wife's sofa, and a parlor table, all of which the family brought to the White House after Pierce was elected president in 1852. Many of the family's personal effects are also on display, including Pierce's top hat and shaving set and a Bible that belonged to his son, Benny. The house has been moved from its original location on nearby Montgomery Street; it now sits on the site where the town's Reverend Timothy Walker built his first log cabin.

ROCHESTER

From the late 1760s, apple orchards, dairies, and milling villages began to fill the valleys east toward Rochester. The discovery of iron deposits created the neighboring towns of **Gilmanton Ironworks, Loudon, Pittsfield, Barnstead,** and **Strafford.** Rochester was granted in 1623 but not incorporated for another century, in 1722. The town on the Cocheco River grew, with tanneries and factories that produced shoes, wooden boxes, woolen blankets, bricks, and other goods in great demand by a developing nation. Four railroads conveyed Rochester's and Dover's products to market. Rochester's commercial prominence is evident in the **McDuffee Block** (South Main Street), built for retail and office space by businessman John McDuffee in 1868. A mansard roof completes the largely Second Empire design. The **Parson Main Monument** in Central Square honors Reverend Amos Main, who was parson here from 1731 to 1774 and was beloved by both the townspeople and the local Indians.

DOVER

Almost coastal, Dover is on the Cocheco River, which flows into the Piscataqua. The water distance from Dover to the sea is but ten miles. Captain John Smith visited the site in 1614, and it was settled in 1623 by William and Edward Hilton at Dover Point. By 1630 a church was established. In the 1650s and 1660s Quaker missionaries visited the town, to their peril. In 1662 the Puritan authorities had three Quaker women tied to a cart, stripped to the waist, and whipped as the cart was pulled through Dover and Hampton. The women returned the following year; by then a third of the townspeople had become Quakers. Dover's Quaker Society, once one of the largest in northern New England, built two meetinghouses before the current **Society of Friends Meeting House** (141 Central Avenue), which dates from 1768. The parents of the poet John Greenleaf Whittier were married here.

In the eighteenth century Dover's main enterprises were fishing, shipbuilding, and harvesting timber for masts. As the region's inland seaport, Dover handled the commerce of Strafford, Belknap, and Coos counties. Cotton mills, first erected on the river in 1815, were the town's mainstay until the Pacific Mills (formerly the Cocheco Manufacturing Company) closed its doors in 1944. The crenelated tower of the company stands on Washington Street. At their peak, Dover's downtown cotton mills employed thousands of workers and produced some 60 million yards of cotton cloth each year. Woolens—including flannels and worsteds—were the specialty of **Sawyer's Mills** (Route 108 and Spaulding Turnpike), founded in 1824 and held in the Sawyer family until 1899. Most of the nineteenth-century mill buildings have been renovated and converted to offices and small factories. The flatiron **Hosea Sawyer's Block** (Portland and Main streets) was built in 1825, with stores on the ground floor and apartments above. **St. Thomas' Episcopal Church** (Locust and Hale streets) was built of local stone in 1891.

Established by the 1915 bequest of Annie E. Woodman, the **Woodman Institute** (182–190 Central Avenue, 603–742–1038) is devoted to the study of the natural history, art, and history of this region. There are three properties on the site: two substantial brick houses of the early nineteenth century and the relatively ancient **Damme Garrison,** a fortified house constructed of square oak logs in 1675. The institute displays collections of Indian artifacts, minerals, local furniture, and military items.

DURHAM

Linked to the sea by the Piscataqua and Great Bay, Durham drew settlers from England and Boston in the 1630s. The French commanded a series of Indian raids against Durham, from 1675 to the early 1700s, with great loss of life and homes—the Durham raids were among the most punishing of the French and Indian raids against the British. The town persevered, and peacetime brought a spurt of shipbuilding and trading as merchants took advantage of their link to the Atlantic and proximity to Boston. Durham's John Sullivan led one of the early acts of rebellion against the Crown when he commanded a party that seized a load of arms and ammunition from Fort William and Mary in December 1774. Sullivan, who went on to become a general and three-time governor, lived in a house built in 1740 at 23 Newmarket Road (private). Town history exhibits by the local historical association are upstairs in the old **Durham Town Hall** (Main Street and Newmarket Road).

South of Durham, in **Newington**, is the **Old Meeting House** (Nimble Hill Road), the oldest meetinghouse in the state. Built in 1712, it is still used for services by the Congregational church. Further down the road is the **Old Parsonage,** a ca. 1725 saltbox house now operated as a museum by the Newington Historic Society (603–436–7640). The museum displays a variety of seventeenth and eighteenth century furniture.

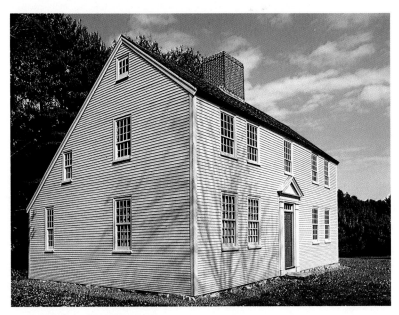

Newington's ca. 1725 Old Parsonage, now a museum.

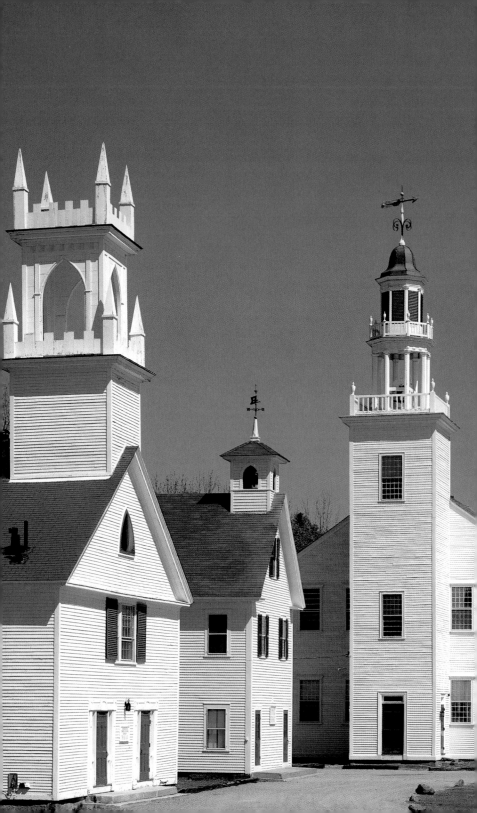

WESTERN
AND
NORTHERN NEW
HAMPSHIRE

OPPOSITE: *In December 1776, Washington, New Hampshire, became the second town in the newly formed United States to rename itself in honor of General George Washington.*

In the 1730s, about a century after settlement had begun on New Hampshire's coast, large numbers of other pioneers began to arrive in western New Hampshire. Most of the newcomers were from Massachusetts and Connecticut, where farmland was becoming insufficient to support the burgeoning population. They farmed the fertile Connecticut River Valley, the richest agricultural land in a colony of thin, rocky soils. At Charlestown—founded about 1740 by Massachusetts families under the authority of that colony—the reconstructed Fort at No. 4 provides a good glimpse of the frontier life of the early Connecticut Valley settlers.

The French and Indian War slowed the settlement of the region somewhat. Although there was no major fighting here, the Valley was constantly on the alert for raids—one historian estimates that about fifty people were either killed or kidnapped during the war. Because the French instituted a policy of paying Indians for English captives—who could be held for a profitable ransom—men, women, and children from the valley were kidnapped and carried off through the wilderness, often at great hardship, to French posts.

The conclusion of the French and Indian War in 1765 brought on an explosion of growth in the region. Its budding sophistication was symbolized by the establishment in 1769 of the first college in New Hampshire, Dartmouth College, in Hanover, on the river. Its founder, like many of the new college's neighbors, was from Connecticut.

The western settlers remained linked by the river to their old colonies, to which they had closer ties than to their capital at Portsmouth. In addition, the Connecticut River settlers were Puritan farmers, with an independent outlook, whereas Portsmouth was dominated by an Anglican elite, whose close religious ties to the Church of England were mirrored by equally close commercial ties to English merchants. Tensions between the new settlements and the old colony increased in the two decades before the Revolution. When the Portsmouth government dispatched officials to oversee the rural courts, the outsiders were denounced as "a swarm of pettifoggers." Even common devotion to the cause of independence could not unite the old and new sections. When the revolutionary government at Exeter issued a state constitution in 1776 the westerners howled in protest, demanding that the document be put to a popular vote, which eventually it was. From 1776 to 1782 a portion of the valley regarded itself as entirely independent. In

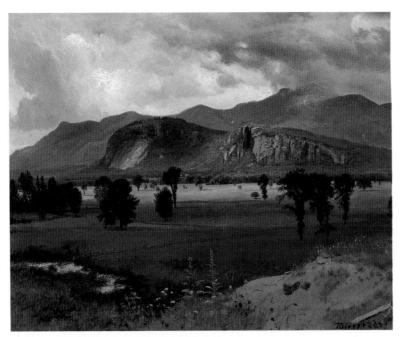

The great natural beauty of New Hampshire, as depicted in Albert Bierstadt's ca. 1862 Moat
Mountain, Intervale, New Hampshire *(detail).*

1781 33 Connecticut Valley towns (along with 17 from the Merrimack Valley) opted to join the newly formed republic of Vermont,
and made preparations to resist New Hampshire's claims by force,
until the matter was settled by the intervention of Congress.

Northern New Hampshire was sparsely settled at the time of
the Revolution. Development was hindered by the harsh terrain
and climate of the White Mountains, the northern extremity of the
Appalachian chain, consisting of three principal ranges, the Franconia, Carter-Moriah, and the Presidential, which is the tallest.
Overlooking Franconia Notch, one of several deep passes through
the mountains, is the well-known geological formation, the Old
Man of the Mountain.

In the mid and late nineteenth century the great natural beauty of the White Mountains led to the development of popular
resorts in such towns as Bethlehem, Fabyan, and Bretton Woods.
While some visitors came to New Hampshire to hunt (for black
bear, beaver, rabbit, racoon, fox) and to fish in lakes and rivers,
others came to write, paint, and sculpt—among the state's seasonal

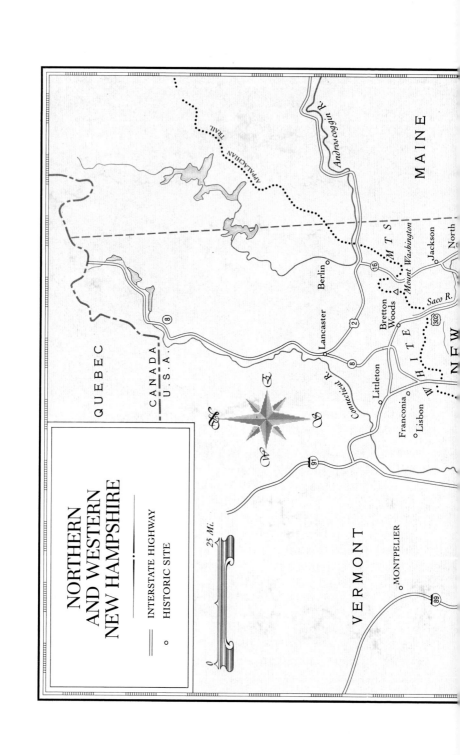

NORTHERN
AND WESTERN
NEW HAMPSHIRE

— INTERSTATE HIGHWAY
○ HISTORIC SITE

25 Mi.

VERMONT

○ MONTPELIER

QUEBEC

CANADA
U. S. A.

Lancaster

Berlin

Littleton

Franconia
○ Lisbon

Bretton
Woods

Mount Washington

Jackson

North

Saco R.

Connecticut R.

Androscoggin R.

APPALACHIAN TRAIL

W H I T E   M T S

MAINE

NEW

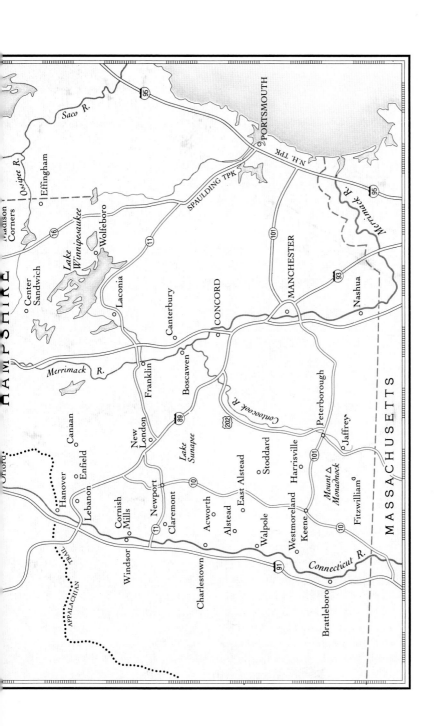

residents were the landscape painters Thomas Cole, Albert Bierstadt, and George Inness—all of whom worked in the North Conway area. The region remains one of the most popular, and rugged, recreational areas in the country. Looping through the
Whites, the Appalachian Trail takes hikers through some of the
most challenging terrain on the trail—freezing winds above the
timberline on Mount Washington, New Hampshire's tallest peak at
over 6,000 feet, have been clocked at 200 miles per hour.

Rich forests of the farthest frontier, the North Country and
Coos County, attracted lumbermen in the early nineteenth century. Small mills gave way to large-scale operations in the second
half of the century. One northern lumber mill processed seven and
a half miles of lumber a day. Since that time, the commercial capital
of the northern lumber region has been Berlin.

This chapter begins in southwestern New Hampshire at
Keene, proceeds up the Connecticut River Valley to the North
Country, and then heads south through the White Mountains to
the area around Canterbury and its Shaker community.

KEENE

Founded in the 1730s, Keene developed into a string of cabins
along Main Street before being abandoned a decade later, in the
face of Indian attacks. The town was resettled in the 1750s. Surviving from the eighteenth century is the **Wyman Tavern** (339 Main
Street, 603–357–3855), site of the 1770 founding meeting of Dartmouth College. Isaac Wyman, who built the tavern in 1762, led a
band of Patriots south to Boston, Massachusetts, in April 1775 after
the battles of Lexington and Concord. The New Hampshire men
participated in the Battle of Bunker Hill.

From a log-cabin settlement, Keene grew into a renowned arts
and crafts center: Pottery was made here beginning in the 1790s
and glass in the early 1800s. The site of **Hampshire Pottery Works**
is marked on Main Street.

Glassmaking began in New Hampshire in the town of Temple,
where a factory was founded in 1780, employing Europeans
schooled in the art of glassmaking. Others followed in **Stoddard,
Suncook, South Lyndeborough,** and the largest of them, in Keene.
The site of the **Keene Glass Factory** is marked on Washington
Street. The Historical Society of Cheshire County's **Colony House
Museum** (104 West Street, 603–357–0889) occupies the 1819

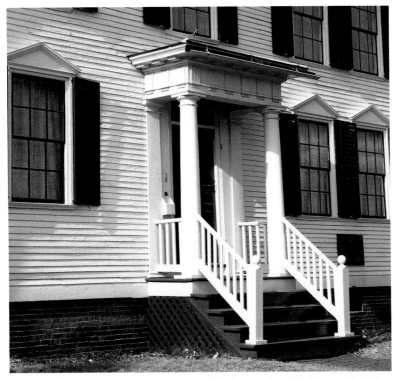

In 1770 Keene's Wyman Tavern was the site of the first meeting of the Dartmouth College trustees.

house of Keene's first mayor, Horatio Colony. Among its displays of native glass and pottery are green and amber Keene Glass bottles and flasks and examples of Hampshire pottery, developed in 1871 and prized by collectors. The home and many possessions of Mayor Colony's grandson, also named Horatio, are on display at the **Horatio Colony House Museum** (199 Main Street, 603–352–0460). The 1806 Federal style building displays Colony's collections of walking sticks, Buddhas, Oriental carpets, paperweights, and cribbage boards.

Textile manufacturing was also part of the local industrial scene—Keene flannels were regarded as particularly fine—as well as shoemaking and woodworking. By the turn of the century, five furniture factories were in operation, and Keene chairs were famous along the Eastern Seaboard. Products were conveyed to major markets on the Boston and Maine Railroad.

The industrial past is responsible for some of the handsomest buildings in Keene—the Second Empire **Colony's Block,** on the town's Central Square; the **Faulkner and Colony Mill** (now converted to stores), on West Street; the **Cheshire Railroad Maintenance Shops and Roundhouse,** on Gilbo Avenue.

Among the earliest industries of nearby **Fitzwilliam** were yarn-making and woodworking; granite quarrying became important in the late nineteenth century. The chief site, on the green, is the 1817 **Fitzwilliam Meeting House.**

JAFFREY

In the valley below Mount Monadnock, Jaffrey attracted many summer visitors in the nineteenth century, including Ralph Waldo Emerson, who wrote the poem "Monadnock" after climbing the mountain in 1845. The sturdy, foursquare **Old Meeting House** in Jaffrey Center was built between 1775 and 1799. Behind the meetinghouse is the 1801 grave of Amos Fortune, a slave who bought his freedom, set up a tannery, and endowed the local church and school. Also buried there are author Willa Cather and Hannah Davis, who patented wooden band boxes; she died in 1863. The **Stone Brothers and Curtis Mill** (Main Street) was built in 1872 as a textile factory; an addition dates to 1897.

East of Keene is **Harrisville,** a nineteenth-century industrial community that survives virtually intact from its milling heyday. It is one of the few towns of this type in the nation that imparts so complete a sense of that time. **The Harris Mill,** built over its source of power, Goose Creek, in 1830, is at the village center. The stone **Cheshire Mills** are recognized by the square-towered central building. A sorting house, storehouse, tenements, and other worker housing complete the factory district; beyond are private residences, churches, and public buildings also incorporated in Harrisville's historic district.

WALPOLE

The town of Walpole was granted as "No. 3" in 1736. It was the site of the first bridge across the Connecticut River, built in 1785. The bridge was replaced in 1840 and again in 1904. There are several

fine Greek Revival houses (private) along Main Street, as well as
the Walpole Academy building, built in 1830. It now houses the
Walpole Historical Society (Main Street, 603–756–3602).

STODDARD

Settled in 1769, Stoddard developed into a glass-manufacturing
center in the nineteenth century. The first of three glass factories
opened in 1842, producing bottles for the popular Saratoga
Springs mineral water, medicines and elixirs, and flasks. Stoddard
glassmaking figured among New Hampshire's major early industries until 1873, when competitors' cost-efficient technologies
forced the factories to close. The town's **Congregational Church**
(Route 123), crowned by a crenelated belfry, was built in 1835.

Northeast of Walpole in the village of **Drewsville,** the Gothic
Revival **St. Peter's Episcopal Church,** built in 1836, faces the
village green.

ALSTEAD

The first paper mills in New Hampshire operated here on the Cold
River in the early 1790s. Alstead was established in 1772 as a New
Hampshire town but switched allegiance to Vermont a decade
later; within a few months it rejoined New Hampshire. Nineteenth-
century milling brought a measure of prosperity. North of the
river is the **Universalist Church** (Route 123), built in 1844. South
of the river, across from Milot Green, the town erected the domed,
granite **Shedd-Porter Memorial Library** in 1910.

CHARLESTOWN

In Charlestown itself, Richard Upjohn designed **St. Luke's Episcopal Church,** on Main Street. Constructed in 1863, it is notable for
its wooden construction and slate roof.

Fort at No. 4

Granted in 1735 by the Massachusetts Bay Colony as "No. 4,"
Charlestown was New England's northwesternmost settlement during the long period of the French and Indian wars. In 1744 the
settlers built a stockade, enclosing log houses and lean-tos, a watch-
tower, barn, smithy, and other buildings. The French and their

Indian allies attacked in 1747, but the fort held. During the Revolution, John Stark used the town as a military base for his 1,500-man expedition to Bennington.

The Fort at No. 4 has been reproduced on a twenty-acre site north of Charlestown. Fortifications and living quarters appear as they originally did; within the museum are furnished houses and exhibits of colonial and Indian artifacts. Costumed staff visit with the public and demonstrate skills of the early eighteenth century.

LOCATION: Route 11. HOURS: June through August: 10–4 Wednesday–Monday; first two weeks of September: 10–4 Saturday–Sunday; mid-September through mid-October: 10–4 Wednesday–Monday. FEE: Yes. TELEPHONE: 603–826–5700.

ACWORTH

Up the Cold River is the 1821 **United Church of Acworth,** one of the most beautiful churches in the state, looking out over the town from a rise on the common. Built by Elias Carter, the church has a superb bell tower with a Palladian window. Renovations made in 1886 harmonize with the original structure.

CLAREMONT

When settlers arrived here from Connecticut in the 1760s, they dammed the Sugar River and built a saw- and gristmill. The town soon had an iron foundry, a shoe factory, and a woolen mill. Sheep raising spread throughout the nearby valleys, and in 1846 the big Sugar River Manufacturing Company merged with another firm to become the **Monadnock Mills** (Water Street). For the next century they produced high-quality textiles, particularly quilts. Paper milling grew in the 1860s, at the same time that machine manufacturing came to Claremont, attracting workers from Poland, Canada, and Russia. Original factories and mill housing still line the riverbanks.

The oldest Episcopal church in New Hampshire is the 1773 **Union Church** (Old Church Road), the work of master carpenter Ichabod Hitchcock. The box pews within the church are original,

OPPOSITE: *The United Church of Acworth, built in 1821 by Elias Carter.*

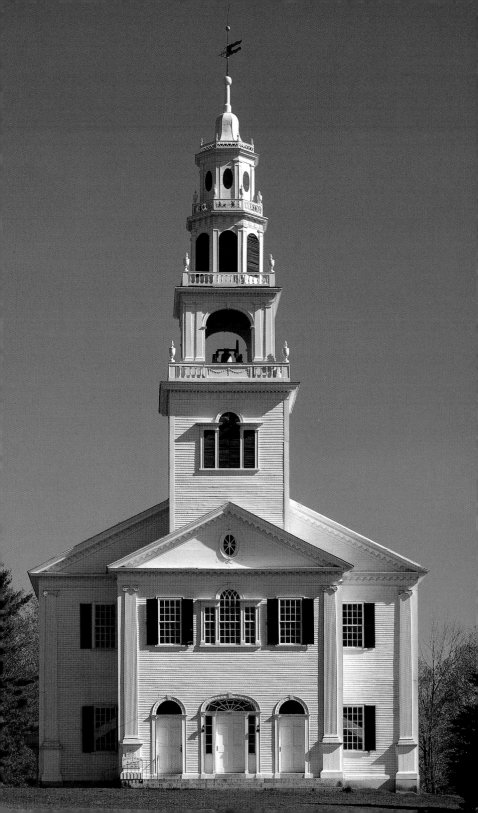

as are the stables behind it. Also in Claremont is the state's oldest Roman Catholic Church, **St. Mary's** (Old Church Road), built of brick in 1823.

East of Claremont is the former fur-trading post of **Newport,** quickly industrialized due to its proximity to the Sugar River. The **Dexter Richards and Sons Mill** (Sunapee Street), built in 1905 on the river, is among the most handsome of New England's industrial buildings, with patterned brick walls and a campanile-like tower. On South Main and Church streets is the 1822 Federal-style **South Congregational Church.**

Newport was the hometown of Sarah Josepha Buell Hale, author of the verse "Mary Had a Little Lamb." Born in Newport in 1788, Hale, a schoolteacher, edited *Godey's Lady's Book* and became a champion of women's rights.

On the high land across Lake Sunapee and the mountains of the same name is **New London,** home of **Colby-Sawyer College** (Main Street, 603–526–2010). Among its founders was New Hampshire's governor Anthony Colby; his daughter Susan was the school's first principal. Chartered in 1837 as the New London Academy for young women, the academy was actually coeducational when its doors opened in 1838 and remained so until it became a junior college for women in 1928. In 1975, the school's name was changed to Colby-Sawyer College and it began granting baccalaureate degrees. Today the college occupies a number of fine buildings on Main Street. New London's **Historical Society** (Little Sunapee Road, 603–526–6564) has restored several buildings from 1800 to 1830—a house, barn, carriage house, schoolhouse, general store, meetinghouse, and smithy.

Spanning New Hampshire and Vermont near Cornish on the Connecticut River is the **Cornish–Windsor Bridge,** at 460 feet the longest covered bridge in the United States. Just south of the bridge is the **birthplace of Salmon Portland Chase** (private), a two-story frame house on Route 12A. Born into a large family of lawyers in 1808, Chase studied at Dartmouth and in Washington. As a young lawyer, he often defended the rights to freedom of runaway slaves. After practicing in Ohio, Chase went on to become senator and governor of that state and to help found the Republican Party. He was a presidential possibility in 1860. Abraham Lincoln named Chase secretary of the treasury and in 1864 appointed him chief justice of the Supreme Court.

THE SAINT-GAUDENS NATIONAL HISTORIC SITE

When artists took to the hills of Cornish around 1900, they were following the lead of one of the country's foremost sculptors, Augustus Saint-Gaudens. Brought to America from Ireland in 1848 at the age of 6 months by his French father and Irish mother, Saint-Gaudens grew up in New York, attending public schools and working as a cameo cutter. He later studied sculpture at Cooper Union and the National Academy of Design. In 1867 he traveled to France, where he studied at the Ecole des Beaux-Arts. He won commissions in Rome and returned to New York, where others came his way, including a monument to Civil War hero Admiral David Farragut for New York's Madison Square. Critics noted Saint-Gaudens's ability to invest heroic sculpture with individual character. Stanford White, the most celebrated architect of the day, created a pedestal for the Farragut statue, and the two men embarked on an exciting collaboration that helped redefine public sculpture. Other notable Saint-Gaudens works include the Diana

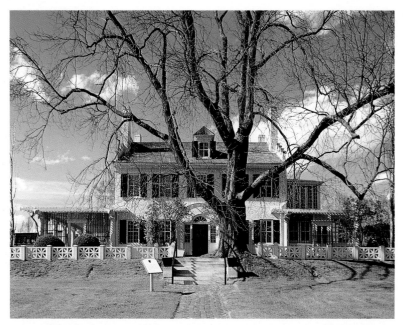

The sculptor Augustus Saint-Gaudens executed many of his major works while living in this house near Cornish.

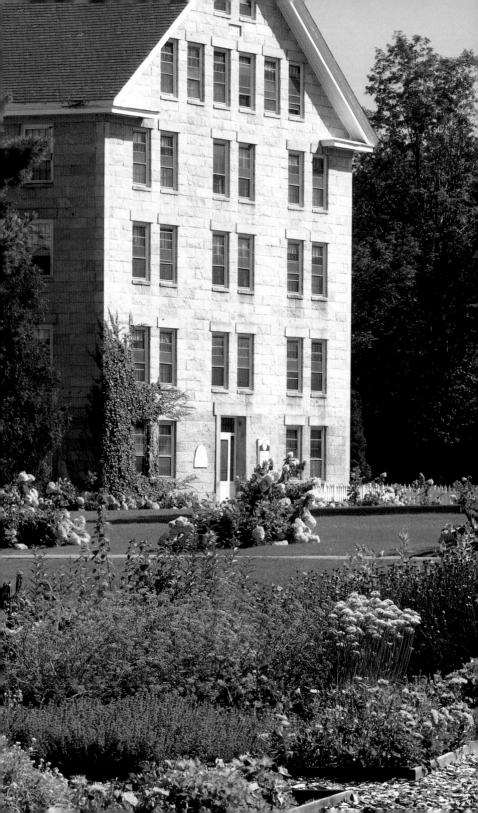

for the roof of the original Madison Square Garden (the sculpture is now in the Philadelphia Museum of Art) and memorial statues of Mrs. Henry Adams (in Rock Creek Cemetery, Washington, DC) and Robert Louis Stevenson (in Edinburgh, Scotland).

In 1885 Saint-Gaudens rented a former inn (called Huggin's Folly) on the Connecticut River; a few years later, he bought the 1805 Federal-style structure and began renovation, making a studio in the hay barn and landscaping the grounds. He named the property Aspet, after his father's French birthplace, and lived and worked there—summers at first, then year-round—until his death in 1907. Some of his finest reliefs and statues were executed here, including standing and seated portraits of Abraham Lincoln. Saint-Gaudens attracted many colleagues in the arts to his studio, and they too were moved by the countryside. The Saint-Gaudens house, appointed with family possessions, is open to the public, along with the studio, stable, gallery, and gardens. Much of the artist's work is on view.

LOCATION: Off Route 12A, two miles north of the Cornish–Windsor Bridge. HOURS: June through October: 8:30–4:30 Daily. FEE: Yes. TELEPHONE: 603–675–2175.

LEBANON

The prolific architect Ammi Burnham Young was born here in 1798. Thirty years later he designed the town's **First Congregational Church,** overlooking the green. For much of the nineteenth and early twentieth centuries Lebanon was a busy mill town—mills along the Mascoma River processed wool until the 1940s.

LOWER SHAKER VILLAGE

This remarkable village was an active Shaker community from 1793 to 1923. Thirteen Shaker buildings are preserved in the village itself, and there are seven others in the area. At its peak in the 1850s the community had 350 adults and 100 children in residence. In the nineteenth century Shaker communities were a haven for homeless children and adults wandering the countryside. The village supported itself by selling seeds, medicinal herbs, brooms, buckets, tubs, and woolen goods (it kept a herd of 3,000 merino sheep).

OPPOSITE: *The Great Stone Dwelling in the Shaker Village at Enfield, designed in 1837 by Ammi B. Young, is the largest structure ever built by Shakers.*

The most important building in the village is the **Great Stone Dwelling,** designed by Ammi Burnham Young and built between 1837 and 1841. The largest building ever constructed by the Shakers, it was the dwelling for the Church Family, the 150 adults who formed the core of the community.

The **cow barn,** built in 1854, is the only wooden Shaker cattle barn still standing. The upper two floors remain unchanged. The 1820 **West Brethren Shop** and the 1819 **East Brethren Shop** were workshops. Other structures in the village include barns; laundries; dairies; the ministry shop, where the elders lived and worked; and a stone machine shop. The **Sacred Feasting Grounds,** a large field surrounded by trees, is where the Shakers held outdoor ceremonies. A **museum** displays Shaker artifacts, including early sulfur matches (a Shaker invention), furniture made in the village, and seed-sorting boxes. The village offers many demonstrations of weaving, box-making, dying, and basketmaking and maintains large herb and vegetable gardens.

In 1923 the last residents of the village, seven sisters and one brother, moved to the community at Canterbury, which is still active today. The village was sold to a Roman Catholic teaching order. In 1985 the order sold the village to the private group that currently manages it as a museum of Shaker life. Some buildings in the village have been converted to modern shops and inns and are not part of the restoration proper.

LOCATION: Route 4A, Enfield. HOURS: Mid-May through mid-October: 10–5 Monday–Saturday, 12–5 Sunday; mid-October through mid-May: 10–4 Saturday, 12–4 Sunday. FEE: Yes. TELEPHONE: 603–632–5533.

CANAAN

Incorporated in 1761, Canaan was settled by people from Norwich, Connecticut. Although a great fire in the 1820s leveled most of the downtown area, mile-long Canaan Street, bordering the west side of Canaan Street Lake, looks much as it did in the early nineteenth century. The first historic district formed in New Hampshire, this road, once called Broad Street, is lined with handsome Federal and Greek Revival buildings—the 1791 **Old Meeting House,** with its original bell clock; the 1828 Gothic Revival **Old North Church;** and the ca. 1840 **Canaan Historical Museum** (603–523–4202), with exhibits of Shaker artifacts, tools, old scientific and medical equipment, and other items of local history. The museum building was formerly an academy and site of one of the first integrated schools in the country. (Canaan was one of the stops along the underground railroad.) The town was a popular summer resort in the late nineteenth and early twentieth centuries.

DARTMOUTH COLLEGE

The farming village of **Hanover,** granted in 1761, and Dartmouth College, founded eight years later, grew together. Hanover continues to be a college town—education, medical facilities, and research fuel the local economy, and the college enlivens the cultural life of the entire area.

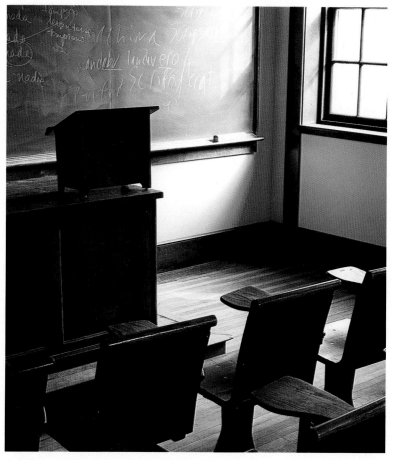

A classroom in Dartmouth College's 1829 Wentworth Hall.

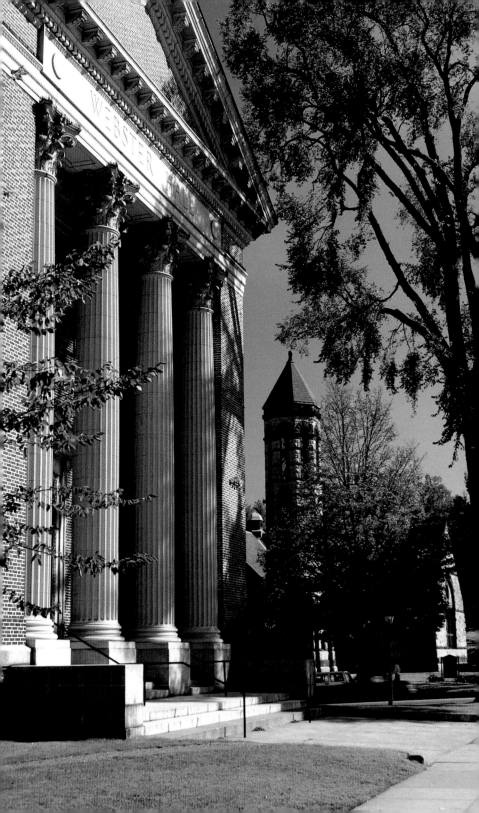

The college was founded when Eleazar Wheelock, a minister who operated Moor's Indian Charity School in Connecticut, decided to move the school to New Hampshire and start a companion institution for English youth. He sent two of his pupils, Samson Occom and Nathaniel Whittaker, to England to raise funds for his educational endeavors. The Earl of Dartmouth made a generous donation for the education of Native American youth, but some of the money was used to found the college for English boys, which Wheelock named after the Earl. Wheelock chose Hanover for the site when the town offered him 3,000 acres, labor, and cash. Governor John Wentworth bestowed a royal charter to officially establish the school. Wheelock called the first meeting of the college trustees at the Wyman Tavern in Keene. Classes commenced in 1770.

Confusion over the precise legal status of the college and the powers of its president and trustees culminated in the famous Dartmouth College case, argued before the Supreme Court in 1818 by Daniel Webster, a Dartmouth graduate. (In his arguments Webster uttered one of his memorable phrases: "It is . . . a small college, and yet there are those who love it.") The case had wide, but temporary, ramifications for the course of American business, because the Court decided that the royal charter was a contract and that the state of New Hampshire could not interfere with its terms. For a brief time American corporations enjoyed total immunity from state regulations in the writing of contracts. The Supreme Court later gave the states certain regulatory powers.

On the campus, **Dartmouth Row** is an array of four impressive buildings: the 1829 **Wentworth Hall; Dartmouth Hall,** a 1904 replica of the 1791 original destroyed by fire; the 1829 **Thornton Hall;** and Ammi Burnham Young's 1839 **Reed Hall.** The architect also designed the college's **Shattuck Observatory.** Dartmouth claims one of the state's finest examples of the Romanesque style, **Rollins Chapel,** built in 1886. It's contemporary, **Wilson Hall,** on Wheelock Street, mirrors the style. A newer building, the 1928 **Baker Memorial Library,** imitates Philadelphia's Independence Hall. While teaching at Dartmouth, the noted Mexican artist Jose Clemente Orozco painted a series of frescoes in the library. Near it, at 30-B Main Street, is one of Hanover's oldest houses, the **Webster Cottage,** built in 1780 and named for Daniel Webster.

LOCATION: Main and Wheelock streets. TELEPHONE: 603–646–1110.

OPPOSITE: *Dartmouth's Webster Hall is named for its famous alumnus, Daniel Webster.*

North of Hanover are fertile meadowlands and farming villages that define the rural New England ideal—**Lyme, North Dorchester, Piermont,** and **Haverhill.** In **Orford,** the **Orford Street Historic District** consists of a tree-lined roadway with houses built between 1773 and 1839. Architectural styles range from Adamesque to Greek Revival. The town architecture took an exuberant Victorian turn in its 1854 **Congregational Church.** Route 302 passes through **Lisbon,** where charcoal was made for the area's iron industry. The **Old Coal Kiln,** one of many that burned pine scrap from nearby lumber mills, stands on Route 302, about two miles north of the Route 117 junction.

FRANCONIA

The New Hampshire Iron Factory Company began operations here in 1790; its production peaked during the Civil War years. Cast-iron Franconia Stoves were famous, as were locally made farm tools. A **stone iron furnace** stands south of the junction of routes 18-116 and 117. Summer visitors to Franconia included some of the nineteenth century's best-known writers.

The Robert Frost Place

The poet Robert Frost came to Franconia in 1915, at the age of 40, and bought a simple white clapboard farmhouse set on a ridge overlooking the Franconia Valley. He spent five years here, writing poetry and farming the land, then sold the house, returning every summer as a renter. The years he lived here were productive ones: in 1915, Frost had yet to be published in this country; by 1920, he had published three books and won a Pulitzer Prize. The house, built in 1859, is now a cultural center, featuring poetry readings, workshops, a poet-in-residence, and exchange programs. Two rooms are given over to a museum of Frost memorabilia, including his writing desk and signed first editions, and an audio-visual presentation describes the poet's life and work. On the grounds, a trail winds for half a mile through woods and fields; fifteen of Frost's poems are engraved on plaques along the way.

> LOCATION: Ridge Road. HOURS: June: 1–5 Saturday–Sunday; July through August: 1–5 Wednesday–Monday; September through mid-October: 1–5 Saturday–Sunday. FEE: Yes. TELEPHONE: 603–823–5510.

OPPOSITE: *The porch of Robert Frost's farm, with its view of the Franconia Valley.*

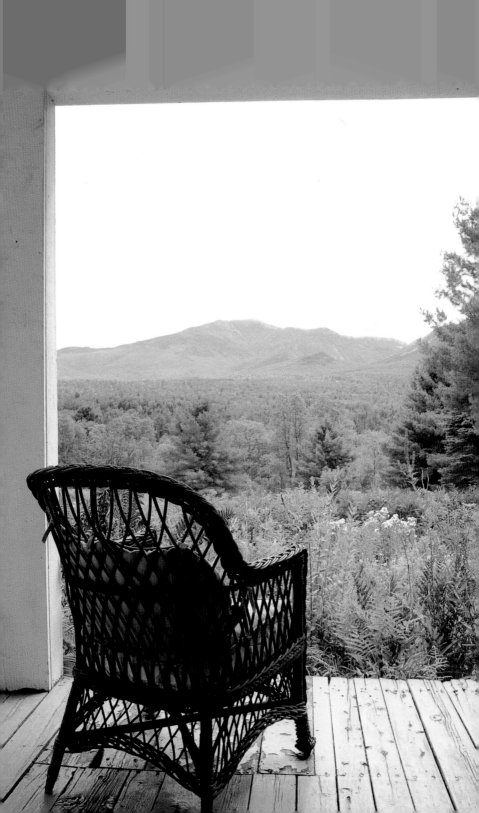

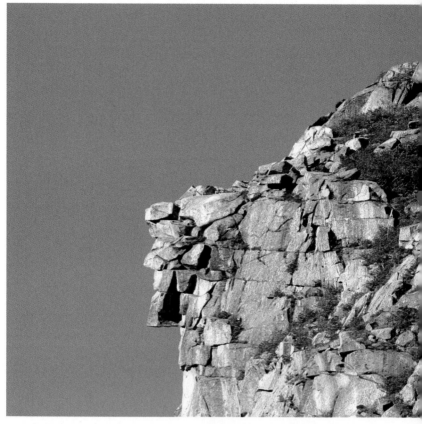

The Old Man of the Mountain, a series of granite ledges in the White Mountains, juts into the

The **Old Man of the Mountain** (Route 93, Franconia Notch State Park), a famed New England landmark far to the northeast, is a series of five granite ledges that resembles a craggy human face in profile. The "face" measures forty feet from chin to forehead and protrudes from cliffs 1,200 feet above Profile Lake. Nathaniel Hawthorne, who set some stories in the White Mountains, immortalized the Old Man in "The Great Stone Face." Among other well-known visitors to the area was Daniel Webster, who is said to have remarked about this monument: "Men hang out their signs indicative of their respective trades: shoemakers hang out a gigantic shoe; jewelers, a monster watch . . . but up in the mountains of New Hampshire, God Almighty has hung out a sign to show that there He makes men."

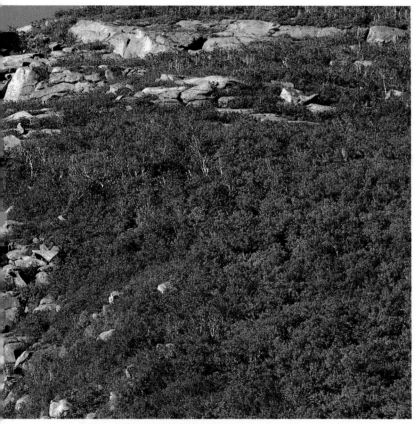

landscape at Franconia Notch State Park.

BRETTON WOODS

The town of Bretton Woods lies in a glacial plain at the base of Mount Washington. The White Mountains cut off the valley from easy contact with Portsmouth until the 1790s, when a rough and winding road was cut through Crawford Notch, a cleft in the mountains. The Notch had been discovered by accident in 1771 by Timothy Nash while tracking a moose. A year later (with the help of a block and tackle), he and a companion brought a horse through the Notch, proving that, with difficulty, it could be traversed. According to local lore a young woman lost her life here in 1778 when her lover abandoned her and left for Portsmouth. She followed him and froze to death before she could catch up.

Inns operating as early as 1800 received sportsmen, tourists, artists, and writers—Nathaniel Hawthorne came, as did Ralph Waldo Emerson and Henry David Thoreau. In the late nineteenth and early twentieth centuries Bretton Woods took its place with Newport, Bar Harbor, and Saratoga as a fashionable resort. One of the great attractions of the area was the **Mount Washington Cog Railway,** which opened in 1869. It was an audacious task to lay such steeply graded track, but the engineers succeeded—cog-wheeled, steam-powered cars have chugged up and down the mountain for over a century. Railroad magnate Joseph Stickney opened the lavish **Mount Washington Hotel** (Route 302, 603–278–1000) in 1902. It was an immediate sensation. Billed as the largest wooden building in New England, the hotel remains in business. In 1944 it was the site of the Bretton Woods Conference, which established international monetary policies for the post–World War II period, including the use of the U.S. dollar as the basis of international currency exchange.

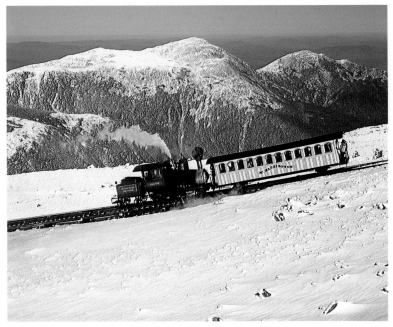

Started in 1869, the Mount Washington Cog Railway still carries passengers up and down the mountain.

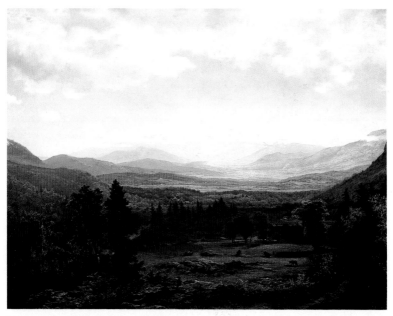

Mount Washington, New Hampshire, *by Alexander Wust, ca. 1869 (detail)*.
OVERLEAF: *The Mount Washington Hotel, opened in 1902, still welcomes visitors to its spectacular setting at the foot of the Presidential range.*

LITTLETON

One of New Hampshire's oldest inns, its three-story Doric columns towering above Littleton's Main Street since 1848, is **Thayer's Hotel.** Across the street is the late-nineteenth century **Community House.** The 1894 **Town Building** contains the local opera house as well as the town hall; in addition, it has served as the courthouse, jail, and fire station.

In the Victorian age, every proper parlor was filled with various games and amusements, including stereoscopes. In the United States, most of these double-picture viewers were manufactured here at the **Kilburn Brothers Factory** (43 Cottage Street). The factory, which operated from 1867 to 1909, is now apartments.

LANCASTER

Settled in the 1760s, Lancaster grew into a manufacturing center in the 1800s, with mills and factories along the Israel River. It also

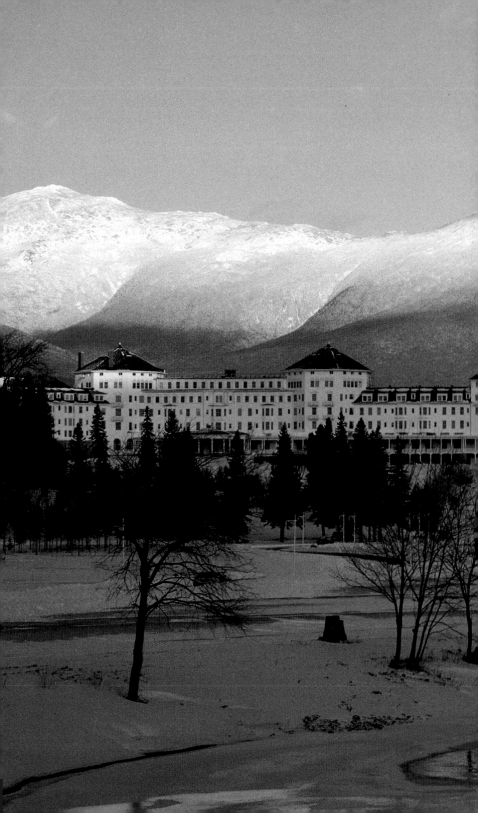

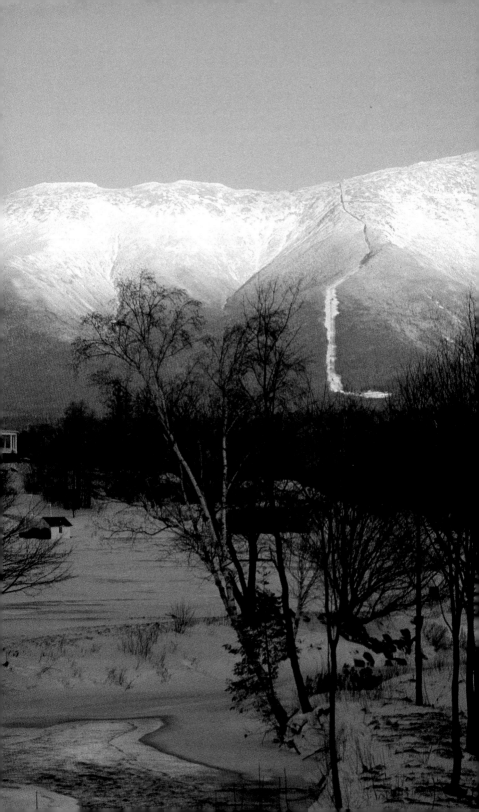

became an important transportation link in New Hampshire's northern reaches, as a major railroad junction in Coos County. At **89 Bunker Hill Street** (1885) is one of northern New England's rare Eastlake houses, trimmed with ornate brackets, braces, and openwork friezes that carpenters achieved with special saws and lathes. Also of architectural interest are the **Coos County Courthouse** (Main Street), with its mansard tower, and the Gothic Revival **St. Paul's Episcopal Church** (Main Street), built in 1875 of board and batten. In 1835, Lancaster lawyer John Sullivan Wells built a Greek Revival house (140 Main Street, private) of local granite; the result is a striking juxtaposition of classical columns and rough stone. The 1780 **Wilder-Holton House** (226 Main Street, 603–788–3004), the first two-story house in Coos County, may have been a rendezvous point on the underground railroad. Its rooms and collections of pewter, stoneware, and local antiques are on view.

Above Lancaster and **Stark,** known for its **Union Church** and **covered bridge,** both built in the 1850s, Coos County is sparsely populated, much as it was two centuries ago when it was known chiefly to hunters and fishermen, Indian, French, and English. Such towns as **Colebrook, Pittsburg,** and **Clarksville** were part of the frontier claimed by both the United States and Canada in territorial disputes that did not stop with the Revolution. In 1832 these most independent of settlers formed their own Republic of Indian Stream. The state of New Hampshire formally annexed the territory in 1840.

BERLIN

Coos County's anchor city is Berlin, on the edge of the White Mountain forests and straddling the mighty Androscoggin River. It was the last town settled in Coos County. In 1825 two farmers began a logging operation here as winter work. This was the beginning of a logging and milling industry that would make Berlin into "The City that Trees Built." By midcentury Berlin had a small sawmill that was later greatly expanded to become one of the largest in the East. About twenty-five years later came a shift to pulp and paper production. A small pulp mill was started in 1877 and a large mill was built later, but the process was not profitable and had to be abandoned. About 1881 the sawmill company and a competitor both put up newsprint mills, using wood pulp with rags added for strength. Paper towels were also manufactured. With the start of the pulp and paper mills, the demand for labor brought a flood of immigrants—French-Canadians mainly, along with some Scandinavians, Russians, Irish, Germans—and Yankees. In 1881 the Berlin Mills Company gave land on Main Street for the Stick-style **Congregational Church of Christ.** Russian immigrants built their own Eastern Orthodox church, the **Orthodox Church of the Holy Resurrection,** complete with onion domes (20 Petrograd Street). **St. Anne's Catholic Church,** at 58 Church Street, was built by a French-Canadian congregation.

The **Berlin Public Library** (Main Street, 603–752–5210) has an exhibit of stone implements made by the region's Indians as long as 7,000 years ago. The Indians hollowed out a cave on Mount Jasper to obtain the stone for their tools.

Due south through the White Mountains is the village of **Jackson,** a lonesome wilderness settlement until it emerged in the late nineteenth century as a resort. Below Jackson in **North Conway** is the eclectic Victorian **North Conway Depot** (603–356–5251). Built in 1874 by the Portsmouth Great Falls & Conway Railroad, the twin-towered station saw regular passenger-train service until 1961. Its nineteenth-century layout is intact, with Ticket and Telegraph Office, women's and men's waiting rooms, Baggage Room, and upstairs offices. The station's telegraph and telephone equipment, baggage wagons, benches, and other furnishings are original, as is the brass-and-iron clock, still wound weekly. Out on the tracks are forty-five railroad cars, including Pullman sleepers, and six nineteenth- and twentieth-century locomotives. Equipment on the grounds includes the water spout used to fill steam locomotives, hand-operated gates, and early electric crossing signals. There is a specially designed stand from which fast-moving trains snatched mailbags. Also on the grounds are the century-old **Roundhouse,** a **garage** for locomotive repair, and an 1870s **Freight House.** The Conway Scenic Railroad operates out of the station, taking passengers on an eleven-mile tour of Mount Washington Valley.

North of the village of **Madison Corner** is a survivor of the Ice Age, a large erratic boulder measuring eighty-three by thirty-seven by twenty-three feet and weighing an estimated 7,650 tons. One of the largest known erratic boulders, it was deposited here by a glacier (Route 113).

EFFINGHAM

One of the state's finest early-nineteenth-century houses is here, **Squire Lord's Great House** (Route 153, 603–539–4803), built in 1822 by the successful merchant Isaac Lord. The twenty-room house features a ballroom, hand-carved woodwork, imported wallpapers, and an elliptical stairway that rises to the cupola. It is part of a cluster of historic houses (private) on **Lord's Hill.**

CENTER SANDWICH

The 1869 **Durgin Covered Bridge,** named for the miller who built it, is the fourth to span the banks of the aptly named Swift River—floods washed away the earlier bridges. The 1850 **Elisha Marston House,** typical of this farming country, is a simple Cape Cod structure with subtle Greek Revival decoration. The Sandwich Historical Society, which owns and administers the house, displays rooms of period furniture and rotating exhibits (Maple Street, 603–284–6269). The **Brick Store** (Route 109) served as Sandwich's general store and post office from its construction in 1845 until it closed in 1985; the building now houses a silversmith's shop.

Throughout the lake region are towns that established themselves in the mid-1700s with farming, often only on a subsistence level. Those located near fast water could put in mills and start up industry on a modest scale: within the fertile triangle formed by Conway, Center Sandwich, and Wolfeboro are **Ossipee, Moultonborough,** and **Madison,** handsome survivors of New Hampshire's colonial days. In Moultonborough is **Castle in the Clouds** (Route 171, 603–476–2352), the lavish 6,000-acre estate of millionaire shoe manufacturer Thomas G. Plant. Designed by Plant himself, and built primarily of stone, the buildings reflect an eclectic set of influences: Norman, English, Japanese, Norwegian, and Swiss Chalet. The interiors display Plant's desire for a house that was both luxurious and supremely modern and efficient, featuring conveniences highly uncommon for the time (1913).

WOLFEBORO

Located at the southern end of Lake Winnipesaukee, Wolfeboro benefited from a philanthropist, John Brewster, who in 1886 endowed the **Brewster Free Academy** (52 South Main Street, 603–569–1604) for any student—regardless of age, race, or sex—"of

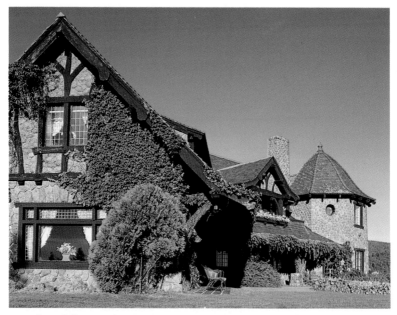

Located on a hilltop 750 feet above Lake Winnipesaukee, the eclectic Castle in the Clouds was designed by millionaire shoe manufacturer Thomas G. Plant.

good moral character." Brewster also built the **Municipal Building** (South Main Street), a sprawling Romanesque structure noted for its clock and bell tower. In 1768, John Wentworth, New Hampshire's last royal governor, built a lakeside estate here. The Wolfeboro Historical Society maintains the 1778 **Clark House,** the 1826 Pleasant Valley **Schoolhouse,** and a **Fire Museum,** all on South Main Street (603–569–4997).

The natural history of the region is explored in the **Libby Museum** (Route 109 North, 603–569–1035). Specimens of a variety of flora and fauna are on display; other exhibits include Abenaki Indian tools; artifacts from the site of Governor John Wentworth's summer home, which is currently being excavated; nineteenth-century farm and home implements; and a 350-year-old dugout canoe that was raised from nearby Rust Pond. The museum was built in 1912 by Henry Forest Libby, a retired Boston dentist, to house his collection of mounted specimens. The stuccoed frame building features a Greek-style portico, handsome mahogany doors, and a view of Winter Harbor on Lake Winnipesaukee.

LACONIA

Laconia was once part of nearby Gilmanton (chartered in 1727) and Meredith. Mills operated on a canal built in 1800, and railroad lines linked the town to Concord and Boston by 1848. The Laconia Car Shops opened in 1859 for the manufacture of railroad cars; other factories produced nails, hosiery, knitting machinery, and starch. The **Belknap-Sulloway Mill** (Beacon Street East, Mill Plaza), distinguished by the weathervane atop its cupola, went up on the Winnipesaukee in 1823; it now houses a cultural center. Across from it is the larger **Busiel-Seeburg Mill,** a hosiery factory constructed in two stages, in 1853 and 1878. On Court Street is Laconia's **South Baptist Church,** its doorway dwarfed by a central gabled tower. The **Boston and Maine Railroad Station** (Church and Pleasant streets), with its splendid porte-cochere, opened in 1892. The **Gale Memorial Library** (North Main Street, 603–524–4775), built in Romanesque Revival style in 1901, contains a museum.

Daniel Webster, perhaps New Hampshire's best-known public figure, was born in 1780 on a farm outside **Franklin.** The two-room farmhouse known as the **Daniel Webster Birthplace** (off Route 127, 603–934–5057), is a replica of the original, containing books and furniture from the days of Webster's youth.

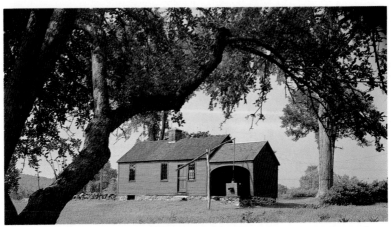

Daniel Webster was born in this farmhouse near Franklin in 1782, while his father was serving in Washington's army.

CANTERBURY SHAKER VILLAGE

A few years after she arrived in the Hudson River Valley from England to found the Shaker religion in 1774, Mother Ann Lee dispatched two followers to New Hampshire's Canterbury Hills. Here they established a thriving community, one of two still in operation in the United States. In Canterbury, 22 buildings remain of the 100 that graced the original 4,000-acre community, including houses, barns, workshops, mills, and a schoolhouse.

By the early 1800s the Canterbury Shakers numbered about 300, and the community was augmented by converts throughout the nineteenth century. The men and women worked together, farming (herbs and seeds were their specialties) and making textiles and a variety of farm and household implements—all of them for sale. The Shakers were inventors, dedicated to improving the condition and quality of their labor. Self-sufficient to a degree, the group relied on its own tinsmiths, cooks, cabinetmakers, weavers, and broommakers. Many ailments were treated by the community's own nurses, using medicinal herbs, but the Shakers did not forbid the use of outside doctors.

The first building in the Canterbury village was the **Meeting House,** raised in 1792. Like all Shaker architecture, it shows the sect's concern for order and simplicity. Next came the **Dwelling House,** with an impressive row of dormers beneath its chimneys and cupola. The last surviving brick structure is the 1838 **Trustee's Building.**

LOCATION: Route 93, Canterbury. HOURS: May through October: 10–5 Tuesday–Saturday. FEE: Yes. TELEPHONE: 603–783–9511.

A small island in the Merrimack River, in what is now the town of **Boscawen,** was the scene of an early episode of frontier violence. Hannah Dustin was brought here after being kidnapped by Indians from her home in Haverhill, Massachusetts; two others were taken captive with her, and her baby was killed before her eyes. When night fell, the three slew and scalped their captors and escaped down the river in a canoe. The incident is commemorated in a marker on the bypass of routes 3 and 4 in Boscawen; a nearby footbridge leads to the island (now known as Dustin's Island), where a statue of Dustin stands.

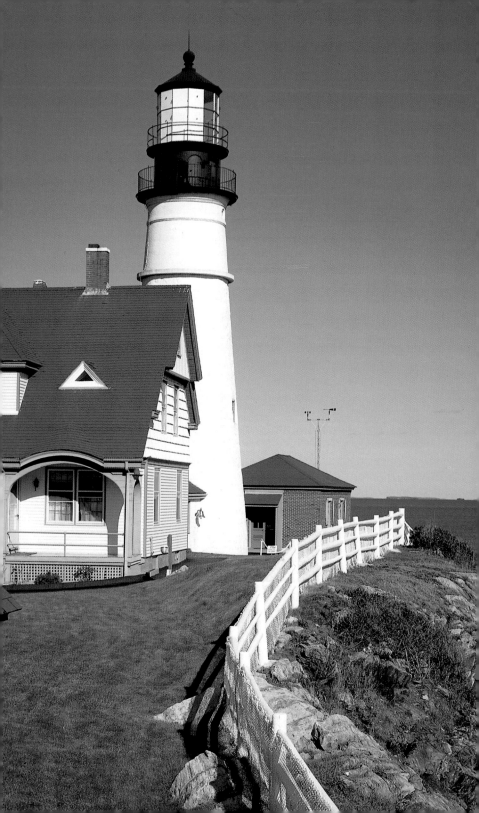

SOUTHERN MAINE

The northeasternmost corner of the United States gave chilly reception to its first transatlantic visitors. The Vikings probably were the first to sail into Maine's waters, about AD 1000. Sixteenth-century explorers scouted the coast, seeking Norumbega, a mythical land of riches much like the El Dorado sought by Hernando Cortes in Mexico at about the same time. Though the explorers never found the Norumbegan paradise and pots of gold, they did discover a more beautiful and—winters excepted—a more hospitable country than they might have expected from the Algonquin name for the place, Land of the Frozen Ground.

No one knows when European fishermen first began making semipermanent camps on the Maine coast to dry their fish, repair their boats, and trade for furs with the Indians. The kings of France and England both granted patents for Maine (the French in 1603 and the English in 1606). The first English settlement in Maine of which there is any record was established in 1607 at the mouth of the Kennebec River. Led by Sir George Popham, these colonists, many of them parolees from English jails, built the first English vessel constructed in America but disbanded after their first winter, the likes of which they had never felt in England.

Exploring the Maine coastline in 1614, Captain John Smith exulted over the natural abundance of "Lobsters . . . Fruits, Birds, Crabs," and "such excellent fish as many as their Net can hold." In 1622 two Englishmen eager to harvest Maine's abundance, John Mason and Sir Ferdinando Gorges, obtained a charter to the sixty-mile strip of coast between the Merrimack and Kennebec rivers and to all of the interior land between them. A 1629 division gave Gorges the land between the Piscataqua and the Kennebec. He planned to create large estates, along feudal lines, but a set of misfortunes, including the wreck of a new ship that was to carry him to America, prevented him from re-creating on this rugged coast a little England of colonial nobles and sturdy peasants. Maine continued as the domain of a tough lot of fishermen and traders.

Massachusetts assumed judicial control over Maine in 1652, and in 1677 Gorges's grandson sold the patent to Massachusetts. (Maine would remain part of Massachusetts until 1820.) The origin of the name of the province is obscure—it may have been so called to distinguish it, the mainland, from the offshore islands. In 1641, the English crown chartered its first city in America at the site of present-day York, Maine. That did not mean, however, that Maine belonged to England alone: The French, allied with Indians,

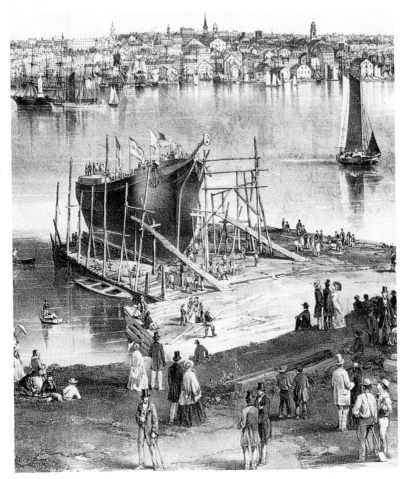

The Old Fishing Docks, Portland.

fought for their claims, and the Dutch came to fleetingly stake out some territory of their own.

From the 1670s to the end of "Queen Anne's War" in 1713, southern Maine was wracked by a series of wars with the Indians, marked by brutality on both sides. In those decades, the Indians succeeded in reclaiming much of their old land from the English. Entire settlements were abandoned, and streams of impoverished refugees descended on the towns of eastern Massachusetts, where they subsisted on official and private charity. The settlement at Wells survived only by transforming itself into a virtual fortress. In the thirty years of peace after Queen Anne's War, the coast and portions of the interior were rapidly resettled. French territory east of the Penobscot River came into English possession at the end of the French and Indian War in 1759, and the French formally surrendered their interest in the Treaty of Paris, signed in 1763. Except in the far northern borderlands (where the French language still can be heard), Maine became indisputably English.

At the end of the French and Indian War, Maine was still the least developed part of New England, with just fifteen incorporated towns and a population of roughly 20,000, about half that of New Hampshire, and a third of the population of Rhode Island. Fishing and farming settlements dotted the coast between Kittery and the Kennebec River. A primitive road ran parallel to the coast up to the Kennebec. (John Adams, travelling along it in 1771, called the trip "vastly disagreeable.") The interior was settled only to a distance of about twenty miles from the shore, with some deeper settlements along the rivers.

Southern Maine saw no fighting during the Revolution, with the notable exception of the British raid on Falmouth in 1775, in which the town was virtually destroyed. Most of the fighting in the state took place farther north. After the Revolution, Falmouth was rebuilt and renamed Portland. Despite a burgeoning population and some discontent with the policies of the state government in distant Boston, Maine would not become a separate state until 1820. It was admitted to the Union as part of the Missouri Compromise—Maine entered as a free state, Missouri as a slave state. Abolitionist groups formed in Portland and other cities as early as 1830, and Maine sent about 70,000 men to fight for the Union. Hannibal Hamlin, Abraham Lincoln's vice president during the war, was a former Maine governor and U.S. senator.

Industry developed rapidly after the war, when the railroads joined overseas shippers in getting Maine's huge timber harvests to market. The lumber, paper, and pulp industries, granite quarrying, iron and copper mining, and ice harvesting all contributed to the state's economy in the nineteenth century, as did its maritime pursuits—lobstering, cod fishing, sardine canning, and whaling.

This chapter covers the southern corner of Maine, beginning at Kittery and then following a route north along the coast, describing along the way the industrial cities of Berwick; Saco and Biddeford; Portland, Maine's most important urban center; and Brunswick (the site of Bowdoin College).

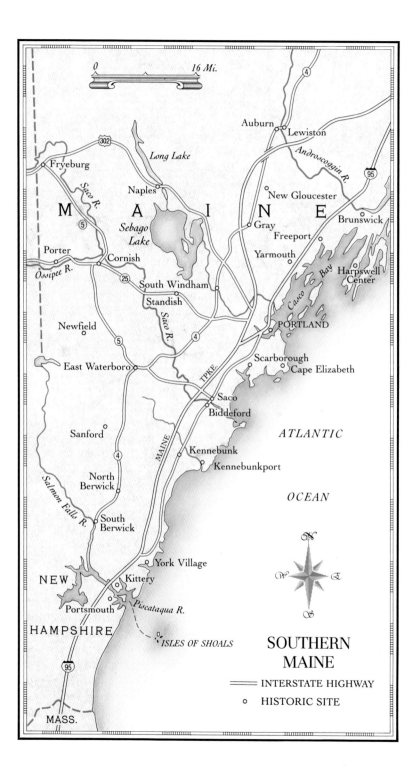

0   16 Mi.

4

Auburn Lewiston
302   Androscoggin R.
Fryeburg   95
           Long Lake
M Naples A   New Gloucester I N E
Saco R.   Gray   Brunswick
5   Sebago   Freeport
            Lake   Yarmouth   Casco Bay Harpswell
Porter   Cornish   Center
Ossipee R.   25
                     South Windham
                     Standish   PORTLAND
Newfield   Saco R.   4
           5   TPKE.   Scarborough
East Waterboro   Cape Elizabeth
                                              ATLANTIC
                                   Saco
                                   Biddeford
Sanford   OCEAN
           4   MAINE   Kennebunk
North   Kennebunkport
Berwick
Salmon Falls R.
           South
           Berwick
NEW   York Village
           Kittery
           Portsmouth   Piscataqua R.
HAMPSHIRE
                        ISLES OF SHOALS

                        SOUTHERN
                        MAINE
           95
                        ═══ INTERSTATE HIGHWAY
MASS.   ∘ HISTORIC SITE

KITTERY

Shortly after Kittery's founding in 1647, the British began building ships in this port city on the Piscataqua River. English warships were constructed here until 1776, when a Continental Navy ship, the *Raleigh,* was launched. In 1777, the *Ranger* sailed out of a Kittery shipyard under the command of John Paul Jones. (A monument to the Revolutionary War hero stands on Route 1, in the center of town.) The *Ranger* proceeded to France to bring news of Burgoyne's surrender, where she received the first official salute given the American flag by a foreign warship. Then, disguised under various flags, the *Ranger* confounded and waylaid British shipping vessels, adding to the war effort at home. She was captured by the British in 1780 and added to their navy.

Kittery remained active in shipbuilding after the Revolutionary War. In 1800 the U.S. Navy established the Portsmouth Naval Shipyard, which today continues to service ships and submarines on a number of Kittery's islands. Submarine construction began at the shipyard with the 1917 *L8.* Seavey Island, the original shipyard site (not open to the public), is almost entirely an historic district with eighteenth-century warehouses and other industrial structures and the Greek Revival residence quarters of naval officers. The **Kittery Historical and Naval Museum** (Rodgers Road, near routes 1 and 236, 207–439–3080) interprets Kittery's and the country's naval shipbuilding history, as well as the history of the community and the lives of the townspeople, through models of ships from the eighteenth century to the present, dioramas, photographs, and paintings. Special exhibits display the museum's assorted artifacts, including early examples of lighting, physicians' instruments, and other trade tools.

Fort McClary

The rise in the land at Kittery's Point, the oldest section of town, was officially ordered fortified in the early eighteenth century against the French, Indians, pirates—and to protect boats from the taxes and duties imposed by the government of New Hampshire. The initial breastwork that made up the fortification was named Fort William in honor of Sir William Pepperrell, a distinguished Maine colonist, justice of the peace, and loyalist. Fort William was garrisoned at the time of the Revolution and renamed Fort McClary in honor of Major Andrew McClary, a casualty of Bunker

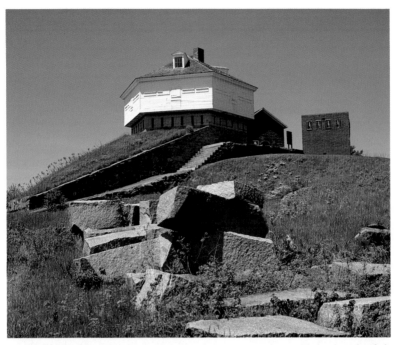

The hexagonal blockhouse of Fort McClary, perched on a granite point that has been fortified for nearly three centuries.

Hill. The fort was considered too well fortified for British attack during the Revolution; it was garrisoned during the War of 1812, Civil War, Spanish-American War, and World War I, when it was equipped as an observation post.

Fortification was improved in three major efforts, the first ca. 1808, next in 1844, and again in 1864, during the Civil War. The hexagonal blockhouse, probably built during the middle construction, is composed of a cut-granite first story on a mortared fieldstone foundation, topped with the traditional overhanging second story of squared logs. Maine's Bureau of Parks and Recreation administers the fort's surviving structures: the brick magazine, barracks' foundation, and granite wall from the first phase of improvements ca. 1808; the blockhouse and rifleman's house from the 1844 additions; and the granite powder magazine, unfinished perimeter walls, and two caponiers from the final modifications.

LOCATION: Kittery Point Road, off Route 103. HOURS: June through September: 9–5 Daily. FEE: None. TELEPHONE: 207–439–2845.

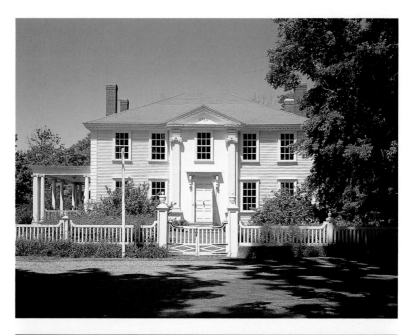

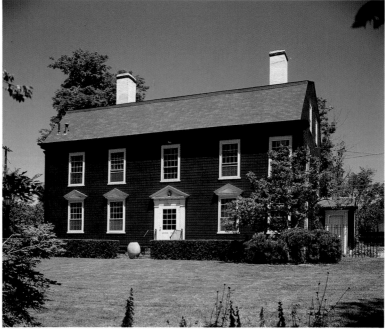

The **First Congregational Church** and **Old Parsonage** (Pepperrell Road) are survivors from the early eighteenth century. The church was incorporated in 1714, and the present building—the oldest church building in the state—dates from 1730. The Old Parsonage, now a parish house, was built in 1729.

Nearby is the **William Pepperrell House** (Pepperrell Road, private), built in 1720 as the residence of a Welsh lumber magnate and shipper who first settled on the Isles of Shoals before building this house. His son was named a baronet for leading the attack on the French fort at Louisbourg in King George's War in 1745. The house was remodeled by successive generations of Pepperrells into the structure seen today. Pepperrell died in 1759; in 1760, Lady Pepperrell took advantage of her wealth and built herself a stately and fashionable Georgian mansion. The **Lady Pepperrell House** (Pepperrell Road, private) overlooks the Piscataqua River and Portsmouth Harbor. A hipped roof covers the projecting center pavilion, which is flanked by two-story Ionic pilasters surmounted by a closed pediment. Dentil molding beneath the roof line encircles the house. The porch, fence, and grape arbor are additions from the 1920s. Nearby is a picturesque graveyard with a number of nineteenth-century headstones.

Also on Pepperrell Road is the 1870 **summer home of William Dean Howells** (private), author and editor of *Atlantic* magazine. Howells bought the house in 1902 and spent his summers here, writing and gardening, until 1912. He wrote from his "barnbry," stables he had moved from a corner of the lot and converted to a library, which his son later turned and attached to the house. Howells was publisher and friend to such literati as Henry James and Samuel Clemens, both of whom were guests here. In 1979, Howells's heirs donated the house to Harvard University.

ISLES OF SHOALS

Maine and New Hampshire share the Isles of Shoals. Lying nine miles off the coast, the handful of islands (Duck, Appledore, Smuttynose, Malaga, and Cedar belong to Maine) have a richer history than their barrenness suggests. Credited to Captain John Smith for discovery, they were originally called Smith's Islands and were home to all-male settlements of fishermen until 1647, when a man

OPPOSITE: *The stylish Georgian Lady Pepperrell House, above, and the gambrel-roofed Sir William Pepperrell House, below.*

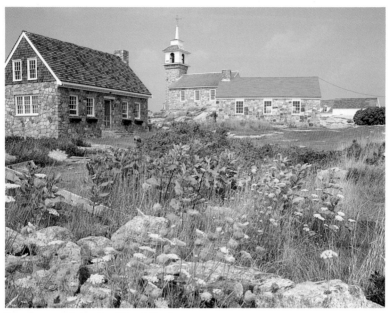

Stone houses and churches, Isles of Shoals.

named Reynolds battled the General Court of Massachusetts for the right to live with his wife and livestock on the island. It was decided that the woman could stay but the livestock had to go, for fear of disrupting the open-air fish drying and curing. That decision brought families to the Isles of Shoals, primarily to Appledore and Star islands. The islands gained a reputation for decent government, righteous churches, and outstanding education; mainlanders were known to send over their children for schooling. In 1715 the village of Gosport was settled on Star Island, and the islands thrived on whaling and fishing plus a healthy trading business with Spain.

The islands' vulnerability to British attack precipitated the settlers' relocation to the coast at the time of the Revolution. Afterwards, the islands were repopulated, but this time gained a reputation for rum, shipwrecking, and pirating.

Tales of ghosts, pirate treasure, and shipwrecked Spaniards proliferated, but by the 1820s the coast had exerted a proper civilizing influence over the islands. In 1847 Thomas Laighton of Portsmouth, New Hampshire, established the first summer hotel on Appledore Island and then another on Star Island. Through the early twentieth century the islands attracted intellectuals and artists, counting among their visitors Nathaniel Hawthorne, John Greenleaf Whittier, James Russell Lowell, and Frances Hodgson Burnett. An 1873 double murder on Smuttynose Island, which led to one of the last penal executions in Maine, revived images of the islands' post-revolutionary reputation and most likely aided their decline.

The islands are open to the public for day trips; ferries run regularly from Portsmouth, New Hampshire (603–431–5500).

YORK

Originally settled in the 1630s, the coastal village of York (incorporating York Corner and York Harbor) has a beautifully maintained historic district along both sides of the York River. The town was known earlier as Gorgeana, after its founder, Sir Ferdinando Gorges, before it was renamed in honor of the county in England.

The townspeople defended themselves against a series of Indian raids by raising a series of garrison houses at strategic points. A garrison house is often characterized by its bulky overhanging second story, but other configurations were used as well. The function of the house, providing a stronghold for both defense and offense, overshadowed any strict adherence to one specific form. The **MacIntire Garrison** (Route 91, private) was constructed ca. 1707 but architecturally recalls the seventeenth century. Its sawn log walls, nearly eight inches thick, are covered in dark clapboard siding, giving the structure a dark, seemingly impregnable mass. This garrison house has a second-story overhang and a large central chimney, which was rebuilt in 1909.

In the 1760s, York merchant and civic leader Jonathan Sayward bought a 1718 Georgian house, enlarged it, and filled the rooms with Queen Anne and Chippendale furniture, paintings, and porcelain. (The story goes that Sayward furnished his house with spoils from an expedition he led against the French in 1745.) Later Sayward generations and subsequent owners kept the house and its furnishings intact. The **Sayward-Wheeler House** (79 Barrell Lane Extension, York Harbor, 207–363–2709) now belongs to the Society for the Preservation of New England Antiquities.

During the Revolution, patriotic local citizens staged their own version of the Boston Tea Party, seizing a shipment of tea from an English sloop rather than pay taxes on it. Residents were also early industrialists—the town's 1811 cotton mill is among the oldest in the state. After the Civil War, York was a popular summer resort.

The **Old York Historical Society** (York Street and Lindsay Road, 207–363–4974) administers a complex of seven historic buildings dating from the mid-eighteenth century. The society's offices and library are housed in the George Marshall Store, a mid-nineteenth-century · general store overlooking Hancock Wharf. Some of the society's collections of furniture, textiles, and books belonged to York's earliest families. Tours of the society's properties, listed below, begin from **Jefferds Tavern** (Lindsay Road). Built in 1750 by Captain Samuel Jefferds, the tavern serves as a visitor center with exhibits and crafts demonstrations.

The 1719 **Old York Gaol** (Jail), one of the oldest public buildings in the country, was originally the King's Prison for the District of Maine. With fieldstone walls nearly three feet thick, it was used as a jail until 1860. In addition to the dungeons and cells used for

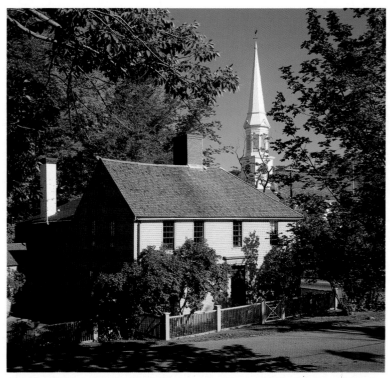

A pre-Revolutionary York landmark, the putty-colored Emerson-Wilcox House.

felons and debtors, the gaoler's quarters may also be viewed, furnished according to the household inventory of 1790.

The 1742 **Emerson-Wilcox House** has been many things—post office, tavern, tailor's shop, and private house several times over. It is now a museum of local history and crafts, displaying the country's most comprehensive collection of crewelwork bedhangings; twelve period rooms showcase furniture made in the region.

York's 1745 **Old Schoolhouse,** one of the oldest one-room schoolhouses in Maine, is furnished with original desks, benches, and books as well as exhibits on early schooling in the area. The **John Hancock Warehouse,** named for the Patriot who owned it, is the earliest commercial building in York, built in the mid-1700s. Interpretive materials illustrate river commerce and maritime trade of the region. The Society also administers the 1732 **Elizabeth Perkins House** (South Side Road at Sewall's Bridge). The former home of York's pioneer preservationist reflects the eclectic tastes of a family of collectors of the Colonial Revival period.

SOUTH BERWICK

The town of South Berwick, settled in 1623 on the Salmon Falls River near the Maine–New Hampshire border, figures prominently in Maine's agricultural and industrial history. In 1634 a shipload of the first cows in the state was unloaded on the banks of the Salmon Falls River, thus beginning dairy farming in the area. The first sawmill in Maine was established in 1634 on the falls, downriver from South Berwick village. The town is perhaps best known in New England for the **Berwick Academy,** a highly regarded secondary school dating to 1791.

The **Sarah Orne Jewett House** (5 Portland Street, 207–384–5269) is named for the noted New England author. Built in 1774, the house, which belonged to Jewett's grandfather, brought elegance to South Berwick—its hipped roof, dormer windows, and pediment doorway separated it from its simpler colonial neighbors. The house's interior is elaborate; local legend has it that three ships' carpenters spent 100 days carving the wainscotting, cornices, and door moldings. Jewett's sea captain grandfather and physician father lavishly appointed the house with imported furniture, tapestries, porcelains, and silver.

OVERLEAF: *Hamilton House, which was the setting for one of Sarah Orne Jewett's novels. It faces the Piscataqua River.*

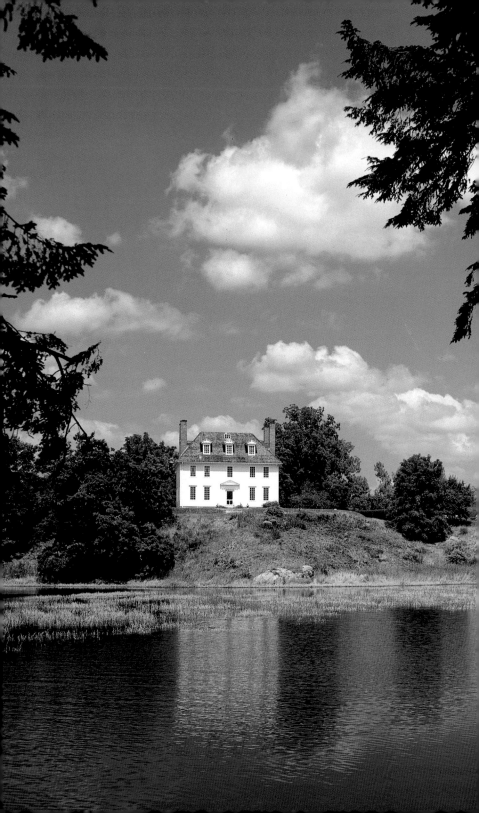

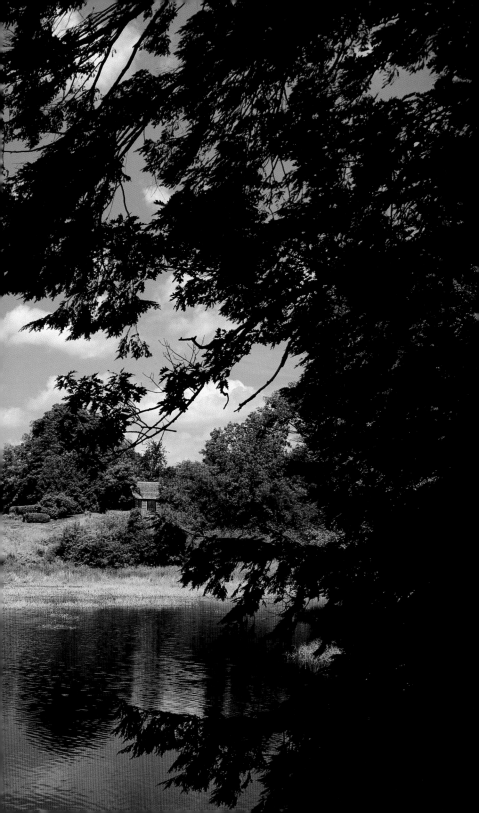

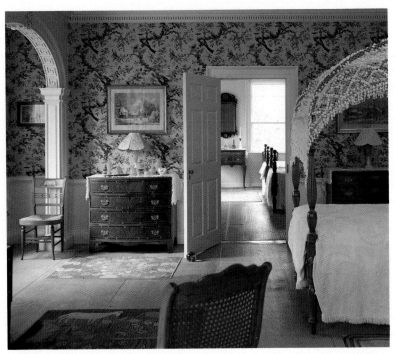

The master bedchamber of Hamilton House contains such fashionable turn-of-the-century appointments as Currier & Ives prints, bird-and-vine wallpaper and a fishnet bed canopy. The chest to the left of the doorway was made by a Piscataqua-area craftsman in the late eighteenth century.

Jewett set her Revolutionary War romance, *The Tory Lover,* in **Hamilton House** (Vaughan's Lane, off Route 236, 207–384–5269), which is dramatically sited on the Piscataqua River just outside the town of South Berwick. Colonel Jonathan Hamilton built the house on the river bluff in 1785. It passed to other owners and survived changes in the local economy from timber to shipping, farming, and manufacturing. In the 1840s the Hamilton estate was a sheep farm. Emily Tyson, a friend of Sarah Orne Jewett's, bought the house at the turn of the century and became one of the country's first patrons of historic house restoration. Tours of the property include the main house, the gardens, and the summer house.

The Old Berwick Historical Society is located in the **Counting House** (Route 4, 207–384–8041), an 1830 brick cotton mill. Local collections include a Jewett family library, Gundalow models, and historic papers.

NORTH BERWICK

The English settlers of North Berwick were fur traders in the 1630s and held on to their town when other settlements were abandoned during the upheavals of the French and Indian Wars. A veteran of those wars, Thomas Hobbs, Jr., built the **Hobb House,** a small inn on Wells Street, in 1763. Quaker Winthrop Morrell built his own two-story farmhouse in 1763, and his family has kept it for centuries. Known as the **Old Morell House,** it, like the Hobbs House, is privately owned.

In the nineteenth century, manufacturing dominated North Berwick's economy. Manufacturers specialized in plows and other farm tools, as well as sleds and toboggans. The **Hussey Plow Company** (Dyer Street, 207–676–2271), a family business since 1835, has turned its original store front and factory into a museum, displaying early agricultural equipment.

SANFORD

At the foothills of the White Mountains, Sanford was named for Peleg Sanford, a seventeenth-century governor of Rhode Island whose stepfather held the original deed to this verdant land. Sawmills and gristmills were operating on the Mousam River as early as 1740. After the Civil War Sanford became a major textile-manufacturing center. Woolen blankets and heavy cotton robes were local specialties. Later, Sanford mills became the automobile industry's major supplier of plush upholstery fabrics. One of the town's industrialists, Thomas Goodall, provided his workers with housing and recreational facilities and built the public library, the town hall, hospital, and baseball stadium. Goodall's **1871 Victorian house** is at 232 Main Street (private).

The **Emery Homestead** (Lebanon Street, private) dates from the 1830s and is an excellent example of "continuous architecture," with main house, barns, sheds, and other structures attached.

KENNEBUNK

Kennebunk's history as an important shipbuilding center is evident in its great variety of nineteenth-century houses. Ranging in style from Colonial to Queen Anne, from somber Federal to exuberant Gothic Revival, the houses were home to the shippers, shipbuilders, and sea captains who populated the town. Among the residences are the **James Smith Homestead** (Route 35, private), a mid-eighteenth-century Georgian farmhouse; the **Bourne Mansion** (8 Bourne Street, private), perhaps the finest Federal house in Maine; and the **Wedding Cake House** (Summer Street, private), a Victorian steamboat fantasy, supposed to have been a sea captain's extravagant gift to his new bride.

The **Brick Store Museum** (117 Main Street, 207–985–4802) began in an 1825 brick dry-goods store built by local merchant and shipowner William Lord and has expanded to fill three connected nineteenth-century buildings. Rotating exhibits pertaining to local social and maritime history are held in the first-floor galleries; on the second floor is a formal gallery of Federal-period furniture, portraits, and paintings of ships. Books, manuscripts, and personal effects of the Maine writer Kenneth Roberts and the novelist and playwright Booth Tarkington are also on display.

The museum also operates the 1803 **Taylor-Barry House** (24 Summer Street), built by the architect and builder Thomas Eaton for a prominent local family of shipmasters and shipowners. The Federal style house features a hipped roof, and the interior retains its original woodwork, moldings, and in the hallway, stencilling attributed to the itinerant stenciller Moses Eaton. Rooms are furnished with original pieces and are decorated in the Federal and mid-Victorian styles. The studio of Edith Barry, a twentieth-century painter, is at the rear of the house. Exhibits on local artists and authors are occasionally held in the house.

KENNEBUNKPORT

Nestled between Cape Porpoise Harbor and the Kennebunk River, this village began as a fishing and shipbuilding center. The historic district (along North and Maine streets and Ocean Avenue) is rich with houses from the eighteenth and nineteenth centuries, showing a stylistic progression from Colonial to Federal, Greek Revival, Gothic Revival, Italianate, and Second Empire. At the close of the nineteenth century, when shipbuilding was on the wane, Kennebunkport emerged as a summer resort. The most conspicuous evidence of the town's resort life is the 1889 **Kennebunk River Club,** a rambling Shingle-style clubhouse on Ocean Avenue, beside the river as it approaches the sea.

OPPOSITE: *A collection of Oriental export Rose Medallion porcelain is kept in the dining room of the Taylor-Barry House, just off the stencilled entrance hall.*

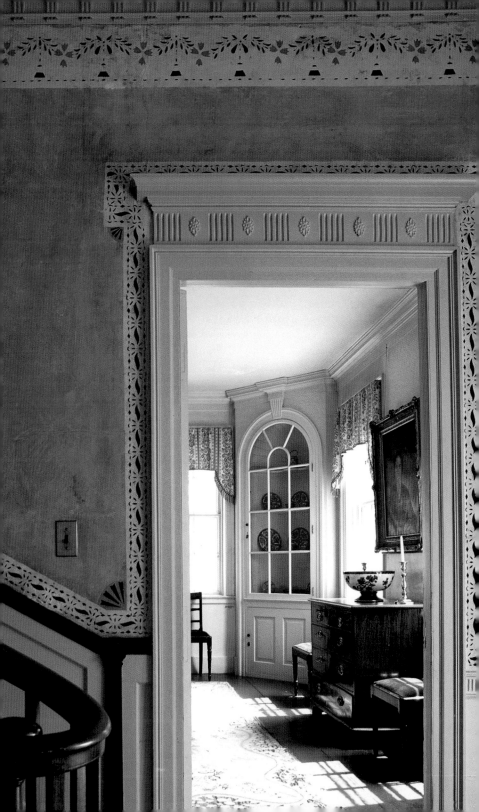

Among the notable houses are **White Columns** (Maine Street. 207–967–2751), an outstanding Greek Revival house with a monumental Doric colonnade topped by a bold pediment. The house was built in 1853 by Charles Perkins, a merchant who sold supplies to the big clipper ships as well as investing in their cargoes. He and his wife, Celia Nott Perkins, moved into the house as newlyweds; an interpretive tour of the house draws heavily from the detailed diaries Celia kept throughout her life there. The house retains all the original wallpaper, carpets, and furnishings, including a painting of the Perkins's daughter, Lela, by Kennebunkport artist Hannah Skeele and two magnificent embroidered crazy quilts made by Celia Perkins.

The three-and-a-half story Federal-period **Captain Lord Mansion** (corner of Green and Pleasant streets) was built from 1812 to 1815 by Captain Nathaniel Lord, a wealthy shipbuilder. The house features an octagonal cupola and a widow's walk. Charles P. Clark, president of the New York–New Haven Railroad and a grandson of Lord, used the house as a summer residence in the late nineteenth century; it is now being operated as an inn.

One of the country's best preserved gristmills is the **Perkins Tide Mill** (Mill Lane). Built in 1749, the mill, powered by tidal waters, remained in operation for nearly two centuries, finally shutting down in 1939. It is currently occupied by a restaurant.

The **Clark Building** (North Street, 207–967–2751) contains a small marine museum displaying artifacts of the shipbuilding era, such as ship models, paintings, tools, and anchors. The building formerly housed the offices for the Clark shipyards.

BIDDEFORD

Divided by the Saco River, the twin towns of Biddeford and Saco became Maine's first major industrial area. The first sawmill was constructed in 1653, and the nineteenth century brought vast brick mills, which still dominate the downtown area. The products of these mills—textiles, textile machinery, lumber, and flour—supplied a large domestic and foreign market.

A **monument** at Leighton's Point in Biddeford commemorates the explorer Richard Vines, who spent the winter in this area in 1616. Permanent settlement was established on June 25, 1630. The **Biddeford Historical Society** (270 Main Street, 207–282–9165), which resides at the McArthur Library, holds the town's records from 1653 to 1855. The library houses local genealogies, mill histories, and historic memorabilia—including photographs and architectural records of the region. The Society also administers the **First Parish Meeting House** (3 Meeting House Road), erected in 1759 and renovated in 1840, which may be seen by appointment.

SACO

Sharing Biddeford's industrial history, Saco is also home to the **York Institute Museum** (371 Main Street, 207–282–3031). Established in 1867, the museum houses a superb collection of Maine fine and decorative arts. The adjacent 1881 **Dyer Library** has a large collection of Biddeford and Saco records, including early newspapers, city records, and personal papers.

Nearby on Elm, North, and Upper Main streets are accomplished examples of Federal-period architecture interspersed with the later dwellings of textile-mill owners and workers. Several fine Greek Revival houses (all private) line the side streets.

SCARBOROUGH

On a peninsula just south of Portland is the small town of Scarborough. Its oldest structure, built in 1684, is the **Richard Hunniwell House** (Black Point Road, 207–883–8427), named for its owner, a captain during the Indian wars of the late seventeenth century. The modest shingled house and herb garden are typical of the period.

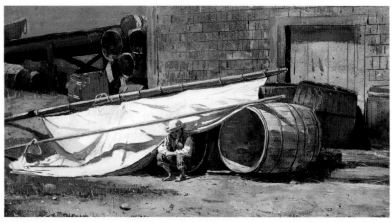

Winslow Homer, a longtime resident of Scarborough, painted many scenes of Northern New England such as the 1873 Boy in a Boatyard *(detail).*

In 1884, the artist Winslow Homer moved to a carriage house in Prout's Neck, an area of Scarborough, making it both home and studio until his death in 1910. The house, a modest structure built about 1870, offers vast views of the Atlantic that recall the artist's well-known paintings of the sea. The house has changed little since Homer's tenure and remains in his family.

In the Dunstan area of Scarborough is the **Scarborough Historical Society Museum** (Route 1, 207–883–6159). Housed in a 1911 brick building used as a generator house for trolley cars, the museum's collections include records of the town's early families, as well as their household items and tools, and fifteen murals by Roger Deering representing Scarborough's early history beginning in 1630.

On the Dunstan Landing Road a **millstone marker** identifies the birthplace of Rufus King, a signer of the U.S. Constitution, and his brother William, Maine's first governor.

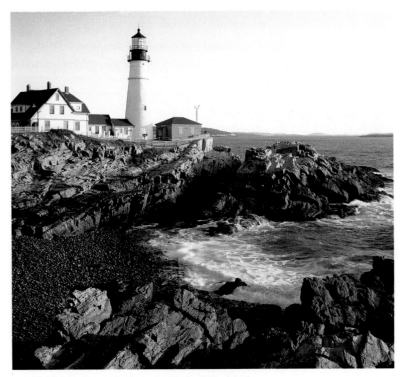

Rising above Maine's rocky shore: the Portland Head Light.

CAPE ELIZABETH

Jutting out into the Atlantic, Cape Elizabeth is the site of two of Maine's lighthouses—the **Portland Head Light,** built in 1790, and **Two Lights,** made of cast iron in 1874. Probably the best-known lighthouse on the eastern seaboard, the Portland Head Light is practically unchanged since George Washington ordered its construction. Off the cape is Richmond's Island, where an early-seventeenth-century trading post and fishing station has been preserved as an archaeological site.

PORTLAND

Beginning in 1623, the Casco Bay Peninsula attracted a series of French and English settlers who fought with one another, with Indian tribes and pirates—and with the brutal winters. The fragile European settlements hung on for nearly a century, occupied in fur trading, fishing, and lumbering. A hardy Massachusetts contingent arrived in 1715 and fortified the site with stone garrisons. By 1770, the place had gained a name—Falmouth—and some prosperity, from shipbuilding, as well as stepped-up exports of fish, furs, and lumber. White pines from the nearby forests became sturdy masts for the British Navy. From the West Indies came molasses to be distilled into rum.

During the Revolution, in October 1775, British ships dropped anchor in Casco Bay and opened fire, nearly leveling the town. Even in ruins, Falmouth was too important to abandon, and a few hundred colonists stayed on through the Revolution.

The town was gradually rebuilt after the war, and as Portland—so named on July 4, 1786—it grew into one of the Atlantic seaboard's major commercial centers. The nineteenth century saw fortunes made from the shipyard, railroad, textile, and lumber industries. By the 1850s, a dozen shipyards were launching trade vessels bound for Russia, India, and Europe. One of the first sugar refineries in the United States was the Portland Sugar Company, opened in 1855. A heavy manufacturer, the Portland Company, made train locomotives and other large industrial equipment for an international market. By the late 1860s, Portland ranked among the top U.S. ports—fourth in imports, fifth in exports. There was also the business of government: Between 1820 (when Maine joined the Union) and 1831, Portland was the state capital. Immigrants arrived from Scandinavia, Ireland, Italy, and Great Britain.

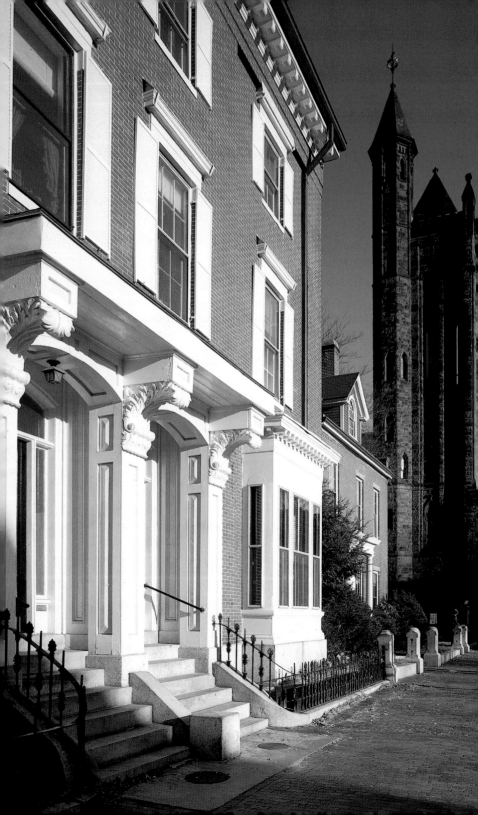

During the Civil War, strongly abolitionist Portland sent 5,000 troops and a fleet of gunboats to the Union. Shortly after the war the city experienced the disaster that has visited so many others: On July 4, 1866, a fire swept out of a tiny boat-house to engulf entire blocks of buildings. One third of Portland was destroyed, altering the development of many of the city's districts. Fore, Middle, and Exchange streets were the hardest hit by the fire. Whereas many of the buildings on the waterfront side of Fore Street survived, leaving architectural examples of Colonial, Federal, and Greek Revival buildings intact, the rebuilding of the devastated Exchange Street provided an array of later architectural styles. The fire accelerated Congress Street's transformation from residential to commercial development, which in turn opened the Eastern and Western promenades to residential building. The Western Promenade became Portland's affluent residential neighborhood, exhibiting the popular Victorian style of the day.

Along the historic waterfront and Portland's older residential streets are houses, churches, and commercial buildings that survived the fire. The **Tate House** (1270 Westbrook Street, 207–774–9781), a handsome Georgian residence built in 1755, belonged to George Tate, "mast agent" for the Royal Navy. Tate's job was to oversee the selection of trees, primarily white pine, used for masts on the king's ships. Mast production and trade helped establish Portland as a center of commerce after suitable timber from Portsmouth, New Hampshire, grew scarce. Tate lived in the house from 1755 to 1794. His son has the distinction of being the only American to become a first admiral in the Russian navy.

The building is unusual for its clerestory, an indented, windowed exterior wall rising above the second story. Inside, the first floor contains fine wood panelling, wide stairways, and tall chimney breasts: The central chimney serves eight fireplaces. The interior is furnished to exhibit the style customary to a wealthy eighteenth-century official. Letters and artifacts relating to Tate's son and collections of pewter and iron kitchen utensils are also displayed.

The Wadsworth-Longfellow House

Boyhood home of American poet Henry Wadsworth Longfellow, this house was the first brick house built in Portland. In 1785 General Peleg Wadsworth, the poet's grandfather, ordered the

OPPOSITE: *A quiet street in Portland. State Street Church rises to the right.*

bricks from Philadelphia and succeeded in having the first story built before running out of them. Perhaps the shortage was due to inexperience with the new building material—the first story has sixteen-inch-thick walls, twice as thick as usual. The second story was built in 1786 with the second shipment of bricks. The top story and Federal style roof of this primarily late Georgian three-story house were completed in 1815 after a fire destroyed the original roof. The changes in the brick patterns from story to story provide evidence of the building's history.

Henry Wadsworth Longfellow's family moved to the house in 1807, when he was an infant. There he grew up with his seven brothers and sisters, his parents, and his aunt. Both the Wadsworths and the Longfellows were descended from *Mayflower* Pilgrims, and his upbringing reflected the family's emphasis on education and moral purpose. Longfellow moved away to attend Bowdoin College in 1821 but returned frequently for lengthy visits. The house was given to the Maine Historical Society in 1901 by Anne Longfellow Pierce, the poet's sister. Wadsworth and Longfellow family furnishings, mementoes, and portraits, as well as an eighteenth-century kitchen are on display.

> LOCATION: 487 Congress Street. HOURS: June through mid-October: 10–4 Tuesday–Saturday. FEE: Yes. TELEPHONE: 207–772–1807.

Founded in 1822, the **Maine Historical Society** (485 Congress Street, 207–774–1822) is the fourth oldest such organization in the United States, ranking behind those of Massachusetts (1791), New York (1804), and Rhode Island (1822). Located behind the Longfellow House, its galleries and extensive collections cover genealogy and local and regional history.

At the turn of the nineteenth century, the Federal style of architecture gained in popularity, as evidenced by the buildings of Portland. The **Joseph Holt Ingraham House** (51 State Street, private) was built in 1801 for the prominent businessman and silversmith who is credited with the development of State Street; he later lost his wealth in the War of 1812. The house, which was designed by famed New England architect Alexander Parris, has undergone major changes, leaving the fanlight and cornice the only remaining

OPPOSITE: *A genealogy in sampler form, made by Elizabeth Mountfort of Portland in 1820, from the collection of the Maine Historical Society.*

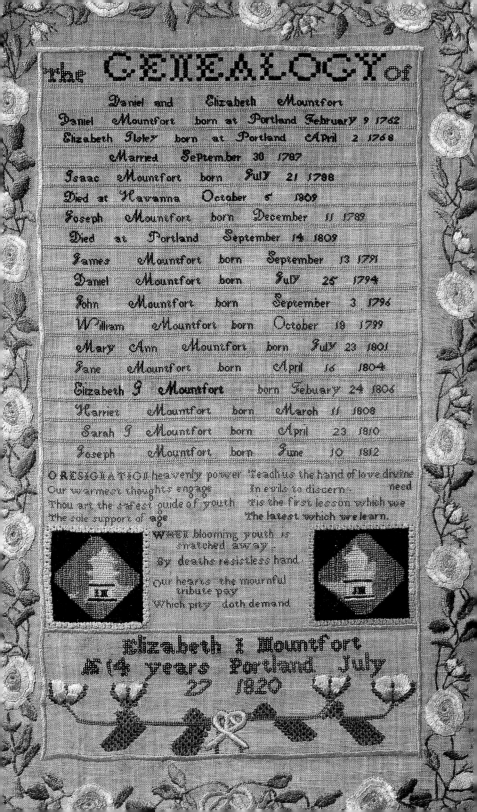

the GENEALOGY of

Daniel and Elizabeth Mountfort

Daniel Mountfort born at Portland February 9 1762

Elizabeth Ilsley born at Portland April 2 1768

Married September 30 1787

Isaac Mountfort born July 21 1788

Died at Havanna October 5 1809

Joseph Mountfort born December 11 1789

Died at Portland September 14 1809

James Mountfort born September 13 1791

Daniel Mountfort born July 25 1794

John Mountfort born September 3 1796

William Mountfort born October 18 1799

Mary Ann Mountfort born July 23 1801

Jane Mountfort born April 16 1804

Elizabeth I Mountfort born Febuary 24 1806

Harriet Mountfort born March 11 1808

Sarah I Mountfort born April 23 1810

Joseph Mountfort born June 10 1812

O RESIGNATION heavenly power   Teach us the hand of love divine
Our warmest thoughts engage   In evils to discern: need
Thou art the safest guide of youth   'Tis the first lesson which we
The sole support of age   The latest which we learn.

WHEN blooming youth is
snatched away.

By deaths resistless hand.

Our hearts the mournful
tribute pay

Which pity doth demand

Elizabeth I Mountfort
Æ 14 years Portland July
27 1820

Federal details. Parris also designed the **Richard Hunnewell House** (156 State Street, private). Built in 1805 for Colonel Hunnewell, a participant in the Boston Tea Party, this Federal mansion was remodeled in the 1920s by John Calvin Stevens, who enlarged it and added the front portico and Palladian window.

McLellan-Sweat House

This house remains an outstanding example of Federal architecture and a tribute to the expectations of a growing city and young country. The three-story brick mansion was built from 1800 to 1801 by John Kimball, Sr., for Major Hugh McLellan, a mariner and founding businessman of Portland. However, the Embargo of 1807 so set back the McLellan fortune that in 1815 the house was sold to Asa Clapp for about a quarter of the cost of its construction. The house was again sold in 1880 to Colonel Lorenzo de Medici Sweat, whose wife bequeathed it to the Portland Society of Art on her death in 1908.

The exterior of the McLellan-Sweat House now boasts its original ochre color, complementing a Palladian window and porticoed doorway with fanlight and sidelights in Federal style. Inside, the optimism of the times is depicted in the dining room mantel ornamentation: A goddess of plenty rides a chariot accompanied by a cupid and cornucopia. Both the interior and exterior of the mansion highlight the attention to detail and scale inherent in Federal styling. The Portland Museum of Art arranges tours through the unfurnished house, focusing on its architectural elements and plan.

LOCATION: 103 Spring Street. HOURS: By appointment. FEE: Yes. TELEPHONE: 207–775–6148.

The **Park Street Row** (88–114 Park Street), the largest rowhouse structure to be erected in Portland, was originally built in 1835 as twenty townhouses forming a U-shape around a park. The remaining fourteen attached brick houses gracefully carry Greek Revival details such as the cast-iron railings that unite the second-floor balconies. Begun as a real estate venture, the complex was sold by the stockholders before completion. Although the project was finished by the individual buyers, it remains a tribute to the forward thinking of its originators.

Morse-Libby House

A dramatic departure from the elegant Federal and restrained Greek Revival houses in Portland is the 1860 Morse-Libby House, better known as the **Victoria Mansion**—the style of the mansion a tribute to the Victorian age of opulent decoration and to the Queen herself. Ruggles Sylvester Morse, a Maine native, earned his fortune in the hotel business in New York, Boston, and New Orleans. He hired the architect Henry Austin to design this mansion in the grand manner of the South. The house was intended to be a summer home, away from the heat of New Orleans, where Morse lived at the time, but with the onset of the Civil War, he and his wife moved to Portland permanently.

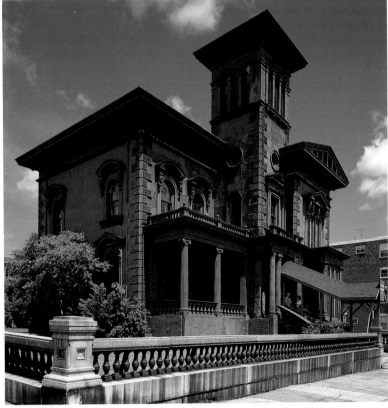

A stone villa, complete with Tuscan tower: Portland's Victoria Mansion, also known as the Morse-Libby House.

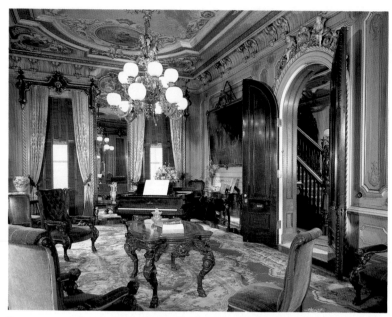

Extravagant window treatments, ceiling and wall decoration, and suites of furniture in the Morse-Libby House display the fashionable excess of the Rococo Revival.

A fine example of the Italian Villa style, the Victoria Mansion dominates the corner of Park and Danforth streets. A central square tower rises above two stories, a prominent cornice on one side, a classic pediment on the other. The pediment is echoed above the second-story windows on the one side while heavy hood-molds trim those on the other.

Within, the house displays a panoply of ornamentation: extravagant carvings, etched and stained glass, vibrant paintings and frescoes, medallions, cherubim, and richly appointed light fixtures. The painted and carved walls and ceilings, thought to be designed by Gustave Herter of New York, were executed by numerous artisans. A mahogany staircase ascends from a base flanked by bronze torch bearers; hand-carved chestnut panelling adorns the dining room walls; gilt, damask, satin, rosewood, mother of pearl, and marble accent the craftsmanship throughout. Most of the furnishings are original to the Morse household and reflect the taste and wealth of a Victorian entrepreneur.

Morse died in 1893; the house and furnishings were purchased from his estate in 1894 by Joseph Ralph Libby, a Portland merchant. In 1940, after more than a decade of abandonment, the house was bought by Dr. William Holmes and his sister, Clara, who subsequently donated it to the Victoria Society in 1943. LOCATION: 109 Danforth Street. HOURS: June through August: 10–4 Tuesday–Saturday, 1–4 Sunday. September: 10–1 Tuesday–Saturday, 1–4 Sunday. FEE: Yes. TELEPHONE: 207–772–4841.

Neal Dow Memorial

Built in 1829, this mansion was home of reformer Neal Dow and a center of political activity focusing on temperance, abolition, prison reform, and women's rights. A brigadier general in the Civil War, twice the mayor of Portland, a state legislator, and presidential candidate on the Prohibition ticket, Dow was internationally known for his temperance work. Portland's prosperous rum trade was an affront to Dow, and his response was the Maine Law, which in 1851 prohibited the making and selling of alcohol in the state. He spent much of his life touring the U.S. and abroad to promote his reforms. Dow's son bequeathed the home and furnishings to the Maine Woman's Christian Temperance Union, which maintains it as a memorial to Dow and as their headquarters. Rooms display furnishings original to the house from various periods, as well as paintings, portraits, silver, ornamental ironwork, and family memorabilia—including a set of china emblazoned with Dow's picture, a gift to his wife.

LOCATION: 714 Congress Street. HOURS: 11–4 Daily. FEE: None. TELEPHONE: 207–773–7773.

At 387 Spring Street stands a fine example of mid-nineteenth-century Gothic Revival architecture, a style made popular by American architect Andrew Jackson Downing and reflecting the prevailing romanticism of the day. Designed by Henry Rowe, the John J. Brown House, also known as the **Gothic House** (private), has a central gable with bargeboards and a porch with a Tudor arch, above which sits a simple tracery window. In 1971 the house was moved a half-mile to this location to preserve it from destruction.

The 1866 **Leonard Bond Chapman House** (90 Capisic Street, private) is notable for its mansard roof and concave tower. Chapman was a local historian whose collection of documents forms the foundation of the Maine Historical Society's library holdings on Portland's history.

Portland's oldest church is **First Parish Church** (425 Congress Street), also the city's first stone public building. This Colonial-Federal style structure was built in 1825–1826 on the site of "Old Jerusalem," the parish's wooden meeting house where Maine's constitution was drafted by the Constitutional Convention in 1819. The parish itself dates back to 1674 and its current members work to keep the church as it was when it was built; the pulpit, minister's chair, lighting fixtures, communion table, and even the pulpit Bibles date to the 1820s.

The **Portland Observatory** (138 Congress Street, 207–774–5561) sits on Munjoy Hill, where George Munjoy settled as early as 1659 and where victims of the 1866 fire dwelt in tent cities. The observatory was built in 1807 as a signal tower; a system of signal flags alerted citizens to approaching ships, and ships in distress could be spotted. The tower was closed at the turn of the century and reopened in 1939 as a historic site. The octagonal tower rises 221 feet above sea level, affording panoramic views of the harbor and the White Mountains; visitors climb 102 steps to reach the top.

Also on Munjoy Hill lies the oldest cemetery in Portland, the **Eastern Cemetery** (Congress at Mountfort streets). Chartered in 1688, it dates from the time when Portland was called Falmouth. Many of Portland's prominent citizens were buried here from 1670 to the late 1800s.

The 1828 **Mariner's Church** (368 Fore Street) brought Greek Revival architecture to Portland, though embellished with Federal style cornice and fanlight. The church was part of an unusual scheme: The large, columned structure housed shops on the ground floor—their rent financed the church and its missions—while the church maintained its chapel on the third floor. Built in the dock area of this rum-trading town where temperance was on the rise, the church meant to serve and educate the seamen. The building stands mostly unchanged, with shops operating on the ground floor, but the church is no longer used for worship services.

Another Portland church noted for its architecture is the **Chestnut Street United Methodist Church** (17 Chestnut Street). Designed by Portland architect Charles A. Alexander and built in 1856, it is an early example of Gothic Revival architecture.

At 32 Thomas Street, the 1878 **Williston-West United Church of Christ** stands in its high Victorian Gothic splendor, designed by Francis Fassett and later altered by his onetime partner John Calvin Stevens. Stevens also built the parish house, in 1904. This church is noteworthy not only for its outstanding ecclesiastical architecture but also as the home of the Young People's Society of Christian Endeavor, begun here in 1881. The society sparked the Sunday school movement, providing religious education tailored for children.

The **U.S. Customhouse** (312 Fore Street), a grand edifice in the Second Empire style, is a reminder of Portland's nineteenth-century prosperity. The massive building occupies a complete block on the waterfront, its mansard-roofed towers rising above two stories of New Hampshire granite, topped by an encircling balustrade. The interior chandeliers, woodwork, painted and gilded ceilings, and marble floors remain as elegant as when they were new; both within and without, little has been altered since the building was completed in 1871.

Eighteen hundred buildings were lost in the Great Fire of 1866 and for months many of the 10,000 homeless victims lived in emergency shelters and tent camps, eating in soup kitchens. The **Portland Fire Museum** (157 Spring Street, 207–775–6361, ext. 201), housed in the 1837 granite Greek Revival Fire Station No. 4, documents the history of firefighting in Portland and the Great Fire of 1866, using photos and artifacts.

Portland Museum of Art

As the oldest public art museum in the state, founded in 1882, the institution's original facilities include the 1800 McLellan-Sweat House and the 1911 L.D.M. Sweat Memorial. In 1983, the opening of the Charles Shipman Payson Building, designed in the Postmodern style by Henry Nichols Cobb of I. M. Pei & Partners, increased the museum's space tenfold and provided its current home. Five levels of galleries hold the museum's collections of American and English silver, Chinese art, Federal-period furnishings, American primitives, glass, maritime art, and paintings from the eighteenth century to the present. The core State of Maine Collection includes works by artists such as Charles Codman, Andrew Wyeth, Benjamin Paul Akers, Marsden Hartley, and Peggy Bacon, all of whom lived or worked in the state. The Charles Shipman Payson Collection of Winslow Homer paintings is also part of this core collection. Gallery space is provided for traveling exhibitions of fine and decorative arts.

LOCATION: 7 Congress Square. HOURS: 10–5 Tuesday–Saturday, 12–5 Sunday. FEE: Yes. TELEPHONE: 207–775–6148.

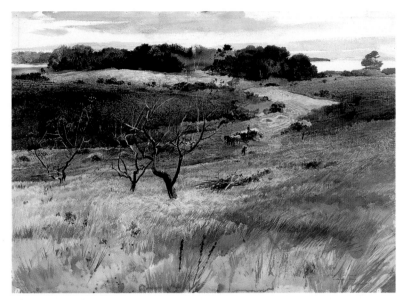

The 1941 Broad Cove Farm, *and other Andrew Wyeth paintings of the Cushing area, are in the Portland Museum of Art (detail).*

Fort Gorges was begun in 1858 on Hog Island, at the entrance to the city's harbor, and served as Portland's principal Civil War fortification. The fort is a massive hexagonal granite pile, typical of defensive military architecture of the time. Ironically, even before its completion in the 1860s, Fort Gorges's architecture was already obsolete. During both world wars, the U.S. Navy stored equipment and ammunition here.

Local architect George M. Harding, practicing in Portland from the 1850s to the 1870s, designed three prominent buildings on Middle Street, known as the Woodman, Rackleff, and Thompson blocks. The buildings were some of the earliest commercial structures built in Portland after the devastating fire of 1866, which explains their homogeneous character. The **Woodman block** (133–141 Middle Street) was the first of the three, built in 1867. Its rounded mansard roof, the most prominent Second Empire feature, tops an Italianate arrangement of windows and ground floor arcade. The cast-iron storefronts on the ground floor were made locally by the Portland Company. Harding put his name at the base of one of the pilasters. The first floor arcade and window arches of the **Rackleff block** (129–131 Middle Street) echo those of the Woodman; the facade, however, sits one foot lower. The flat roof and vertical groupings of windows give this structure a distinctive Italianate expression. Beyond its rounded corner and across the street, the **Thompson block** (117–125 Middle Street) imitates the Woodman block even more closely. Here a flat mansard roof tops a set of windows. A repetitive oak-leaf-and-acorn detail ornaments the building. Together, the blocks exemplify the grand commercial architecture of the late nineteenth century while concretely asserting Portland's viability after the Great Fire.

Another of Portland's outstanding commercial buildings commemorates the life of John Bundy Brown, the city's embodiment of the American Dream. Brown started work as a grocery clerk and died in 1881 the city's leading capitalist, having founded the Portland Sugar Company and the Falmouth Hotel, a favorite society spot. John Calvin Stevens designed the Queen Anne style **John Bundy Brown Memorial Block** (529–543 Congress Street) in Brown's memory. Its richly textured surface, asymmetrical facade, and variegated roofline are typical elements of this style, more often reserved for domestic structures. The **Greater Portland Landmark Association** (207–774–5561) offers walking tours of these areas.

SOUTH WINDHAM

The little town of South Windham is home to one of the finest Georgian residences in New England, the **Parson Smith House** (87 River Road, 617–227–3956), built in 1764 by the settlement's second pastor. The clapboard house has a handsome, if simple interior, with hand-planed panelling and spacious rooms, a showcase for the decorative styles of the day. The Smith family, among South Windham's original settlers, kept the house for almost 200 years, and many of its furnishings belonged to them. The eighteenth-century kitchen is primarily original, with a ten-foot hearth incorporating a later beehive oven. The house is owned and administered by the Society for the Preservation of New England Antiquities.

Babb's Covered Bridge, originally built in 1864 and reconstructed after a fire in 1973, crosses the Presumscot River off River Road, about two miles north of town.

STANDISH

The fine Georgian **Marrett House** (Route 25, 617–227–3956) went up for sale the same year it was built—when the Reverend Daniel

Marrett bought it in 1789, the house was only a few months old. It remained in the Marrett family for over 150 years, and each generation made changes outside and in. As a result, its architecture and furnishings reflect many decades of evolving styles. Among its many fine pieces are a Victorian parlor set, an eighteenth-century Newport card table, and Parson Marrett's standing desk, where he wrote his sermons. Marrett's descendants gave the house to the Society for the Preservation of New England Antiquities.

Reverend Marrett's church was Standish's first parish meeting-house, the **Old Red Church** (Oak Hill Road). The large but graceful frame structure, topped with an impressive cupola, went up in 1804 on land donated by the minister himself. Marrett served as pastor until 1829. Currently owned by the town of Standish, the church holds services in summer. The **museum** of the Standish Historical Society is located on the second floor.

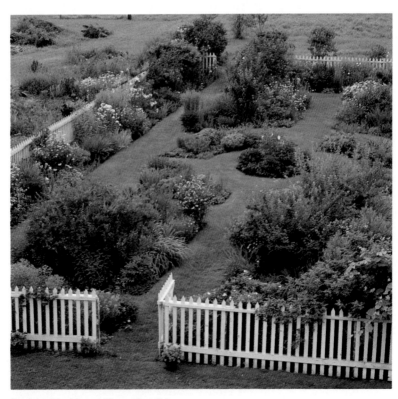

Garden of the Marrett House, Standish.

In nearby **Newfield** is the museum village **Willowbrook** (207–793–2784), an early nineteenth-century compound that includes a schoolhouse, two farmhouses, barns, and sheds.

PORTER

Porter profited from its position downstream from **Kezar Falls,** which powered many woolen mills near the New Hampshire border. Porter also attracted the Bullockites, followers of Jeremiah Bullock, a fundamentalist Baptist. In 1819 the Bullockites built their own church, stark and boxy, now known as the **Porter Old Meeting House** (Colcord Pond Road, 207–625–4667). Until 1900, town meetings were also held here. The historical society has administered the property since 1947.

FRYEBURG

Situated on the fertile Saco River plain, the land called Pequawket by the Indians became one of Maine's first English farming communities. It was later named in honor of Colonel Joseph Frye, who laid out the town lots in 1762.

Two of Fryeburg's earliest residences were incorporated into later structures. The **Squire Chase House** (151 Main Street, private) incorporates the ca. 1767 home of one of the first settlers, Nathaniel Marrill, moved from its original site in 1824. The current structure has been modified by Italianate detailing. The Federal-style **Benjamin Wiley House** (Fish Street, private) also contains an earlier structure, dating from 1772.

NAPLES

Arriving from Massachusetts in 1776, the Perley family acquired farmland around Naples and joined the ranks of the state's most prominent and politically active citizens. Their homestead, originally consisting of 2,000 acres of timberland, includes the 1809 **Perley Farmhouse.**

The **Songo Lock** is a relic of Naples's economic past. Built in 1830, the lock operated for years on the Cumberland–Oxford Canal (off the Songo River), an important trade artery between Portland and points north and west. From the Civil War to the turn of the century, the lock—a massive piece of machinery consisting of a stone frame and wooden gates—conveyed logs to sawmills. It is now used for private boat travel.

YARMOUTH

Sharing Casco Bay with Portland, Yarmouth is now a commuter town, lying just north of the city. A fishing village in the late 1600s, Yarmouth grew into a shipping and shipbuilding center in the nineteenth century. One of its oldest surviving buildings is the **Old Ledge School** (West Main Street, 207–846–6259), a 1738 one-room schoolhouse administered by the Yarmouth Historical Society. The Society also operates a **Museum of Yarmouth History** housed in the town's Merrill Memorial Library, designed in 1905 by A. W. Longfellow of Boston. Exhibits illustrate the region's heritage.

On the campus of **North Yarmouth Academy** (123 Main Street, 207–846–9051) are the Greek Revival **Russell** and **Academy** halls. Russell Hall was built in 1841; Academy Hall went up five years later. The town's **Baptist Meeting House** sits on an elevation above Hillside Street. Renovated twice since it was built in 1796, the church now blends Federal, Greek Revival, and Gothic Revival styles. A twentieth-century treasure is the **Grand Trunk Railroad Station** (57 Main Street). The small, ornate station was built in 1906, when Yarmouth was a stop on the Boston-to-Bangor rail line. It is now a shop.

FREEPORT

An eighteenth-century farming and fishing village, Freeport grew industrially in the 1800s. The **Freeport Historical Society** (45 Main Street, 207–865–3170) is housed in an 1830 brick house furnished with reproductions of nineteenth-century furniture and crafts. The Society also administers the **Pettengill House and Farm,** an eighteenth-century saltbox house on a 140-acre saltwater farm. Characterized by their proximity to the sea, saltwater farms combined agricultural and marine activities—their farmers used salt marshes as pasture land and supplemented their income with shipping and fishing. The farm also includes three outbuildings.

NEW GLOUCESTER

In the early 1700s sixty citizens from Gloucester, Massachusetts, established themselves in Maine in a settlement they named after their old home. Rebuilt after attacks during the French and Indian Wars, New Gloucester grew rapidly on a primarily agricultural basis after the Revolutionary War. Many of its white farmhouses and gray barns are over 200 years old.

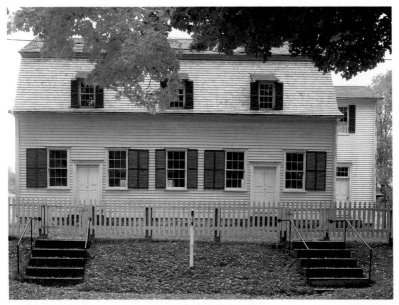

ABOVE *and* OVERLEAF: *Shaker Meetinghouse, near Sabbathday Lake and New Gloucester. The blue paint on the interior beams is almost 200 years old.*

The **Shaker Village** (Route 26, 207–926–4597), near Sabbathday Lake, is the remnant of the Shaker community founded there in 1783. The village consists of thirteen buildings, all of them exemplifying the Shaker ideal of uncluttered, functional beauty; some of them—the boys' shop, Shaker store, meetinghouse, ministry's shop—and the herb gardens are open to the public. Within the meetinghouse, the **Shaker Museum** displays many examples of the elegantly simple and functional designs for which the Shakers are known. Collections include furniture, textiles, farm tools.

LEWISTON/AUBURN

Known as Maine's twin cities, Lewiston and Auburn are divided by Lewiston Falls on the Androscoggin River. In its village days of the early nineteenth-century, the west bank of the river—the Auburn side—was known as Goff's Corner, for developer James Goff, Jr., whose store became a popular meeting place. The falls were harnessed to power both cities' textile mills and shoe factories. Shoemaking was a particularly big business in Auburn, with the first of the city's twenty-five shoe factories established in 1835.

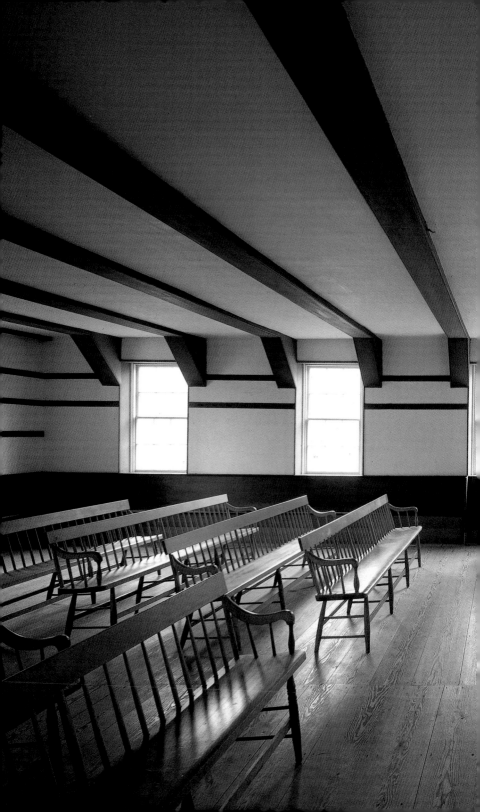

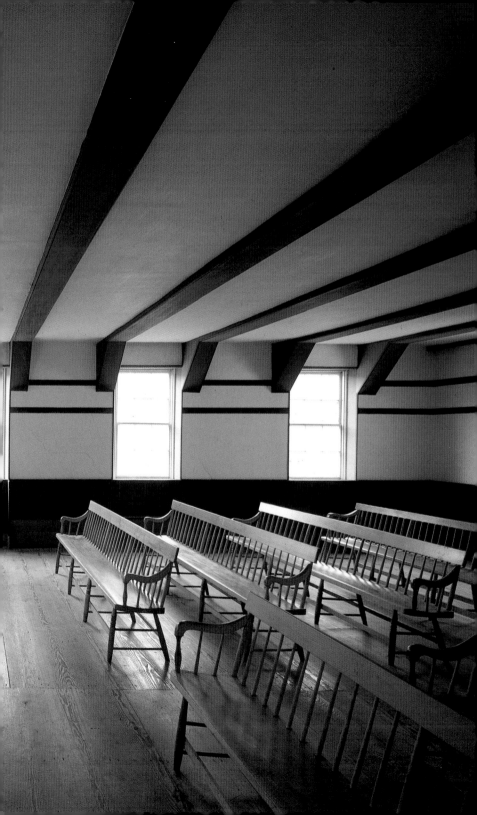

Most of the people employed by the factories after the Civil War were French Canadians, who created a rich bicultural society. The French influence is still felt and heard today, particularly in Lewiston where many family names are French. The neighborhood within Oxford, Lincoln, Cedar, and River streets is known as "Little Canada." Lewiston, on the east side of the river, was settled in the 1770s by Paul Hildreth, from Massachusetts. He built a log cabin on the Androscoggin, and operated the first ferry. Lewiston and Auburn grew steadily, as more arrivals from New England, Europe, and Canada came to work in the mills.

Lewiston and Auburn's historic sites date from the cities' late-nineteenth century industrial heyday and include handsome commercial rows, mills built of granite and red brick, and some grand Victorian houses and churches.

In Lewiston's Little Canada, the brick tenements of **Continental Mill Housing** originally spanned many blocks of Oxford Street. Two of the 1865 buildings survive, at numbers 66 to 82. The site of settler Hildreth's log cabin is now occupied by the **Continental Mill** (Oxford Street), a massive structure combining French Empire and Italian Renaissance styles. No longer an active mill, it is still readily identified by its high towers and long mansard roof. Across the street is the Norman Gothic style **St. Mary's Church,** built of Maine granite in 1907. The 1882 **Dominican Block** (141 Lincoln Street, private), a five-story Queen Anne-style building of brick and granite, housed the first school for French Canadians. It was designed by Lewiston's George M. Coombs, one of Maine's busiest architects at the turn of the century.

Coombs also designed the Second Empire **residence of U.S. Senator William P. Frye** (453 Main, private), one of Lewiston's grandest houses. One of Coombs's notable public commissions was the Romanesque **Oak Street School,** featuring elaborate interior woodwork. In 1902, Coombs designed another Romanesque edifice for the city, the public **library** on Park Street. Coombs also left Lewiston its most exotic building, the Shriners' **Kora Temple,** a Moorish, copper-domed structure on Sabattus Street.

The **Grand Trunk Railroad Station** (Lincoln Street) is another important landmark in the city's French-Canadian history—thousands of immigrants arrived in Lewiston at the small, Shingle-style terminal, opened in 1874 on a new branch of the Montreal-to-Portland line. Also of interest are the 1870 **Savings Bank Block**

(215 Libson Street), unified beneath a long mansard roof, and
Lewiston's baroque **City Hall** (Pine and Park streets), ornate and
spired, which was completed in 1892.

In the 1850s Irish immigrants populated the area south of
Oxford and Lincoln streets, where some of their modest houses
may still be seen. The area was also the site of the city's **1854
gasworks,** although a small brick Greek Revival office building and
decorative iron framework that once contained a huge gas tank are
all that remain.

On the quiet southern edge of Lewiston is **Bates College.**
Founded in 1855 as a Baptist seminary, it was named for Boston
benefactor Benjamin E. Bates in 1864, the same year that it became
one of the first coeducational colleges in New England. The
school's oldest buildings are **Hathorn Hall** and **Parker Hall,** both
designed by Gridley J.F. Bryant and both dating to the mid 1850s.

One of the oldest structures in Auburn is the 1827 **Edward Little
Mansion** (Main and Vine, private), the Federal-style home of the
man known as the city's founding father. Little inherited an enormous tract of land and did much to develop Auburn, establishing
the local academy and Auburn's first church.

Auburn's commercial development during the 1870s and
1880s is evident along Main Street. The **Roak Block,** once known
as "the cradle of the shoe industry," was named for Jacob Roak,
shoe manufacturer, banker, and developer. The industrial rowhouse is composed of nine distinct sections, designed to house nine
separate manufacturing operations. Built in 1871, it extends nearly
300 feet in length. Auburn's major textile mill, the 1873 **Barker
Mill** (Mill Street), is a decorative industrial facility, with mansard
roof, brick relief, and pedimented windows.

The city's high Victorian Gothic style is seen in the **First
Universalist Church** (Elm and Pleasant streets). Built in 1876, the
brick structure has a high steeple rising from a white, windowed
tower. Two of Auburn's notable houses, both private, are the
Charles A. Jordan House (63 Academy Street), an 1880 Second
Empire mansion built by architect Jordan for himself, and the 1889
Charles L. Cushman House (8 Cushman Place), designed by
George M. Coombs.

The oldest frame building in Auburn is the **Knight House,**
built on the west bank of the Androscoggin in 1796 by a settler

named Caleb Lincoln. Bought in 1861 by Nathaniel Knight, a butcher, the house stayed in the Knight family until 1918. Knight's brother, John Adams, published a pro-Union newspaper in England during the Civil War called *The London American*. Agricultural implements, household utensils, clothing, documents, and photographs are displayed at the **Androscoggin Historical Society** (207–784–0586) in the County Courthouse, built 1855–1857, at the corner of Court and Turner streets. An 1882 **monument** to Union soldiers of the Civil War stands on the courthouse grounds.

BRUNSWICK

In 1714 a group of Bostonians bought Brunswick in the Pejepscot Purchase (named for the Indians who inhabited the area). Previous settlements had disappeared, partially due to Indian raids, and in Lovewell's War of 1722 another raid depleted the new settlement. By 1727, however, settlement at Brunswick was stabilized, and the town was incorporated in 1739. Its location at falls on the Androscoggin River, with easy access to the Atlantic Ocean, promised industry and prosperity. The first dam across the river was built in 1753; Maine's first cotton mill was erected at Androscoggin Falls in 1809. The falls provided more than power—the waters were full of salmon to be caught, cured, and shipped throughout New England and overseas. Shipping, lumbering, and related industries also flourished, and in 1802 Bowdoin College opened.

The structures in the **Federal Street Historic District** (including Bowdoin College campus and Park Row), built in the early 1800s in a variety of architectural styles, were restricted by a twenty-foot setback and a two-story limit on buildings. The graciously proportioned lots and wide streets further display the town planner's concern with appropriately exhibiting prosperity.

The **Lincoln Street Historic District** is an early example of lot subdivisions. True to his orderly sense of urban growth, Dr. Isaac Lincoln made the lots an even four rods (66 feet) along the street; a few corner lots were six rods and twenty links (112 feet), with setbacks of sixteen links (10.5 feet). The lots were sold within fifteen months and the majority of dwellings built within two years, giving the district an architectural homogeneity indicative of the mid-nineteenth century.

Harriet Beecher Stowe lived at 63 Federal Street from 1850 to about 1852. While her husband, Calvin Stowe, taught Natural and

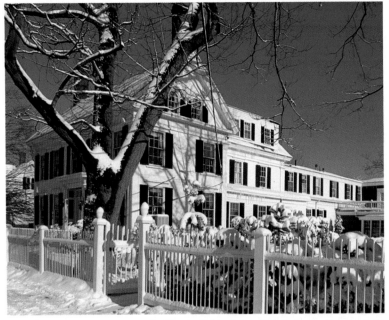

Harriet Beecher Stowe wrote Uncle Tom's Cabin *by candlelight in the kitchen of this rambling Federal house.*

Revealed Religions at Bowdoin College, she wrote her famous work, *Uncle Tom's Cabin*. The 1807 structure where the Stowes lived is now an inn.

St. Paul's Episcopal Church, at 27 Pleasant Street, is a modest 1845 work of Richard Upjohn. The same year, Upjohn designed the **First Parish Church** (Main Street and Bath Road), a more characteristic example of the architect's Gothic Revival style.

The century-old **Pejepscot Historical Society** (159 Park Row, 207-729-6606) owns two Victorian houses notable for their architecture and their residents. The **General Joshua L. Chamberlain Civil War Museum** (226 Maine Street), a simple single-story structure when it was built in 1820, was home to Henry Wadsworth Longfellow when he taught at Bowdoin College in the 1830s. Chamberlain—a Civil War hero at the Battle of Gettysburg, governor of Maine, and president of Bowdoin—moved the house to its present location and enlarged it. Among Chamberlain's guests was Ulysses S. Grant. Restored by the historical society, the house contains period furniture and Civil War mementoes.

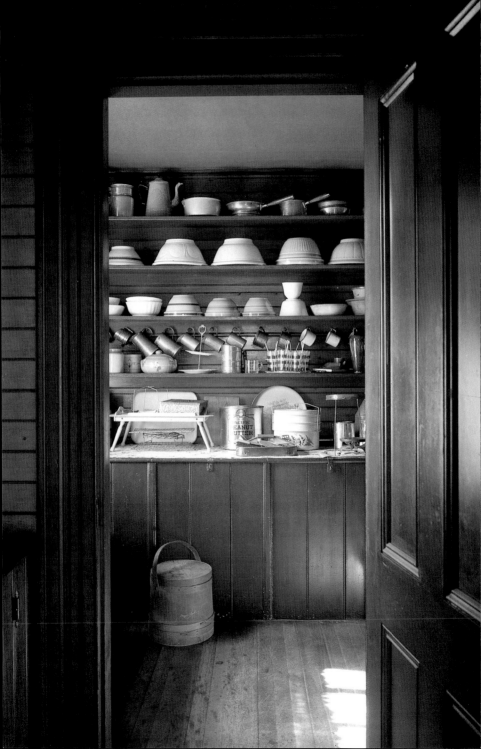

The **Skolfield-Whittier House** (161 Park Row), also administered by the Society, is an Italianate double mansion topped by an eight-sided cupola. It was built in 1858 by George Skolfield, grandson of Irish immigrants who came to Brunswick in 1739, and founder of Brunswick's Skolfield Shipyard in 1801, for his two sons and daughter. The two sides of the house mirror each other, presenting a unified facade, but are split in the rear by an alleyway. Skolfield descendants lived on the south side of the mansion for over 100 years, and in 1982 they donated the house to the Pejepscot Historical Society as a house museum, virtually unchanged since the last half of the nineteenth century. The north side of the mansion, altered extensively in the interior by its successive owners, was purchased by the Society in 1983 and now houses the **Pejepscot Historical Museum.** It contains exhibits on local history, furniture, clothing, household items, and other collections illustrating life in Brunswick from the eighteenth century to the present.

In its seventeen rooms, the south side of the Skolfield-Whittier House Museum reflects three generations of life in Brunswick while remaining true to its Victorian origins. The large drawing room windows are hung with drapes of twill and velvet; also remaining are the twenty-four-candle Belgian chandeliers, an English rosewood piano, delicately needlepointed footstools, and a porcelain French clock with matching vases. The seafaring nature of the Skolfield and Whittier families is documented in paintings of master shipbuilder George Skolfield and the Skolfield ship, *Roger Stewart,* and the display of a ship's barometer used on many Atlantic crossings by Captain Alfred Skolfield. The accumulations of generations of this Yankee trading family add up to a rare trove of nineteenth-century history: Mechanical toys, china-head dolls, pots, pans, books, and ship's logs fill the shelves.

Bowdoin College

Chartered in 1794 and opened in 1802, Maine's oldest college is named for James Bowdoin II, a Massachusetts governor whose son generously endowed the liberal arts institution. Bowdoin College has graduated a number of the country's foremost citizens, among them Franklin Pierce, fourteenth president of the United States; William Pitt Fessenden, secretary of the treasury under Lincoln;

OPPOSITE: *The pantry in the Skolfield-Whittier House contains bowls, tin cups, and other utensils owned by the family.*

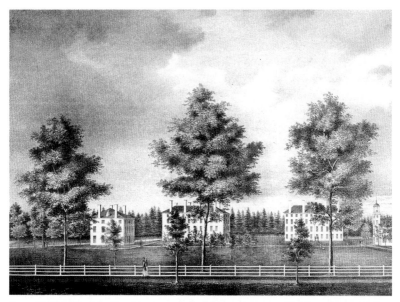

A ca. 1840 print of the Bowdoin campus, viewed from the west, with Massachusetts Hall at left. Newer buildings—and pine trees—have filled in the grounds.

Admiral Robert E. Peary; Nathaniel Hawthorne; Henry Wadsworth Longfellow; and the noted abolitionist and Maine governor John Albion Andrews.

The public is welcome on the handsome 110-acre campus, which is part of the Federal Street Historic District. The representative architecture of the campus includes the work of Samuel Melcher; Richard Upjohn; McKim, Mead & White; Hugh Stebbins; and Edward Larabee Barnes. Guided tours of the campus begin at the Moulton Union (207–725–3000).

Massachusetts Hall, the oldest building on campus, was designed by Aaron and Samuel Melcher and has a cornerstone dating from 1799, when construction began. As a result of financial distress suffered by the college in its early years, the building wasn't completed until 1802. At that time it housed the entire college: eight students, one teacher, and the president. Remodeled in the early 1870s and restored and altered in 1936, the building is currently used for dormitory facilities but maintains its original Federal style exterior.

The **Hawthorne-Longfellow Library,** which contains 725,000 volumes plus a fine collection of rare books and manuscripts, is named for Nathaniel Hawthorne and Henry Wadsworth Longfellow, both members of the class of 1825. On the third floor the library regularly mounts displays from its special collections of Hawthorne and Longfellow manuscripts, books, pamphlets, and memorabilia as well as examples from novelists Kenneth Roberts, Kate Douglas Wiggins, Marguerite Yourcenar, and others.

Peary-Macmillan Arctic Museum

Administered by Bowdoin College, the Peary-Macmillan Arctic Museum commemorates the explorations of Admirals Robert E. Peary and Donald B. Macmillan, another pair of famous alumni, classes of 1877 and 1898, respectively. Peary is best known for his trip to the North Pole; some credit him with being the first man to reach that point. He and his crew sailed from New York in July of 1908 on board the *Roosevelt*, harboring at Cape Sheridan in September and then continuing on sledges in February 1909. Macmillan was his chief assistant on that trip, but his feet froze and he could not complete the journey. When Peary, by his account, reached the Pole on April 6, 1909, his camp consisted of himself, Matthew Henson, and four Eskimos; the others had been sent back as supplies dwindled.

The museum is divided into three sections. The first covers Peary's early career in the tropics and the Arctic with documents, photographs, navigational instruments, and other artifacts from his expeditions. Stuffed musk oxen, polar bears, seals, and a walrus are exhibited on a platform above the gallery.

Peary's famous trek to the North Pole in 1908 to 1909 is covered in the second section of the museum, with in-depth exhibits depicting the methods and equipment he used. Highlighted artifacts include Macmillan's North Pole log and one of five sledges Peary took to the Pole. The box in which Peary carried his navigational equipment, Macmillan's snowshoes, and their pickaxes, guns, and fur garments are also on display. The fur outerwear was Peary's adaptation of Inuit fur clothing worn in North Greenland.

The recent release of Peary's North Pole journal has again cast controversy around his claim to be the first person to reach the North Pole: His navigational errors and extraordinary speed records, in addition to information on Arctic weather patterns, currents, and ice drifts, raise the possibility that Peary missed his goal by as much as sixty miles. However, Peary's Arctic explorations are deservedly commemorated here.

The third part of the museum focuses on Macmillan, whose career included twenty-seven Arctic expeditions, and on the Arctic in the first half of the twentieth century. Inuit soapstone and ivory carvings, bone and antler tools, embroidered and beaded skin clothing, paintings, a full-size kayak, and an egg and bird collection help describe the area and the time. The cameras Macmillan used to capture the Arctic people and landscape are also on display.

Bowdoin alumni have had a strong tie with exploration: In 1869 a Bowdoin professor crewed his ship with students while sailing the coast of Labrador and Greenland. The museum is housed in Hubbard Hall, named for another Bowdoin alumnus and benefactor of both the college and Peary's Arctic adventures. The designer of the museum, Ian M. White, accompanied Macmillan on a trip to the Arctic in 1950.

LOCATION: Hubbard Hall, Bowdoin College. HOURS: 10–4 Tuesday–Friday, 10–5 Saturday, 2–5 Sunday. FEE: None. TELEPHONE: 207–725–3416.

The **Bowdoin College Museum of Art** (207–725–3275), once housed in various campus buildings—including the Chapel, designed by Richard Upjohn—now occupies the Walker Art Building, an 1894 Beaux Arts edifice designed by Charles Follen McKim of McKim, Mead & White. McKim commissioned artwork for the four murals gracing the impressive rotunda to represent the "Four Cities of Art," Athens, by John LaFarge; Florence, by Abbott Thayer; Rome, by Elihu Vedder; and Venice, by Kenyon Cox.

In 1811 James Bowdoin III, first patron of the college and Thomas Jefferson's foreign minister to France and Spain from 1805 to 1808, bequeathed his collection of old master drawings to the school. Today the collection has been expanded to include the Boyd Gallery of American Federal and Colonial portraits, silver, and furniture; the Sophia Walker Gallery, housing American painting and sculpture by John Sloan, Mary Cassatt, Marsden Hartley, Daniel Chester French, and others; the large Winslow Homer Gallery, with memorabilia, graphics, and paintings; a gallery of European painting, sculpture, and decorative arts; and a collection of Mediterranean objects and Oriental ceramics.

The 1849 **Henry Boody House,** now the dean's residence, is named for the college's first professor of rhetoric and oratory. The house, at 256 Maine Street, is conspicuous for its exuberant Carpenter Gothic exterior.

HARPSWELL

On a peninsula just east of Brunswick is Harpswell, a picturesque sea village. **Orr's and Bailey's islands** are off its shores. The **Harpswell Meeting House,** a simple clapboard structure built in 1757, is the oldest surviving meetinghouse in Maine.

After graduating from Bowdoin College in 1877, Robert E. Peary took a job in Washington with the Coast Survey. He took the opportunity to purchase an island in Casco Bay, off the mainland at Harpswell, that he had explored as a youngster. He renamed the island **Eagle Island,** perhaps in token of the first ship that took him to the Arctic, the *Eagle,* and began to build a summer home in 1904. The family spent much time here until Peary's death in 1920, and in 1966 the island was donated to the State of Maine by Peary's daughter. The small, dramatic, rocky island, crossed by nature trails, is accessible from a public landing pier, and the house (207–725–3416) contains Peary family furnishings, photographs from explorations, and mounted animal specimens.

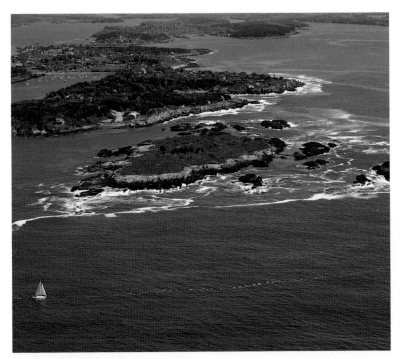

Janquish and Bailey's islands, Casco Bay.

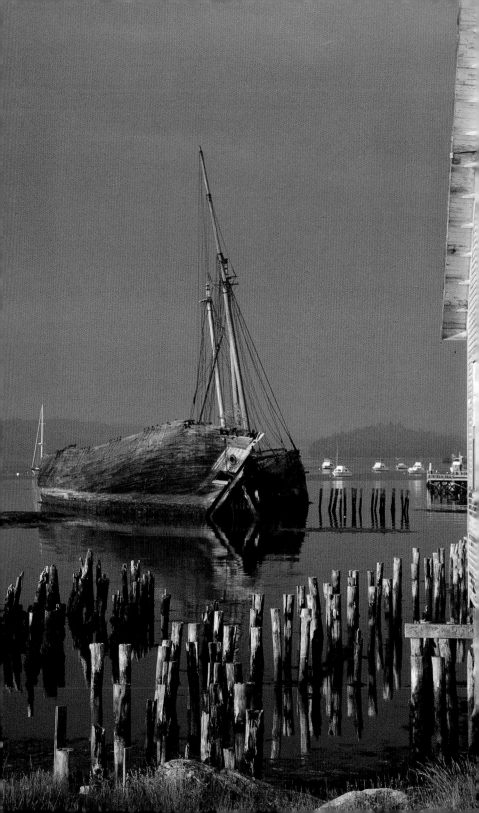

THE
MAINE COAST

OPPOSITE: *Relics of the shipbuilding era, the 1918* Hesper *and the 1917* Luther Little, *in Wiscasset's harbor.*

The Maine coast has long been known as one of the most beautiful landscapes in America. In 1734 a Massachusetts visitor wrote that "All that Coast appears to be full of commodious Rivers, Bays, Harbours, Coves, and delightful Islands; the most agreeable part of the *Massachusetts Province,* both for Scituation, Fishery, Lumber-Trade, and Culture; and highly worthy of the Publick Care." More than a century earlier, the explorer Samuel de Champlain called the mouth of the Penobscot River "marvelous to behold," with its "numerous islands, rocks, shoals, banks, and breakers on all sides." Marvelous it was, but dangerous as well: Champlain had several mishaps on this coastline.

The first attempt to put down a permanent European colony in the New World took place in far northern Maine—one of the least hospitable places for such an endeavor. The French established a colony on the St. Croix River in 1604, but the pioneers had to give up after just a year. In the international tangle of royal land grants, the territory from Pemaquid to the St. Croix River was part of the colony of New York, granted to the Duke of York in 1664. However, a 1667 treaty ceded the land between the Penobscot and the St. Croix to France. It was soon occupied by the colorful Baron Castin, who lived as a local potentate among the Indians, marrying an Indian woman and carrying on a profitable trade in furs. Castin led Indian raids against the English during King Philip's War but was burned out of his house by an English attack in 1688. The land between the Penobscot and the St. Croix became England's after the French and Indian War.

During the Revolution, the coast of Maine was the site of the war's first naval battle—a small affray in which the people of Machias seized an English boat, the *Margaretta*—and an American naval disaster on a much larger scale. A fleet of forty-four Massachusetts ships attempted to take Fort George at Castine, and all of them were destroyed. One of the participants in the debacle was Paul Revere. In the finger-pointing that followed, Revere was accused of insubordination, unsoldierly conduct, and cowardice, but he was acquitted in a court martial. During the War of 1812 the British captured Castine, rebuilt Fort George, and made it their coastal strongpoint—they controlled the coast from Penobscot to the east throughout the war.

The spectacular scenery along the coast is actually a drowned mountain range, the creation of an ice age 13,000 to 15,000 years ago, when the ocean level was 300 to 500 feet lower. An ice sheet

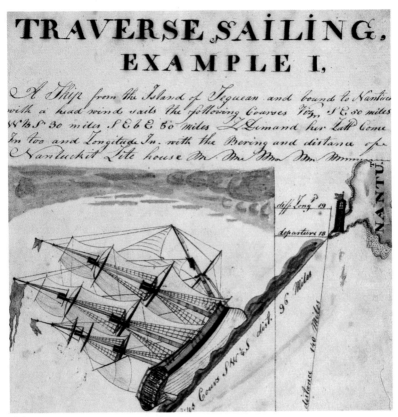

Detail from an 1805 navigation book, hand-written and illustrated by Captain Francis Rittal of Dresden, Maine.

scraped across a bed of volcanic granite, carving and gouging ridges and U-shaped valleys and depositing large "erratic" boulders. As the ice melted, the earth—freed of the great weight of ice—rose, as did the level of the ocean. The granite valleys were flooded, but the peaks remained above water. Somes Sound, 168 feet deep, is the only fjord on the east coast. In the nineteenth century, the beauty of this area attracted some of the country's foremost landscape painters as well as thousands of wealthy summer visitors, who flocked to the fashionable resort at Bar Harbor. Acadia National Park preserves the rugged landscape of Mount Desert Island, which was visited and named by Champlain.

This chapter begins at Bath and makes its way up the coast to Calais on the St. Croix River.

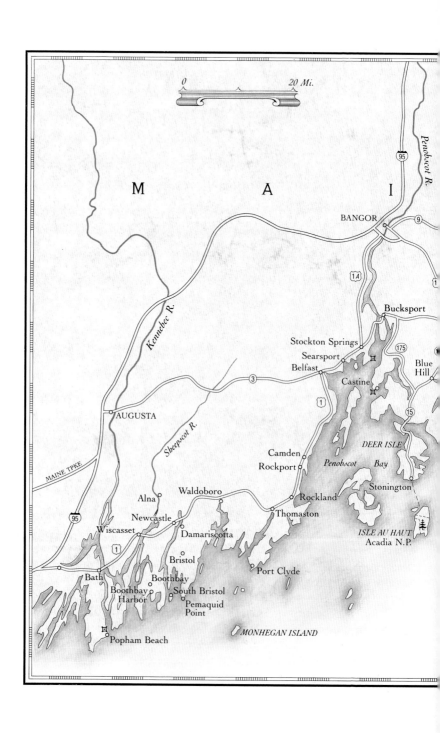

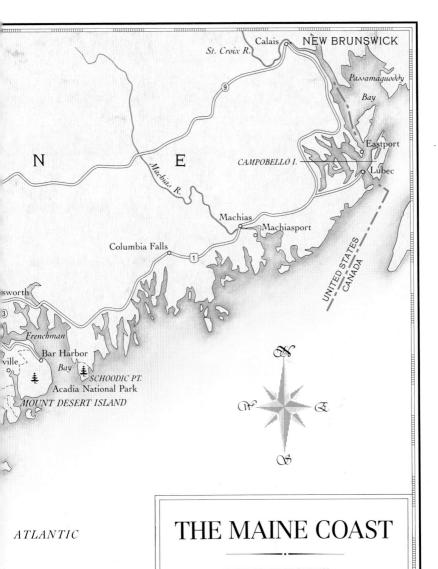

Calais
St. Croix R.
NEW BRUNSWICK
Passamaquoddy
Bay
9
Eastport
N
E
CAMPOBELLO I.
Lubec
Machias R.
UNITED STATES
CANADA
Machias
Machiasport
Columbia Falls
1
sworth
3
Frenchman
Bar Harbor
ville
Bay
SCHOODIC PT.
Acadia National Park
MOUNT DESERT ISLAND

ATLANTIC

OCEAN

THE MAINE COAST

═══ INTERSTATE HIGHWAY
○ HISTORIC SITE
⌕ FORT
♣ PARK

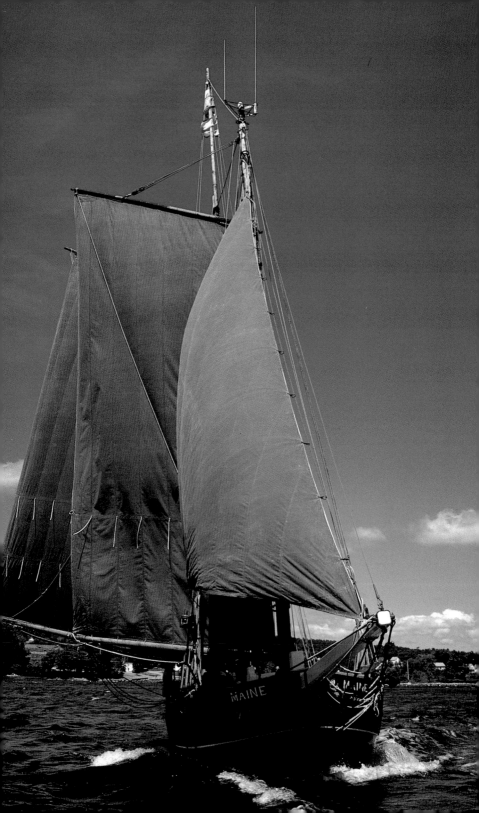

MID-COAST: BATH TO CAMDEN

The road from Bath to Camden passes historic ports and islands, shipbuilding centers, towns built up around sawmills and gristmills, and fishing villages. The path is anything but direct, winding through gently rolling hills and skirting seaside cliffs. Some agriculture is evident, from roadside stands selling squash and corn to blueberries raked up in nearby fields.

BATH

Shipbuilding began early in the Bath area when English settlers christened the thirty-ton *Virginia* near here in 1607. Along the banks of the Kennebec River, Bath became a center for masting, shipbuilding, and trade, accompanying the progress of many Maine coastal towns. Various factors, however, lent the town the strength to survive the Embargo of 1807 and the War of 1812. Bath withstood the impact of the Embargo by building a healthy trade relationship with New Orleans and the east coast of America. Industrial diversification increased Bath's resources as iron founding grew in the early 1800s, and the combination of iron and ships gave the town a very prosperous nineteenth century. Italianate, Greek, and Gothic Revival architectures testify to Bath's heyday, especially in the North End, where prosperous shipbuilders made their homes and the commercial district thrived.

Maine Maritime Museum

In 1762, Bath's first commercial shipyard opened. After the Civil War, trade with foreign countries dropped off and, with it, the building of ocean-crossing vessels. Coastal trading demanded a different type of transport, and two Bath shipwrights, Samuel R. Percy and Frank A. Small, knew how to build fine, wooden schooners, perfect for the new trade routes. From 1896 to the 1920s the Percy and Small Shipyard produced over forty schooners and gained a reputation for building some of the largest and finest wooden ships on the coast.

Today, the history and craftsmanship of Maine shipping and shipbuilding are explored and re-created at the **Museum Shipyard,** on the site of the Percy and Small Shipyard. The *Wyoming,*

OPPOSITE: *A replica of an 1830s double-masted pinky schooner, the* Maine *was launched by Bath's Maine Maritime Museum Shipyard in 1985.*

the largest wooden sailing vessel in America, was built here in 1909. The tradition of fine boatbuilding craftsmanship continues through the museum's apprenticeship program, and visitors can view the apprentices at work on small boats, both specially commissioned and for sale through the museum. Other exhibits at the shipyard include models of classic boats, tools and instruments, dioramas, trade goods, and seamen's possessions. Restored shipyard buildings such as an 1897 paint and trenail shop, an 1899 mill and joiner shop, and a 1905 pitch oven portray the shipbuilding industry, while lobstering and cod fishing are explored at a replica lobster cannery and on board the schooner *Sherman Zwicker* when she is in port.

The museum also operates the 1844 Georgian Revival **Sewall House,** named for the prominent shipping family that bought it in 1898. On view here is a trove of maritime art, scrimshaw, ship models and half models, navigational instruments, and sailors' mementoes, as well as displays on shipbuilding, seafaring families, and famous vessels of the Bath Iron Works.

LOCATION: *Percy and Small Shipyard*, 263 Washington Street; *Sewall House*, 963 Washington Street. HOURS: *Shipyard and House:* Mid-May through mid-October: 10–5 Daily; *House (off season):* 10–3 Monday–Saturday, 1–4 Sunday. FEE: Yes. TELEPHONE: 207–443–1316.

Looming over Route 1, the **Bath Iron Works** (207–443–3311) grew out of an 1826 foundry and remains active in shipbuilding. It is open to the public for launching and commissioning ceremonies.

The 1843 **Winter Street Church** (Washington at Winter Street), merging Gothic and Greek Revival styles, dominates the town green. Its striking design was the work of local builder Anthony C. Raymond. The soaring central steeple and solid temple facade effectively unite the two styles of architecture, presenting one of the finest examples of American Gothic in New England.

The unusual church at 804 Washington Street is the Gothic Revival **Chocolate Church,** named for its brown color. Built in 1846, it has recently been rededicated as an arts center, with performance space and an art gallery.

The **Old Bath Custom House and Post Office** (1 Front Street, 207–443–4282) was designed by Ammi Burnham Young in 1858 while he was supervising architect of the Treasury Department. In the lobby is a model of the Bath waterfront as it appeared in the 1800s. The stone Italianate building stands on the site of the estate of William King, a Bath shipbuilder who became first governor of

Maine. King also owned an **1809 stone cottage,** one of the earliest Gothic Revival structures in America. On Whiskeag Road, it is now privately owned.

POPHAM

South from Bath, Route 209 winds through grassy marshland to the sea. The terminus of the road is **Popham Beach,** named for Sir George Popham, who in 1607 led a band of his fellow Englishmen to this protected harbor. Popham did not survive his first winter in Maine, and his colony disbanded within a year—though not before they had launched the *Virginia,* the first European ship built in the colonies and the vessel that inaugurated Bath's fame.

In 1775, Benedict Arnold set off from Popham on his daring but ill-fated march against the British in Quebec. His expedition, which had a good chance of conquering Canada, came to grief when a message from Arnold to another American officer fell into British hands, spoiling Arnold's element of surprise. Markers chart the 194-mile **Arnold Trail** to Coburn Gore on the Canadian border. From Popham the trail passes through Hallowell, Skowhegan, Solon, Moscow, Stratton, and Sarampus.

Fort Popham, named for the nearby 1607 English settlement, was built to fortify the mouth of the Kennebec River against Con-

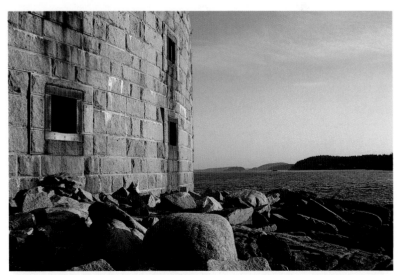

Built in 1861, the granite-walled Fort Popham stands on a strategic site—where the Kennebec River meets the sea—first fortified during the American Revolution.

federate and pro-Confederate European intervention at the beginning of the Civil War. The semicircular granite structure faces the river with thirty-foot walls, broken by two stories of vaulted casemates built to contain thirty-six cannon.

WISCASSET

North from Bath, Route 1 leads straight through picturesque Wiscasset. First settled as a section of the larger town of Pownalborough in the early 1700s, Wiscasset was abandoned during the Indian wars of that time, and resettled around 1730. By 1795 Wiscasset was a town of wealth and prosperity. Its riches came from the post–Revolutionary War lumbering and shipping that aided many of Maine's coastal towns. Along with these towns, Wiscasset was badly hurt by the 1807 Embargo Act and the War of 1812. But during the years of lucrative commerce the citizens of Wiscasset built many large homes and mansions reflecting the wealth and prestige of shipping merchants and lumber barons. Many of these are to be found within Wiscasset's **historic district,** encompassing the village and waterfront.

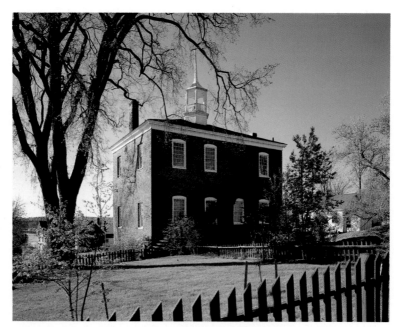

The 1807 Old Academy Building, Wiscasset, above the Sheepscot River.

Nickels-Sortwell House

One of New England's finest Federal houses, this grand three-story house was built in 1807 by Captain William Nickels, a shipmaster and local politician who made his fortune in lumber and shipping. Two-story pilasters frame the porticoed entry and its elliptical fanlight. The interior is notable for the curved three-floor stairway, lit from a skylight, and handsomely carved woodwork throughout.

After Nickels' death in 1815 the house became Wiscasset's best inn, variously known as Turner's Tavern, Mansion House, Belle Haven, and Wiscasset House. It fell into disrepair and was bought in 1900 by Alvin F. Sortwell, then mayor of Cambridge, Massachusetts, and made into his summer home. The Sortwells restored the house and refurnished it to reflect its Federal origins. The house now belongs to the Society for the Preservation of New England Antiquities, which maintains the property as a museum.

> LOCATION: Main and Federal streets. HOURS: June through September: 12–5 Wednesday–Sunday. FEE: Yes. TELEPHONE: 617–227–3956.

Down Federal Street from the Nickels-Sortwell House is the unusual octagonal **Captain George Scott House** (private), built in 1855 by the nineteenth-century shipmaster to plans of Orson Squire Fowler, a phrenologist and proponent of octagonal dwellings. The brick house is in the gracious Italianate style with sandstone and granite window sills and lintels.

The 1807 **Red Brick Schoolhouse** (Warren Street) is also part of Wiscasset's historic district. Used as a school until 1923, it has since functioned in various capacities. The one-time **Customs House and Post Office** (Water Street), now a private residence, has retained its 1870 brick-and-granite Italianate exterior. The **Lincoln County Museum and Old Jail** (207–882–6817) on Federal Street features exhibits on local history that highlight textiles and samplers, photographs of the area, scrimshaw, and Indian artifacts. Two structures make up this site. The jail was built between 1809 and 1811 to accommodate the rowdy seamen and woodsmen attracted to the boom port town. Its walls are built of granite up to forty-one inches thick. The brick jailer's house (1839) was built to replace a previous wooden one that burned down. The kitchen has been restored to its 1840s appearance, and antique farming and carpentering tools are on display in the tool shed. The jail was in use until 1953.

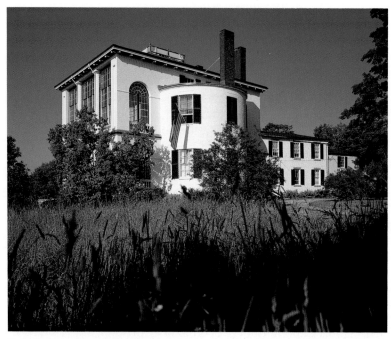

Probably designed to recall a Scottish castle, the Lee-Tucker House is celebrated for its mid-nineteenth-century sea captain's furnishings and freestanding spiral staircase.

Overlooking Wiscasset Harbor, the **Lee-Tucker House,** locally known as **Castle Tucker** (Lee and High streets, 207–882–7364), was built by Judge Silas Lee in 1807. Heavily mortgaged to three neighbors, the house had a variety of occupants until 1858 when it passed to Captain Richard H. Tucker, Jr., third generation of Wiscasset ship captains and owners. He added the portico in 1860 and purchased most of the furnishings now on view. It is still in the possession of his descendants.

Slowly deteriorating in the river harbor are the hulls of two schooners. Side by side, the 1918 *Hesper* and the 1917 *Luther Little* are believed to be the last four-masted schooners built in New England.

FORT EDGECOMB

Just east of Wiscasset, across the Sheepscot River on the tip of Davis Island, is Fort Edgecomb. In the early nineteenth century, Wiscasset's prosperity lay in shipping to and from England and France.

As hostilities between these two countries escalated and England threatened to impound U.S. ships entering French ports, Congress passed the Embargo Act of 1807, which closed all American ports. Built in 1808, Fort Edgecomb was one of many defenses authorized by Congress in response to feared English reprisals. When news of war reached Fort Edgecomb in 1812, the U.S. colors were raised and guns fired, but never in battle. One soldier stationed at Fort Edgecomb in 1814 noted in his diary, "The enemy . . . it is reported are coming with an intent to destroy this fort and Wiscasset," and the British ship *Bulwark* spent that summer harassing the Maine coast. With news of peace in 1815, the guns fired again. The fort was quickly garrisoned in 1864 when the Confederate ship *Tallahassee* sailed into northern waters, but once again, no action was needed.

Today the two-story octagonal blockhouse of massive timber and the semicircular earthworks remain within the stockade, which was reconstructed in 1961. Two stone bastions along the river are connected by a curved stone wall. Harbor seals are often seen here in the Sheepscot River.

LOCATION: Davis Island. HOURS: Memorial Day through Labor Day: 9–sunset. FEE: Yes. TELEPHONE: 207–882–7777.

BOOTHBAY

English settlements sprang up in and around this harbor after Captain John Smith sailed up from Jamestown in 1614 and pronounced it an "ideal" fishing station. The town grew first as a seaport, then as a shipbuilding center. Fishing and shipbuilding are still active in Boothbay, and since the nineteenth century it has been a popular resort.

In 1937 a theater was started to entertain the summer residents, an offshoot of which became the country's first museum exclusively devoted to theater, established in 1957. The **Boothbay Theatre Museum** (Corey Lane, 207–633–4536) occupies the 1784 Federal house of Nicholas Knight, one of the town's first settlers. The museum collections date from the eighteenth century to the present, encompassing American theater scale models, portraits, photographs, playbills, set models, costumes, stage jewelry, and holograph material. South of the village proper is **Boothbay Harbor,** known for its lighthouse, the 1822 **Burnt Island Light Station.**

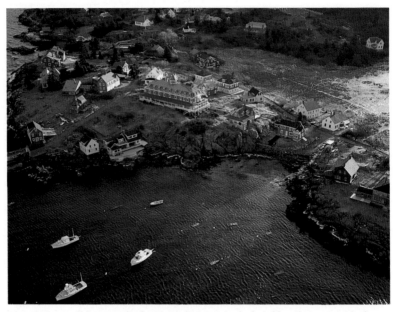

Though the English are credited with its discovery in the late fifteenth century, Monhegan Island was probably visited by Vikings 500 years earlier.

MONHEGAN ISLAND

Situated to the northeast of Boothbay Harbor in the Atlantic Ocean, this island was recorded by John Cabot in 1498. In 1614 Captain John Smith landed here, and his favorable accounts probably hastened settlement, which came in 1625. Abundant fishing has maintained a permanent community here since 1674.

In 1822 Congress appropriated $3,000 to build the **Monhegan lighthouse and keeper's quarters.** First illuminated on July 2, 1824, the light was supervised by a keeper until it was automated in 1959. The lighthouse and its outbuildings are now part of a museum with exhibits on the historical, natural, and economic features of the island. Monhegan Island may be reached from the mainland by ferry from Boothbay Harbor and Port Clyde.

BRISTOL

A center of archaeological activity, Bristol is the location of the **Nahanda Village Site,** a prehistoric coastal Indian encampment. It is believed that the camp was occupied as much as 2,000 years ago, although the majority of the material uncovered dates to ca. 1600. It is probable that this is the Indian village visited by members of the Popham colony in 1607, at which time they recorded the name of the area as Pemaquid. At **Colonial Pemaquid** (Route 130, 207–677–2423), the site of an early-seventeenth-century English settlement, archaeologists have excavated household items, farming implements, stone foundations, and walls.

The settlement is part of a state historic site along with **Fort William Henry,** also on Pemaquid Point. The foundations of the original fort, built by English settlers in 1692 to ward off Indians, pirates, and their French rivals, are here along with a modern replica of the circular, crenelated fort, resembling the stout tower of a medieval castle. Historical artifacts are also on display.

The **Pemaquid Lighthouse** was erected in 1827; its tower was rebuilt eight years later. In 1857 the original stone **keeper's house** was replaced by the present wooden structure, now occupied by the **Fishermen's Museum** (207–677–2494). Maine's 400-year-old fishing industry is illuminated by old charts, photographs, ship models, harpoons, anchors, and nets.

Representative of the eighteenth century is the **Harrington Meeting House** (Old Harrington Road, 207–529–5578). It has

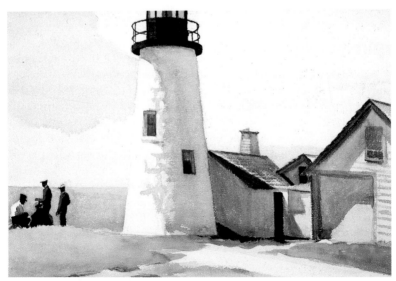

American artist Edward Hopper painted this view of the Pemaquid Lighthouse in the 1920s (detail).

been restored to its 1772 condition, complete with original box pews. That same year, the citizens of Bristol built the **Walpole meeting house** (Route 129) for its sister settlement, **South Bristol.** First a Presbyterian, then a Congregational, church, it reflects superior colonial workmanship inside and out: Even the hand-shaved roof shingles are intact (and still watertight). The pulpit and box pews are original, handcrafted by Bristol cabinetmakers.

Slightly farther out Route 129 is the **Thompson Ice House,** facing a South Bristol pond where ice was harvested for over 150 years, from 1826 to 1986. Ice from this spot was shipped as far as South America. Nine inches of sawdust insulate the double walls. Modern refrigeration has all but ended this Maine industry, which once supplied the nation with 3 million tons of ice each year. The structure is undergoing restoration (1988) and will reopen as a museum.

DAMARISCOTTA

Farther up the Bristol peninsula is Damariscotta, settled on the eastern shore of the Damariscotta River in 1625. Its location at the head of navigable waters encouraged shipbuilding, which brought prosperity to the town in the nineteenth century. A fire in 1845 destroyed most of the town's early buildings, but their replacements, built during the shipbuilding boom, remain intact as the **Main Street Historic District.** Also on Main Street is the one-and-a-half-story **Chapman-Hall House,** built in 1754 by Nathaniel Chapman. Constructed of wood, with a cedar-shingle rooftop and small-paned windows, the house has a central entrance and a central brick chimney. The interior consists of pine panelling and wide-board spruce and pine floors. The house, Damariscotta's oldest surviving building, is open to the public; exhibits include photographs of ships built on Damariscotta River during the period 1754–1820 and small models of ships.

Also in the historic district is the 1802 Federal style **Matthew Cottrill House** (private). Cottrill, an Irish immigrant, became one of Damariscotta's premier merchants. The architect, Nicholas Codd, an Irishman himself, also designed the oldest Catholic church in New England, **St. Patrick's,** on Academy Road in nearby **Newcastle.** Irish immigrants founded the parish in 1796. The steeple houses a Paul Revere bell cast in 1818, the year he died.

WALDOBORO

A German settlement dating from 1748, Waldoboro lies just inland on the Medomak River, protected from the sea while having immediate access to it. Shipbuilding was a major industry here, and five-masted schooners sailed out of local shipyards. Waldoboro's early German heritage resonates in the **Old German Church** (Route 32, off Route 1), built on the Medomak River in 1772. For many years its services were conducted in German.

The **Waldoborough Historical Society Museum** (Route 220, near Route 1) administers a complex of three buildings, including the **Town Pound,** a rough stone corral put up to contain wandering livestock. Such pounds were common throughout Maine in the early nineteenth century; this one, an 1819 renovation of a 1785 original, is a well-preserved example. The museum also maintains a restored country school, farm kitchen, and a collection of shipping memorabilia, tools, documents, and photographs.

THOMASTON

East of Waldoboro the coastal lands open up, rolling gently to the sea. Thomaston, a trading post in 1630, withstood Indian attacks to grow into a town with a lively economy based on shipping, lime

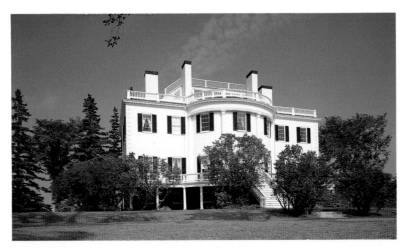

After serving as George Washington's first secretary of war, Henry Knox retired to Thomaston and built Montpelier.

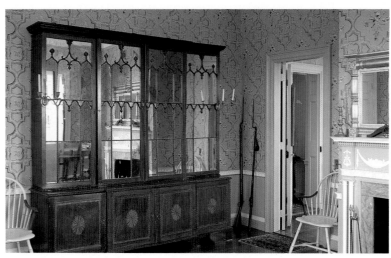

Montpelier's eighteen rooms are furnished with the Knox family's belongings, including a ca. 1785 mirror-fronted bookcase and ca. 1795 Windsor chairs, made in Philadelphia.

processing, and cask making. The town got a champion with the arrival of Major General Henry Knox, honored veteran of Bunker Hill and the nation's first secretary of war.

A replica of Knox's elegant home, **Montpelier** (Route 131, 207–354–8062), is one of Thomaston's best-visited sites. The making of the Federal house was apparently a 1793 collaboration between famed Boston architect Charles Bulfinch and Knox, who specified such details as an oval parlor, flying staircase, and clerestory windows. The original house, completed in 1795, was badly neglected after it was abandoned by Knox descendants in the 1850s, and it was finally razed later that century. The reproduction, exact in countless details, contains many Knox family treasures, including Colonial and Federal furniture.

The houses in Thomaston's **historic district** date from the nineteenth century, when the town was a bustling port. Fine examples of the Federal, Greek Revival, Gothic Revival, Italianate, and Second Empire styles, built by prosperous seafaring families, line the quiet streets of the district.

ROCKLAND

Once part of Thomaston, Rockland was incorporated as its own town in 1854. Marine enterprise naturally figured here long before then—early-eighteenth-century English settlers recorded its local Indian name as "Great Landing Place." Through the 1800s, the town grew with shipbuilding and limestone quarrying; the twentieth century brought the resort business, which, unlike its predecessors, continues to thrive.

Farnsworth Homestead

One of Maine's great houses, this Greek Revival townhouse was built in 1854 by Rockland's most prominent businessman, William A. Farnsworth. It was inherited by his surviving child, the reclusive and eccentric Lucy Farnsworth, who lived to be 96. Although Miss Farnsworth neglected the house, she left behind directions for the family estate and the means to finance them. The result is a fine house, museum, and library complex. The museum's permanent collection is especially strong in American art and the decorative arts of the eighteenth and nineteenth centuries, in addition to holdings of European and Oriental art objects.

LOCATION: 19 Elm Street. HOURS: October through May: 10–5 Tuesday–Saturday, 1–5 Sunday. June through September: 10–5 Monday–Saturday, 1–5 Sunday. FEE: Yes. TELEPHONE: 207–596–6457.

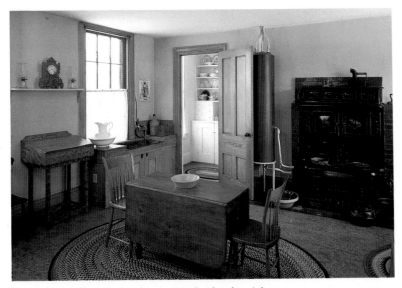

The Farnsworth Homestead kitchen, equipped with a slate sink.

ROCKPORT

Once part of a single municipality with Camden, Rockport has been a separate town since 1891, linked by Route 1. The smaller of the two is Rockport, a longtime exporter of canned sardines, pickled herring, and frozen blueberries. The town also became known for sailmaking and the manufacture of lime used in mortar and plaster. The **Rockport Lime Kilns** produced 2 million casks of the powder in the 1880s and 1890s, when Maine led the country in lime production. A few of the old fieldstone-and-brick kilns still stand on the **Rockport Waterfront.** As the larger coastal towns took over lime production, Rockport turned to the development of its harbor, which remains a favorite among yachtsmen.

CAMDEN

To some, Camden marks the beginning of Maine's mountainous landscape—the local saying is that the town rests "where the mountains meet the sea." To Captain John Smith in 1614, it was the place "under the high mountains . . . against whose feet the sea doth beat." Camden was one of Maine's earliest resorts, attracting seasonal residents as early as the 1830s. By the turn of the century the town was a favorite among the very rich who wanted nothing simple when it came to summer "cottages." One of the grandest of Maine's late-nineteenth-century houses is **Norumbega** (61 High Street, private), built by rags-to-riches millionaire Joseph P. Stearns. His baronial villa and Queen Anne style carriage house are fine examples of the resort lifestyle. The gable-roofed 1904 **American Boathouse** (Atlantic Avenue, 207–236–8500) is another reminder of the country's Gilded Age, when wealthy and often eccentric sportsmen built elaborate shelters for their yachts. In 1926 a prominent seasonal resident, Cyrus H. K. Curtis, publisher of the *Saturday Evening Post,* gave the town the property on which the **Camden Yacht Club** is situated (Bay View Street, 207–236–3014).

The **Conway House** (Conway Road, 207–236–2257) affords a glimpse into Camden's more distant past. The ca. 1770 frame farmhouse still has its brick oven and original hand-hewn woodwork. The house is part of a complex, also including a barn, blacksmith shop, and a museum.

OPPOSITE: *Among Camden's opulent private houses is Norumbega, named for Maine's mythical land of riches.* OVERLEAF: *Seen from Mount Battie, white houses and white boats dot the town of Camden and Penobscot Bay.*

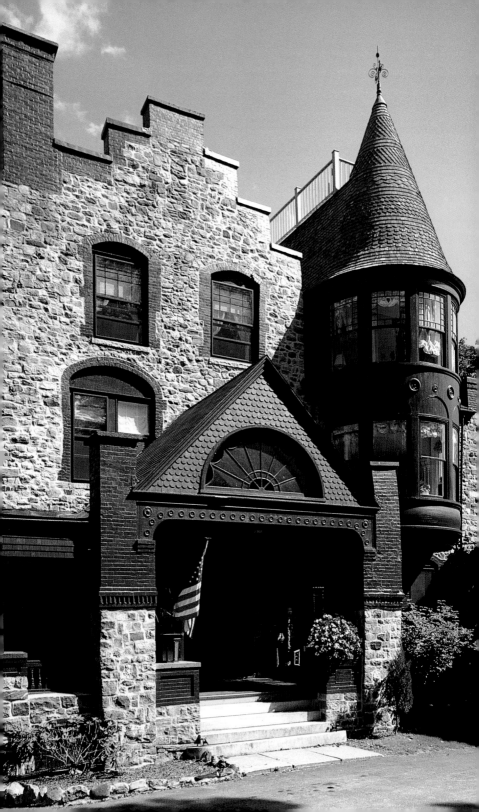

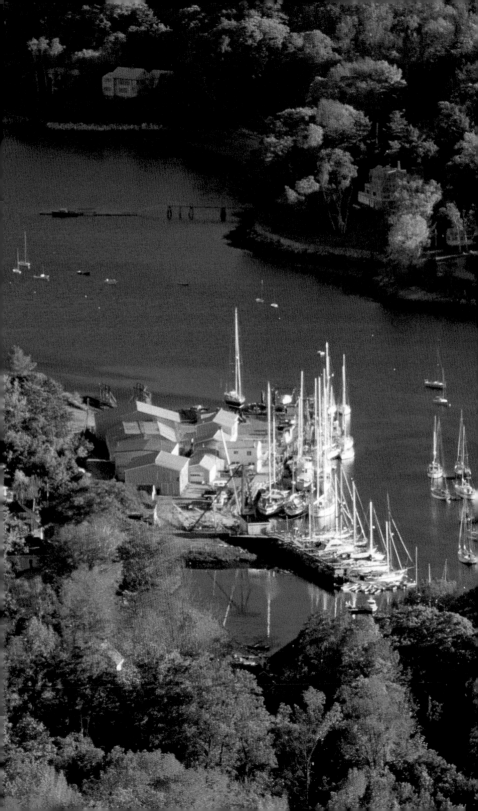

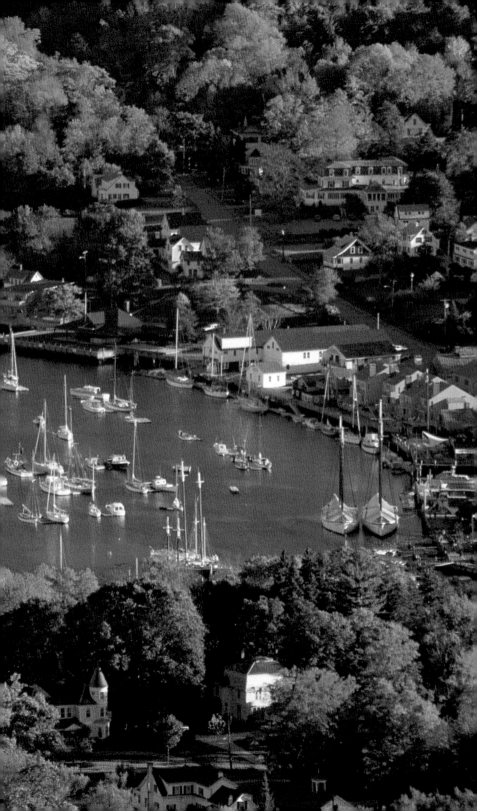

THE   NORTHERN   COAST

The landscape varies in the northern stretch of the Maine coast, from the green farmlands around Belfast to the rocky promontories of Lubec and Eastport to the flat river harbor of Calais. Historians have suggested that these are the coastlands first explored by the Vikings. Certainly they were known to such later adventurers as Samuel de Champlain, John Cabot, and Captain John Smith. East of the resort islands of Deer Isle and Mount Desert, the Maine landscape opens up—it is a rougher, scrubbier land than that which lies to the south. The ocean, too, seems more powerful this far out; the tides here are among the highest in the world.

BELFAST

Named by the Scotch-Irish who landed here in 1770, Belfast is sited on Penobscot Bay. Scattered during the Revolution, the Belfast settlers regrouped and were thriving by the end of the 1780s. Fishing was their mainstay, as well as agricultural enterprises; Belfast is still a major poultry producer. Tied to Bangor by waterways and later by the railroads, Belfast was an important market and port for inland potato growers and lumbermen throughout the nineteenth century. Its prime location on the bay and the Passagassawakeag River encouraged shipping and shipbuilding.

Many buildings survived from this prosperous period in Belfast's **Commercial Historic District** (Main Street). Chief among these are the elaborate 1879 **Belfast National Bank** and the 1878 Gothic **Masonic Temple** by George M. Harding; the 1856 **Post Office and Custom House** (120 Main Street) by architect Ammi B. Young; and the **Waldo County Courthouse** (73 Church Street) by Benjamin S. Dean.

The Federal-style **First Church in Belfast** (6 Court Street, 207–338–2282), built in 1818, is part of the **Church Street Historic District.** The homes of this residential area reflect the affluence of this port city during the 1800s. A fine example is the 1842 **James Petterson White House** (1 Church Street, private). The architect Calvin A. Ryder modified the temple form of the Greek Revival style to create a sophisticated mansion for one of Belfast's leading citizens. In the early 1800s most of the town's wealthy businessmen built their homes on **Primrose Hill,** where Church and High streets come together; from here they could overlook the prosperity they promoted. This grouping of residences is now a historic district. The **Belfast Museum** (66 Church Street) contains items of local history, including ship paintings, antique tools and a ca. 1850 drugstore counter.

SEARSPORT

A few miles up the coast from Belfast is Searsport, settled in the 1760s by soldiers from nearby Fort Pownal. The town took hold quickly, with shipbuilding an established industry by the early 1790s. Set on a rolling green landscape, Searsport seems less bucolic than a serious seaport town, with its heavy granite buildings expressing the confidence that they could match whatever the stormy seas might toss ashore.

Penobscot Marine Museum

Seven nineteenth-century structures form this reminder of Searsport's heritage in the heyday of Maine shipping. Some 250 sailing vessels and 286 sea captains came from this community. The museum complex includes the **Searsport Town Hall** and four sea captain's homes. Three other buildings display navigational and shipbuilding tools, whaling and fishing artifacts, and treasures from the Orient.

LOCATION: Church Street. HOURS: May through October: 9:30–5 Daily. FEE: Yes. TELEPHONE: 207–548–2529.

FORT KNOX

Named for Thomaston's Henry Knox, this fortification was meant to protect the vulnerable and vital Penobscot River Valley during the Maine–New Brunswick boundary disputes with Britain in the 1840s. The enormous structure, measuring 350 by 250 feet, with walls 40 feet thick, took twenty years to complete. Union soldiers trained here during the Civil War. The first of Maine's granite forts, the massive complex was strategically situated on the west bank of the Penobscot, the gateway to Bangor. Original equipment includes ten-inch and fifteen-inch Rodman cannons, and two hot-shot furnaces. The soldiers' quarters, batteries, parade ground, bakery, powder magazines, and storerooms may be toured.

LOCATION: Route 174, Prospect. HOURS: May through October: 9 AM–Dusk Daily. FEE: Yes. TELEPHONE: 207–469–7719.

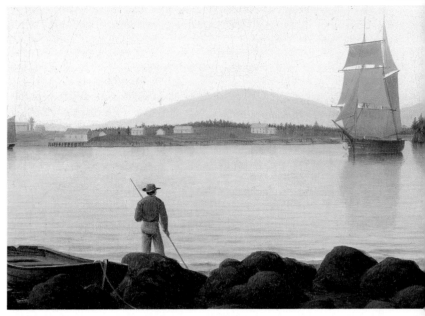

This nineteenth-century view of Owl's Head, a resort village south of Rockport in

CASTINE

Facing Belfast across the Penobscot Bay, Castine is named for the
Baron Castin, who arrived from Quebec in the 1670s to take over
the trading post for France. He did so handily, winning it from the
English, whose first claim on the spot came in 1629, and the Dutch,
who briefly occupied it in the 1670s. Castin's life, as it has been
recounted over the years, was one legendary adventure after another. An impoverished nobleman, he arrived in New France,
determined to claim a royal land grant made to his family. He
befriended the Abenaki Indians, canoeing from Quebec to the
mouth of the Penobscot. Along the way the teenage baron took on
the Abenaki ways and eventually married into the tribe. Castin held
his claim for about twenty years until English colonists won it back
while the Frenchman was off on a fishing trip with his Indian
family and friends.

The British again took over the town of Castine in 1779,
building **Fort George** (Wadsworth Cove Road) to keep their hold
on the strategic Penobscot Bay. Revolutionaries sailed up from
Boston that year, two thousand strong in a fleet of forty-four ships.

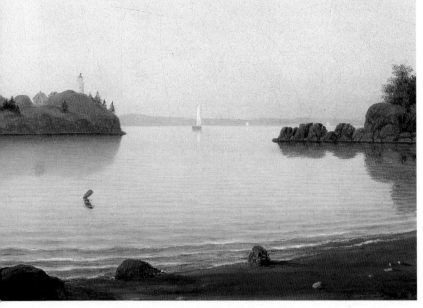

Penobscot Bay, was painted by American artist Fitz Hugh Lane.

A delay in action allowed time for British reinforcements to arrive. None of the American vessels survived—they were either sunk, abandoned, or taken over by the better-prepared British in one of the worst defeats in American naval history. One of the shipwrecks, the *Defense,* is the subject of ongoing archaeological study, and the well-preserved earthwork foundations of Fort George may be toured. Castine is one of the prettiest of Maine's coastal towns, preserving many nineteenth-century buildings along Main and Perkins streets. By the docks on Water Street, at the foot of Main, are several late-eighteenth-century brick commercial buildings. At the end of Battle Street, **Dyces Head Lighthouse,** built in 1828, overlooks the Penobscot River.

The Wilson Museum

This complex on Perkins Street includes the one pre-Revolutionary War house to survive in the Castine area, the ca. 1763 **John Perkins House.** Framed by hand-hewn timbers and constructed with hand-forged nails, the house was occupied by the British during the Revolution and again during the War of 1812. It is now restored

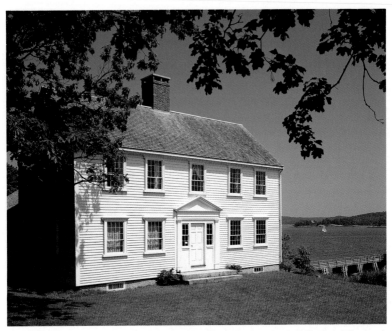

Perkins House, now part of the Wilson Museum complex on Castine's harbor. The town's earliest house, it was designed with a Tuscan front doorway.

and furnished with late-eighteenth-century items. The museum, which is administered by the Castine Scientific Society, also includes permanent exhibitions of prehistoric artifacts from North and South America, Europe, and Africa. Displays follow the growth of the human ability to fashion and use tools. Ship models, farm and home equipment, Victorian-era memorabilia, and local historic items are also on display. Special emphasis is given to the North American Indian tribes native to northern New England. Also on the grounds is a working blacksmith shop.

LOCATION: Perkins Street. HOURS: Memorial Day through September: 2–5 Tuesday–Sunday. FEE: For Perkins House.

SEDGWICK–BROOKLIN

Sedgwick is named for Major Robert Sedgwick, who routed the French from Penobscot Bay in 1654. More than a century later the town was incorporated and grew with fishing and farming. A 1790 boat launching inaugurated shipbuilding. The town's cemetery dates from 1794; the First Baptist Church was built in 1823. Brooklin was chartered in 1859 on land that originally was part of Sedgwick. The Sedgwick-Brooklin Historical Society occupies the 1795 **Reverend Daniel Merrill House** (Route 172, 207–359–8930). The house contains various artifacts from the area's early settlement years, and horse-drawn hearses are on display. Recently moved to the grounds is an 1874 one-room schoolhouse.

At the end of the peninsula, at **Naskeag Point,** a granite marker commemorates a 1778 British raid, apparently provoked by a Patroit who fired upon a passing ship, killing a sailor.

DEER ISLE

Granite quarrying and sardine canning were the founding businesses of Deer Isle, which attracted a resort trade in the late nineteenth century. The high seas lap up to these jagged shores, and legend has it that Deer Isle drew more than its share of smugglers, pirates, and slave runners. Worn memorial stones in the island's cemeteries honor sea captains and sailors lost off the coasts of Africa, China, and Greenland.

One of Deer Isle's earliest houses is the 1775 **Reverend Peter Powers House** (Sunshine Road, private), a gift from the First Congregational Church to its new minister. The islanders found a staunch defender of American independence in Powers, who had been hounded out of New Hampshire by his Tory congregation.

The **Deer Isle–Stonington Historical Society** maintains the 1830 **Salome Sellers House,** which has been restored and furnished with original and period items. Antique farm, quarry, and carpenter's tools are on display in the toolroom. An exhibit building contains displays of ship models, compasses, telescopes, and other local and maritime items.

BLUE HILL

A group from Andover, Massachusetts, settled the undulating western shore of Blue Hill Bay in 1762 and went to work as lumbermen and fishermen. In the nineteenth century, shipbuilding and overseas trade brought some wealth to the town, and the discovery of copper in 1876 ushered in a mining boom. Starting about the same time, granite quarries were opened. Many eighteenth- and nineteenth-century houses, as well as public and commercial buildings, overlook the harbor, forming a historic district that includes the **Holt House** (Water Street), a restored Federal residence. Administered by the Blue Hill Historical Society, it is noteworthy for local memorabilia and its stenciled wall decorations. The carriage house holds examples of early local industries.

Blue Hill's first minister was Jonathan Fisher, who came here in 1796. Fisher was a linguist, printer, inventor, gifted artisan, and painter who built and furnished his 1815 house largely by himself. His house is now open as the **Jonathan Fisher Memorial** (Main Street, 207–374–2757).

ELLSWORTH

Since its founding in 1763, Ellsworth has made the most of the sixty-foot Union River Falls. Sawmills and shipbuilding flourished here. With its spire and colonnade, the **Ellsworth Congregational Church** (Cross Street) has been the focal point of the town since 1846, when the edifice went up on a hill above the Union River. Equally impressive are the pair of **Old Hancock County Buildings,** stout Greek Revival landmarks on Cross Street. Probably the most famous site in Ellsworth is the **Colonel Black Mansion** (West Main Street, 207–667–8671), built by John Black, who came from England at the age of 13 to be the clerk of the great Bingham Estate in

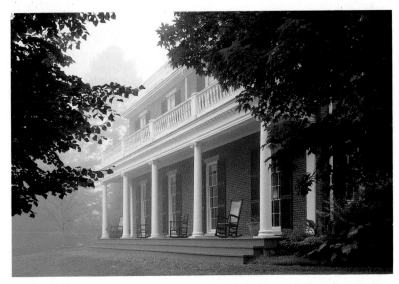

The Black Mansion introduced Georgian formality to the mill town of Ellsworth. OPPOSITE: *Portraits hang over the mansion's beautifully wrought staircase.*

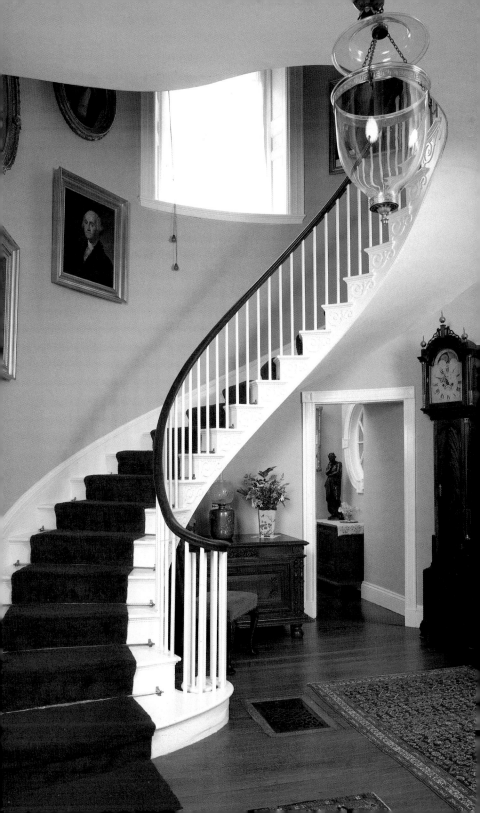

Maine. He became agent in 1810 and later general agent, a position he held until his son was appointed in his place in 1850. Black spared no expense on his stately home, importing its distinctive red bricks from Philadelphia—the 1826 residence could be a Georgian townhouse on Rittenhouse Square. The rooms of period furniture, porcelain, and glass; the carriage house; and the gardens are open.

The Ellsworth **Public Library** occupies the 1817 **Seth Tisdale House,** named for its owner, celebrated locally for his service in the Revolutionary War. The Ellsworth Historical Society on State Street is headquartered in the brick-and-granite **Old Jail,** built as the county jail and sheriff's residence in 1886. The **Stanwood Wildlife Sanctuary** (Route 3, 207–667–8460) includes a Cape Cod–style house built in 1850 by Ellsworth sea captain Roswell Stanwood. It passed to his daughter, Cordelia, an ornithologist and photographer. A bird sanctuary was later established on the grounds. The homestead and sanctuary are open year-round.

MOUNT DESERT ISLAND

Maine has been called the land of a thousands islands, a claim upheld by Mt. Desert's abundance of satellites, many of them with charming names: Burnt Porcupine, Egg Rock, Ironbound, Turtle, Rum Key, Cranberry, Little Duck. Geological forces have formed Mt. Desert itself into perhaps the single most dramatic natural setting in the state, with its hills—one of them a 1500-foot "mountain"—craggy seaside cliffs, lakes, and heavily forested interior. The island, it seems, has always been known for its terrain: the Abenaki Indians who came over from the mainland to fish and gather shellfish on the island called it Pemetic, "the sloping land." When Samuel de Champlain landed here in 1604, he looked to the rugged mountaintops and named it "L'isle des monts deserts," the "Isle of bare mountains."

The first open clash between the French and the English over territory in the New World took place here in 1613, when the English explorer Samuel Argall burned a Jesuit mission and took the survivors captive, selling some into slavery and casting the rest adrift on the open sea. Disputes over the island continued until the English finally gained control of it in 1760, in the French and Indian War. After the Revolution, the settlers prospered on logging, fishing, farming, and shipbuilding.

The transformation of Mount Desert Island from an island of small towns to a popular resort began in the 1850s, with the advent of regular steamboat runs from the mainland. The painter Thomas Cole, founder of the Hudson River School, was one of the first to discover the spectacular scenery on the island; he came here to paint in the summer, and other artists and writers soon joined him. As word of this relatively unspoiled area spread, it became a popular place for wealthy families to escape the discomforts of summer in the city. By the end of the nineteenth century, many of the richest families in the country—the Astors, the Vanderbilts, the Rockefellers—had built summer homes on the island. Referred to somewhat disingenuously as "cottages," many of these houses were more on the order of mansions.

Efforts to preserve the natural beauty of the island began in the early 1900s, when a group of summer residents, led by Boston millionaire George Dorr, began acquiring land. By 1913, they had accumulated about 6,000 acres, which they donated to the federal government. In 1919, this land was made a national park, which has continued to grow as a result of additional donations. Known today as **Acadia National Park,** it now covers some 38,000 acres, encompassing a large area of Mount Desert Island, portions of several smaller islands, and part of Schoodic Peninsula.

The first permanent settlement on Mt. Desert was **Somesville,** a nine-family hamlet established in 1759 by the Massachusetts governor. Somesville's white-painted Victorian houses range in style from the simple to the exuberant, meshing with the scenery as if they had grown from the ground. It is a beautiful spot, probably the first place on the island to be discovered by artists and "rusticators," as the city folk who sought seasonal country comforts and Atlantic air were known. Thomas Cole and Frederic Church, another Hudson River School painter, were among Somesville's visitors in the 1850s.

The **Mount Desert Island Historical Society Museum** (opposite the mill pond, 207–244–3898) is in Somesville, and its collection of maps, deeds, and various artifacts sets forth a colorful local history. The Society maintains a list of landmarks in the island's communities, including **Northeast Harbor, Bernard,** and **Tremont.** In addition, information is available on **Islesford, Southwest Harbor,** and the **Cranberry Isles.**

BAR HARBOR

In its heyday, this scenic town rivaled even fashionable Newport as a mecca for the rich and socially prominent; it remains popular today, and many extravagant and stately houses still stand as reminders of the Gilded Age. Artists and other visitors began coming here in the 1850s, boarding with the villagers. In 1855, the Agamont House was opened as an inn for summer residents, and the local economy began to shift from fishing and shipbuilding to the care and feeding of city folk.

The first summer residence, **Petunia Cottage** (West Street), was built in 1877 for the express purpose of renting to vacationers but was soon bought by physician and author S. Weir Mitchell. Soon, the off-islanders began building their own homes, usually on a grand scale. Many of the houses were designed by prominent Boston and New York architects, and a variety of styles are represented. **Redwood** (Bayberry Lane), built in 1879, is one of the earliest Shingle-style houses in the United States. Other notable houses include the magnificent Colonial Revival **Reverie Cove** (Harbor Lane), built in 1895; **The Turrets** (Eden Street), an 1895 granite cottage done in the Chateauesque style; the 1910 **Eogonos** (Eden Street), designed by Guy Lowell, architect of the Boston Museum of Fine Arts; and **La Rochelle** (West Street), a 1903 French Renaissance mansion. The 1932 **Criterion Theatre,** an art deco movie palace, is one of the finest examples of this style in the country. The history of Bar Harbor is documented in photographs, hotel registers, and other memorabilia in the **Bar Harbor Historical Society Museum** (34 Mt. Desert Street, 207–288–4245).

Abbe Museum

Overlooking the wild gardens of Acadia is the Abbe Museum. A New York surgeon, Robert Abbe amassed great collections of prehistoric artifacts during his summers in Bar Harbor, and in 1926 he built a museum to house them. Most of the exhibits represent Northeast American Indians, including the Passamaquoddy and Penobscot tribes: arrowheads and stone implements, baskets of birchbark and sweet grass, tools and ornaments of bone.

LOCATION: Route 3. HOURS: Mid-May through June: 10–4 Daily. July through August: 9–5 Daily. September through mid-December: 10–4 Daily. FEE: Yes. TELEPHONE: 207–288–3519.

OPPOSITE: *Basketry from the Abbe Museum collection.*

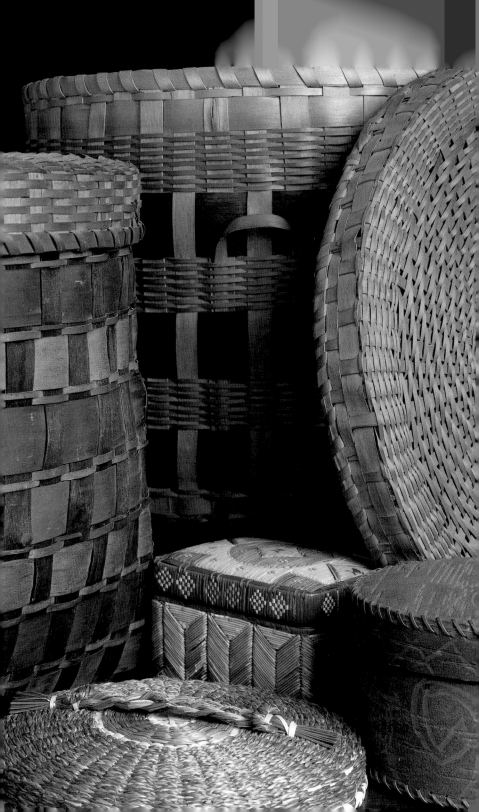

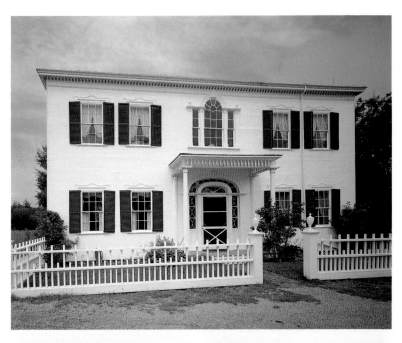

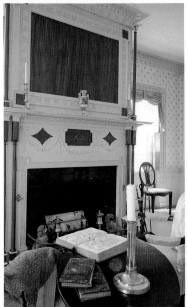

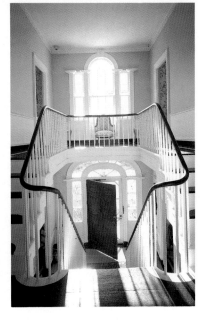

COLUMBIA FALLS

The early nineteenth-century prosperity of Columbia Falls is evident in one of Maine's most beautiful residences, the **Thomas Ruggles House** (Route 1, 207–483–4637), named for the local jack-of-all-trades—Ruggles was a judge, lumber magnate, owner of a general store, and postmaster. His house, built in 1818, is one of understated elegance. Its celebrated flying staircase and detailed interior woodwork, often said to be the work of an English craftsman using a single penknife, are more likely the work of New England woodcarver Alvah Peterson. The delicate woodwork of the 1820 **Samuel Bucknam House** (Route 1, private) is also attributed to Peterson. Bucknam's grandfather, Revolutionary officer John Bucknam, was one of Columbia Falls's first settlers; the **Captain John Bucknam House** (Route 1, private), built in 1792, is one of the oldest in Columbia Falls.

MACHIAS

The small coastal town of Machias was the scene of the first naval battle of the Revolution, in June 1775. The townspeople, stirred by the recent events at Lexington and Concord, refused to supply a British schooner, the *Margaretta*, with lumber intended for British barracks in Boston. The ship's captain, a Captain Moore, threatened to fire on the town if they did not comply. In response, a band of forty townspeople led by Jeremiah O'Brien boarded a British sloop, the *Unity*, and, "armed with guns, swords, axes and pitchforks" (in O'Brien's words), engaged and defeated the *Margaretta*. Captain Moore died the next day of wounds sustained in battle. O'Brien was given command of the *Unity*, which was rechristened the *Machias Liberty* and armed with the *Margaretta*'s guns; a few weeks later, he captured another British schooner.

The townspeople gathered to plan the attacks in the 1770 **Burnham Tavern** (Free and Main streets, 207–255–4432), and the wounded were brought there after the battle. Now a museum, the tavern is furnished with pieces dating from the 1600s to the Revolution; muskets used in the battle are on display, along with other artifacts of local history.

OPPOSITE: *Ruggles House, a treasure box of craftsmanship, is celebrated for its flying staircase and detailed woodcarving.*

Machias was an important railroad center for lumbering communities up north, and a relic of that trade, the oak and iron **Steam Locomotive *Lion,*** is on permanent display at the University of Maine's Machias campus. In service for half a century, the locomotive was retired in 1896.

Nearby is **Machiasport,** first settled by English colonists in 1763 and later a prosperous lumber and shipbuilding center. The Federal style **Gates House** (Route 92, 207–255–8461) has been restored to its 1807 construction and interior decoration. Home to the Machiasport Historical Society, the house includes a museum as well as period rooms and a marine and genealogical library.

EASTPORT

At the tip of Passamaquoddy Bay on Moose Island is Eastport, the easternmost city in the U.S. Settled in 1772, Eastport grew with fishing and sardine canning. The Border Historical Society operates the **Barracks Museum,** which was part of the original officers' quarters and barracks of Fort Sullivan, built in 1808 as tensions rose between England and the U.S. The British invaded Eastport in 1814 and held the town four years—long after the War of 1812 was over. Among the museum's collections are war artifacts, ships' tools, geneological records, and costumes. Remains of the fort's **Powder House** may be seen on Fort Hill, on McKinley Street. (The hill also affords a view of Campobello, site of Franklin Delano Roosevelt's summer home in Canada.) Since before 1794 British soldiers, smugglers, sea captains, and shipwreck victims have been buried in Eastport's **Hillside Cemetery,** on High Street. The town's Federal-style **Central Congregational Church** on Middle Street was built in 1829.

In 1891 a new customs house and post office was built to replace an 1850 structure that burned in an 1886 fire. Much of Eastport's downtown historic district, built after the fire, reflects the Italianate styling popular at the time. Back on the mainland is **Pleasant Point** (207-853-4045), a Passamaquoddy reservation (population about 700), and the **Waponahki Museum.** The museum's exhibits present a pictorial history of the Indians, as well as displaying artifacts, a 100-year-old birchbark canoe, and mannequins in traditional Passamaquoddy dress.

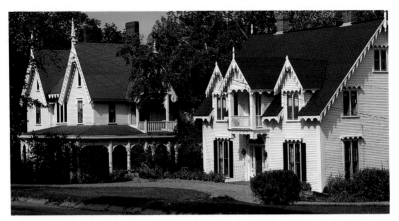

Nineteenth-century houses in Calais.

CALAIS

Calais was established on the St. Croix River in 1809 and steadily grew as word spread among the French and English colonies of its fine forests, fishing, and arable soil. The **Calais Historic District** faces the river from Main Street, with few of its significant buildings predating a devastating 1870 fire. Among those survivors are the Gothic Revival **Gilmore** (316 Main Street, private) and **Washburn** (318 Main Street, private) houses, and a Victorian mansion so outrageously ornate it is known as **Hamilton's Folly** (78 South Street, private), after the man, Thomas Hamilton, who built it and went bankrupt.

In July 1604, Samuel de Champlain and the Sieur de Monts landed on the island of **St. Croix** with a group of eighty Frenchmen, intending to set up a trading post. Had the venture been successful, it would have been the first permanent settlement north of South Carolina, but it was doomed to failure by the harsh winter, lack of drinking water, and an outbreak of scurvy that wiped out half the colonists. The village was abandoned the following year. Foundations and graves have been unearthed by archaeological excavations, but no structures remain standing. St. Croix is not open to the public, but it may be viewed from a small red-granite **enclosure** atop a hill overlooking the island (off Route 1). Brass plaques detail the history of the short-lived settlement.

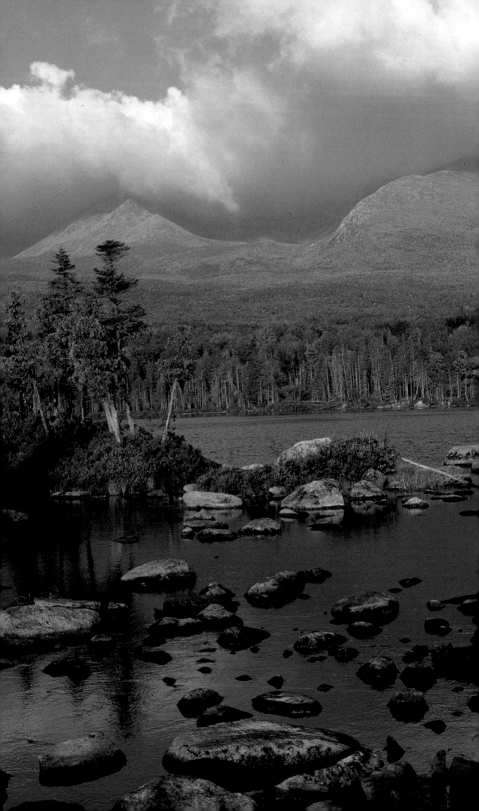

CHAPTER SEVEN

THE
MAINE INTERIOR

OPPOSITE: *Mount Katahdin, from the rivers of Baxter State Park.*

Maine is large—half the size of all of New England—and about 80 percent of it is covered with forests of white pine, balsam fir, basswood, birch, oak, maple, hemlock, beech, and spruce. Mile-high Mount Katahdin, in the center of Maine, is the state's tallest peak. More than 5,000 rivers and streams pour through Maine; lakes and large ponds number 2,500. For thousands of years these waters were fished for salmon, brook trout, and bass by the Indians and in more recent times by sport fishermen. Men of means built great lodges in the woods or stayed at fashionable resort hotels.

The interior was sparsely settled by Europeans, but Indians occupied these lands almost as soon as the glaciers receded, 10,000 to 12,000 years ago. Evidence of human occupation in that era has been found in the vicinity of Chase and Munsungun lakes, which are believed to have been formed by glaciers. Stone tools and animal bones dating from 6,000 to 8,000 years ago have been found near Cobbosseecontee Lake. Of more recent date, from 3,000 to 6,000 years ago, was the culture of the Red Paint people, so called because their burials all contained deposits of a red ochre paint. Little is known of them, despite the many Red Paint graves that have been discovered, beyond the fact that they were skilled artisans. The Indians of the historical period were the Abenaki, of the large Algonquin linguistic group.

French traders generally coexisted peacefully with the Abenaki, trading furs, while the land-hungry English settlers clashed repeatedly with the Indians. The Abenaki, particularly along the coast, suffered tremendously in an epidemic in 1616—estimates of mortality run as high as 75 percent. The series of wars that began with King Philip's War in the 1670s went well for the Indians at first, but their defeat in the French and Indian War in the 1750s broke their power.

In 1786 the state of Massachusetts sold huge tracts of unsettled land in northern Maine to wealthy speculators, notably William Bingham of Philadelphia, who bought 1 million acres and acquired another million from General Henry Knox. At the same time, the surviving Indians of Maine were made wards of the state and lost title to all their lands. Few Mainers regretted any discomfiture of the Indians, but many resented the land policies of Massachusetts and the absentee landowners.

OPPOSITE: *Detail from Frederic E. Church's* Mt. Ktaadin (Katahdin), *painted in 1853.*

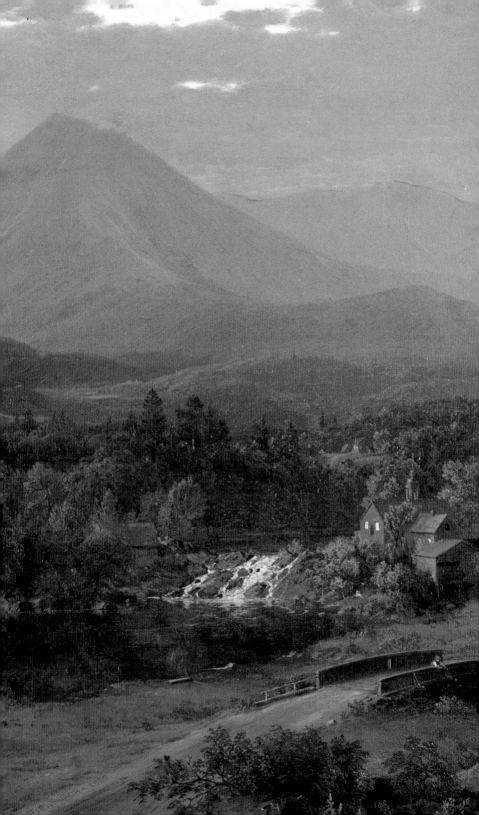

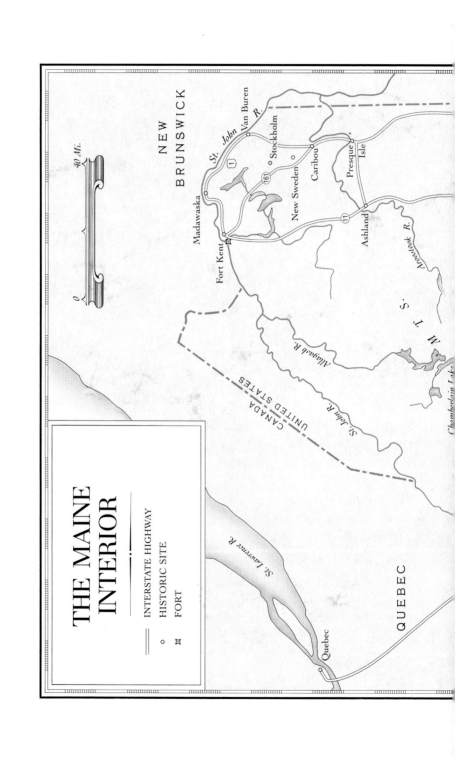

THE MAINE
INTERIOR

═══ INTERSTATE HIGHWAY

o   HISTORIC SITE

⌂   FORT

40 Mi.

NEW
BRUNSWICK

Van Buren

St. John R.

Stockholm

Madawaska

Fort Kent

New Sweden

Caribou

Presque
Isle

Ashland

Aroostook R.

Allagash R.

St. John R.

Chamberlain Lake

M E

CANADA
UNITED STATES

St. Lawrence R.

Quebec

QUEBEC

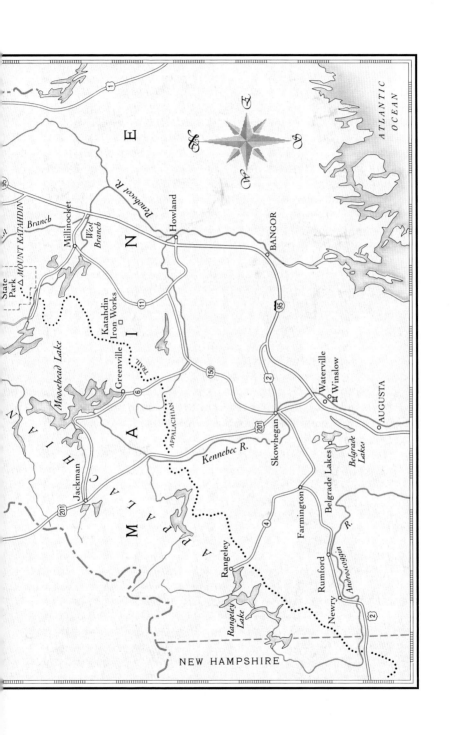

The far northern county of Aroostook is the largest and lone-liest county in Maine. Towns of any size are the exception on these wide-open flat acres. Potato farming is a major industry in this region, and enormous trucks carry the crops southward to markets in Maine, New England, and other parts of the country. Along the green St. John River valley are small farming communities, many of them founded by Acadians, the French Canadians driven from their homes by the English in the late 1700s.

After the Revolution, the United States and Britain anxiously shared the northern border region, competing for its wealth of timber, game, and minerals. Each country trespassed against the other in disputes that lasted over fifty years. Between February and May 1839 there was a confrontation, called the "Aroostook War," which threatened to erupt into violence. Some 10,000 Maine troops massed along the Aroostook River, and the federal govern-ment agreed to send 50,000 more. But before any shooting started, a border was agreed upon by negotiation and formalized in the Webster-Ashburton Treaty.

Maine's great lumber boom began after the Revolution and gathered force through the nineteenth century. Augusta and Ban-gor both prospered as centers of milling and trade in lumber. The Penobscot River carried the harvest of the interior forests to Ban-gor, which, in the middle of the nineteenth century, was one of the world's largest producers of wood products.

This chapter begins with Augusta, the state capital, proceeds northward to Waterville, and then detours to the west. The route then takes up with Bangor, proceeds directly north, and then loops south along the Canadian border to Houlton.

C E N T R A L   R E G I O N

AUGUSTA

Augusta had been settled for over 200 years when it became Maine's capital in 1831. The earliest pioneers did well trading with the Indians for furs, fish, and timber, but they abandoned the settlement around 1700. Settlers returned, however, in the mid-eighteenth century as timber for construction became highly val-ued, and the town developed on both sides of the Kennebec River. Augusta became an active port, sending timber, furs, and other

goods forty-five miles downriver to the sea. One of its chief exports
was ice, harvested from the Kennebec each winter and packed in
sawdust for points south. In 1832 the capital was moved from
Portland to Augusta. Within a decade not only sawmills but cotton
mills as well were adding to the prosperity of the thriving city.

Maine State House

While citizens of Portland made several attempts to move the
capital back to their city, their cause faded in the face of Charles
Bulfinch's impressive structure in Augusta. The architect based the
classical design of Maine's capitol on his earlier one for the Massachusetts State House; the building material, however, was indigenous to Maine: granite from Hollowell. Construction began in
1829 and lasted until January 1832. Its completion was a prelude to
many alterations, additions, and renovations, beginning with a
remodeling of the interior in 1857. Between 1890 and 1891 a
three-story wing was added to the rear of the building according to

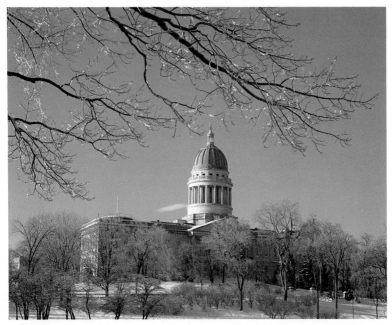

*The Maine State House in Augusta as it has appeared since 1910, when final elaborations
were made on Charles Bulfinch's 1829 original.*

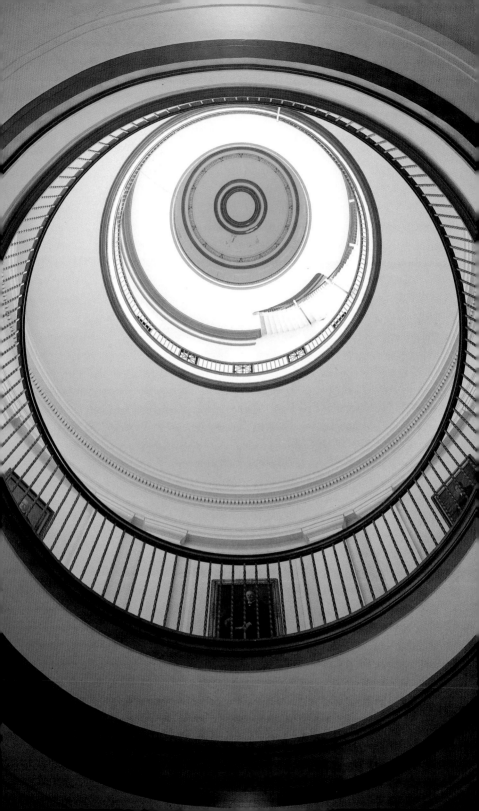

architect John Calvin Spofford's design, attuned to Bulfinch's original plans. Architect G. Henri Desmond paid less attention to maintaining the integrity of the earlier designs; in 1909–1910 he added two large side wings and replaced the original low dome with an almost 200-foot steel dome covered in copper and topped by *Wisdom*, a gold-covered statue sculptured by W. Clark Noble. Bulfinch's mark is still visible in the front Greek Revival portico and its recessed wall. As the demands of civil government varied, the structure that housed it followed suit; the State House reflects its own history. A self-guided tour of the capitol grounds and State House includes temporary exhibits about Maine and local history, dioramas of native wildlife, portraits of governors, and legislative chambers.

> LOCATION: State and Capitol streets. HOURS: 9–5 Monday–Friday, 10–4 Saturday, 1–4 Sunday. FEE: None. TELEPHONE: 207–289–2301.

The **Maine State Museum** (207–289–2301), about a hundred yards south of the State House, offers an excellent overview of the state's natural, industrial, and social history. Curators have devised dioramas of Maine's natural settings, and there is a gem and mineral exhibit. An extensive exhibit, "Made in Maine," presents the history of the state's products and industries. Historical settings of both factory and home display the various crafts of sewing, weaving, furniture making, and shoe making. Principal industrial tools and methods are explained.

Across from the capitol is **Blaine House** (207–289–2301), the Federal-style residence of Maine's governor. As governors' mansions go, the clapboard, green-shuttered house, sitting behind a picket fence, is modest. Sea captain James Hall built it for himself in 1833; the house takes its name from a later resident, James G. Blaine, a Maine congressman who became Speaker of the House, a U.S. senator, a presidential candidate, and secretary of state under presidents Garfield and Harrison. Blaine died in 1893, and in 1919 his descendants gave the house to the state, to be used as the official residence of Maine's governors and their families.

Fort Western (16 Cony Street, 207–626–2385), a 1754 fortification, also served as a store and, in the nineteenth century, as a tenement for factory workers. The main building, a 100-by-32-foot

OPPOSITE: *The three-story Maine capitol rotunda soars 185 feet above the first floor.*

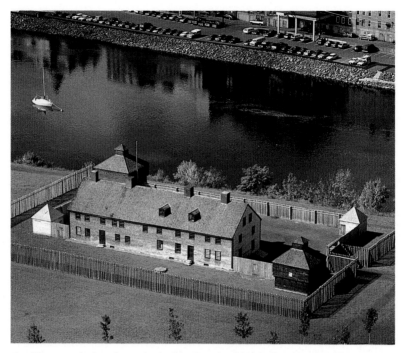

Fort Western, raised on the east bank of the Kennebec River in the mid-eighteenth century.

rectangle of hewn logs covered in shingles and topped by four huge chimneys, is one of the finest remnants of colonial America. Today it is a **museum** that interprets the military, economic, and social history of the Kennebec River Valley.

In 1827 the U.S. government built an **arsenal** in Augusta to defend the frontier at the time of the boundary dispute with England. The arsenal consisted of fifteen buildings, most of them of granite. Ammunition manufactured here supplied the Mexican War, the Civil War, and the Spanish-American War. Ten of the granite buildings survive and are still in use by the state. Known as the **Kennebec Arsenal Historic District,** they are located at the end of Arsenal Street, on the river.

The **Kennebec County Courthouse** (95 State Street) is one of the earliest Greek Revival structures in Maine (1829), with a full Ionic colonnade. Also of architectural interest is the **Old Post Office** (1886), a fabulous Romanesque edifice, and one of the distinguished Victorian buildings on Water Street in downtown Augusta. A central round tower set on a square base is echoed by a rounded tower at each of the building's corners, heavy rounded arches, and ornate dormers with rounded detail. It houses a bank, postal station, and offices.

ALNA

The town of Alna is known chiefly for the village it encompasses, **Head Tide,** located on the Sheepscot River. The lovely siting is the raison d'être of the village: Mills of all kinds operated on the Sheepscot, giving Head Tide an active economy for 200 years, from pre-Revolutionary times into the twentieth century. One of Head Tide's mills produced thousands of cedar shingles every day.

Along the north and south banks of the Sheepscot, within the **Head Tide Historic District,** are the village's eighteenth- and nineteenth-century houses, a store, church, stable, and school. The 1789 **Alna Meeting House** (Route 218) is one of Maine's superior Colonial buildings. The **Schoolhouse,** also on Route 218, is impossible to miss—its tall cupola pokes above the gently rolling landscape. Built in 1795, it is Maine's second-oldest one-room schoolhouse, fifty years younger than York's.

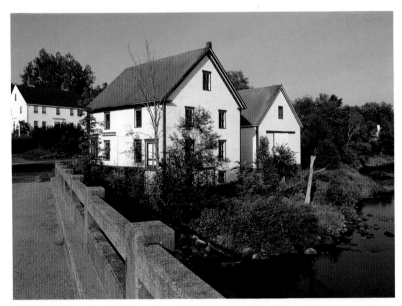

Clustered on the Sheepscot River, one- and two-century-old buildings define the Head Tide Historic District.

East of Waterville, where the Kennebec merges with the Sebasticook River, lies **Winslow,** primarily a farming community. In 1754,
English colonists built **Fort Halifax** on the Sebasticook to protect
their fragile settlements from the French and Indians. The fort was
also a crucial link during the Revolution and a way station for
Benedict Arnold on his ill-fated march to Quebec. Its blockhouse,
believed to be the oldest in the United States until its demise in
1987 floodwaters, is being reconstructed (1988).

WATERVILLE

Just south of Skowhegan, the aptly named Waterville was born on
the Kennebec's Tionic Falls, which drove the town's lumber mills.
River drivers also took advantage of the water's power, sending
logs over the falls to be milled in town.

The Redington Museum

Housed in an 1814 frame house built by one of Waterville's early
pioneers, this well-appointed museum is administered by the Waterville Historical Society and documents the early years of the
town. Asa Redington, a Revolutionary War veteran of George
Washington's elite Honor Guard, built the house with an eye to the
elegance of the time, as evidenced by the spiral staircase, the
original fireplaces, and the woodwork. Five period rooms of the
late eighteenth and early nineteenth centuries contain antiques and
furnishings original to the Redingtons and other pioneering families, including Chippendale and Hepplewhite pieces; a collection
of clocks; kitchen utensils; period children's toys, among them a
Victorian and a Colonial Revival dollhouse; and family portraits.
    The museum's library includes diaries and archives from the
mid-eighteenth century to the twentieth, plus an extensive collection of local newspapers and early photographs. Other exhibits
include displays of early craftsmanship, technological developments in the logging and transportation fields, firearms, Civil War
memorabilia, early business marquees, musical instruments, Indian
artifacts, and period costumes. Adjacent to the museum is the
LaVerdiere Apothecary Museum, housing an extensive collection
of pharmaceutical paraphernalia and furnishings, such as brass
and mahogany cabinets, shelves filled with early patent medicines,

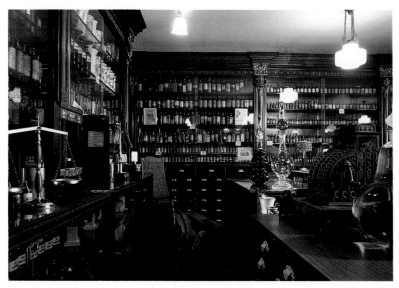

Waterville's authentically furnished and stocked nineteenth-century LaVerdiere Apothecary.

extracts, oils, herbs, and equipment. With an authentic prescription-preparation area and a mirrored fountain backed with stained-glass trim, the museum recalls the soda fountain–drugstore of the nineteenth century.

LOCATION: 64 Silver Street. HOURS: May through September: 2–6 Tuesday–Saturday. FEE: Yes. TELEPHONE: 207–872–9439.

Another particularly picturesque element of the past resides in the **Waterville Opera House** on Castonguay Square. Built at the turn of the century, this well-preserved Colonial Revival structure predates the movie house, harking back to the age of local and traveling theater companies. An early example of Art Deco architecture, the concrete-and-steel **Professional Building** (177 and 179 Main Street), was built in 1923 with stylistic detailing in the reliefs, shield motifs, and low archways.

North of Waterville is some of the most beautiful countryside in Maine—rolling hills, enormous lakes, waterfalls, and streams. Along the waterways grew such mill towns as Hermon, Newburgh Center, Plymouth, Burnham, and Damascus. After 1856, the railroads gave birth to other communities—Fairfield, Shawmut, Anson, and Sidney. **Skowhegan** (an Indian word for "a place to watch fish") was settled in 1771 by two homesteaders, Peter Heywood and Joseph Weston, who brought their families and a few head of cattle from Concord, Massachusetts.

The mid- to late-nineteenth century prosperity of Skowhegan as a regional business center is apparent in its **historic district,** which comprises nearly forty commercial buildings along Water and Russett Streets, as well as Madison Avenue. Virtually all late-nineteenth-century architectural styles are represented here in varying states of renovation. The **Skowhegan History House** (Norridgewock Avenue, 207–474–3140), a dignified, Greek Revival brick residence, is furnished appropriately for its year of construction, 1839. Local documents and artifacts are also on display.

Farther west are fertile agricultural lands, settled for the most part by the English in the 1770s. Highways here roll past fields of corn, potatoes, and pumpkins and past apple orchards. **Farmington,** as its name implies, is a typical farming community on the banks of the Sandy River in the Oxford Hills. The **Little Red Schoolhouse Museum** (Route 2) is complete with desks and books from the last century; built in 1852, it served Farmington's students for over 100 years. It is a visitor center in summer.

Downriver at **Farmington Falls** is the **Old Union Meeting House,** completed in 1827 by a Farmington carpenter, Benjamin Butler. In style the meetinghouse harks back to the eighteenth century, with a steeple in the mode of the London architect Christopher Wren. Used by a variety of denominations before they built their own churches, it now houses the Union Baptist Church. On Holly Road, the **Nordica Homestead Museum** (207–778–2042) pays tribute to the famous opera soprano Lillian Nordica (née Norton). The 1840 Cape Cod–style home, built by her father, was Nordica's home before her mother launched her operatic career. In 1891, Nordica made her debut at the Metropolitan Opera. Her expertise lay in Wagnerian roles, and she in fact studied under Wagner's widow. Nordica spent her last summer here in 1911; she died in 1914. The museum includes concert gowns, programs, stage jewels, music, and other Nordica memorabilia from her career and the family home.

RUMFORD

The largest town in the Oxford Hills, Rumford developed as an industrial and a resort center. The Ellis, Swift, and Concord rivers flow into the Androscoggin, whose powerful falls have driven the town's pulp and paper mills since the late 1800s. The commercial **historic district** reflects the town's fortunes at the turn of the century when Oxford Paper and other companies boosted the local economy. Major downtown buildings, all within sight of the Androscoggin Falls, include the Colonial Revival **Municipal Building,** designed by Harry S. Coombs in 1916; the 1906 Beaux-Arts **Rumford Falls Power Company Building;** the 1910 **Strathglass Building,** also of Beaux-Arts design; and the 1911 Classical Revival **Mechanic Institute.**

The **Strathglass Park Historic District** is an example of an early twentieth-century planned community. Hugh J. Chisolm, a developer for Rumford Falls and the Oxford Paper Company, hired noted architect Cass H. Gilbert to design a residential development for the millworkers. Between 1901 and 1902 fifty-one solid and attractive duplexes, surrounded by gracious lawns, were built on blocks divided by tree-lined avenues. Public services, such as garbage and snow removal, were taken care of by the company. Not until 1948 and 1949 were the lots sold privately.

NEWRY

One of the best-preserved one-room schoolhouses in the country, with its 1895 furnishings intact, is the **Lower Sunday River School** on Sunday River Road in Newry. The town's graceful covered bridge, the **Sunday River Bridge,** was built in 1870. One half of the bridge was assembled on each shore and then settled into place and joined in the center.

The narrow roads and highways heading northwest of Newry toward Baxter State Park seem hardly more than wilderness trails themselves, barely penetrating the heavy forests. But they lead to Maine's lake country. From the mid-1800s, while the sailing set summered at the state's coastal resorts, inland sportsmen stalked moose and fly-fished at Flagstaff and Rangeley lakes. In **Rangeley,** the **Rangeley Lakes Region Historical Society** (Main and Richardson streets) has a large collection of photographs from the resort era. Funds to build the classically designed **Rangeley Public Library** (Lake Street, 207–864–5529) were raised in the early 1900s by summer and permanent residents. The library houses an exceptional collection of material written by—and about—the natural scientist Wilhelm Reich, who fled Nazi Germany and eventually settled in Maine. A student of Sigmund Freud, Reich developed a controversial theory based on a universal biological energy he called orgone. (He named his compound in Maine "Orgonon.") Three miles west of Rangeley is the **Wilhelm Reich Museum** (Dodge Pond Road, 207–864–3443), housed in Reich's observatory. Built of native fieldstone in the Bauhaus style, the building contains his equipment and paintings as well as exhibits on his work. Reich, who died in 1957, enjoyed the region's low humidity and abundant forests, lakes, and mountains, which reminded him of Europe. His study and library are also on view.

THE EASTERN INTERIOR

BANGOR

In his journal of 1604, Samuel de Champlain recorded his impressions of the hilly west bank of the Penobscot River. The land there, twenty-three miles inland and thick with oak trees, struck the French explorer as "pleasant and agreeable," as did the Indians who inhabited the area. It would be another century and a half before a Massachusetts pioneer, Jacob Buswell, settled at the pleasant and agreeable spot that would grow into one of Maine's most rollicking towns. Buswell's community, at first known as Kenduskeag Plantation after the tributary stream that runs through town, made its living by exporting fur pelts and lumber. In about 1800 Bangor got its present name—apparently from the title of a favorite hymn of the town's pastor. Bangor now began to come into its own, with businesses and population expanding even as the War of 1812 brought blockades and other British aggressions.

Harvesting pine and spruce trees upstream from Bangor along a great length of the Penobscot, timbermen floated logs to Bangor mills. From them in the 1850s came an enormous supply of lumber, shingles, clapboards, and lath. Much of that wood went out to sea from Bangor in locally made ships—the river town was an active port with a lively overseas trade. Bangor traded with the West Indies, too, exchanging its large winter ice harvest for their molasses, sugar, and rum.

In the mid-nineteenth century, railroads tied Bangor and its timber goods to all points south. The town boomed as many came

OPPOSITE: *Nineteenth-century buildings on Broad Street, in Bangor's Market Square Historic District.*

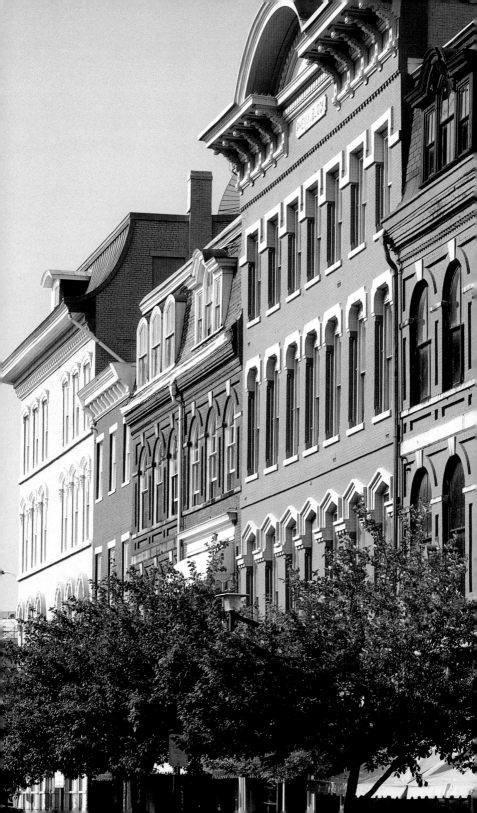

to make their fortunes—in lumber, milling, shipbuilding, and land speculation. The newcomers created an exciting city, full of cultural diversions. And as with most boom towns, the lumberjacks and sailors found no shortage of saloons and brothels.

The citizens built an extremely good-looking town, which is still in evidence, despite the ravages of a 1911 fire and the urban renewal of the late 1960s. The **West Market Square Historic District** consists of two downtown blocks, defined by State, Main, and Broad streets and the Kenduskeag Stream. The first open marketplace in Bangor, it was also where many set up shop in handsome brick and granite buildings—doctors, booksellers, grocers, shoemakers, druggists, hatters. Much of the area was the 1830s design work of Charles G. Bryant, a prominent hometown architect. His best-known commercial commission is **Bangor House** (174 Main), a grand hotel of its day (built 1833–1834), receiving such guests as Ulysses S. Grant, Daniel Webster, and Theodore Roosevelt. It is now an apartment building.

In the same decade Bryant drew up plans for the **City Common,** east of Broadway, and for **Mount Hope Cemetery.** Landscaped with ponds, trees, and pathways, the cemetery was inspired by Mount Auburn in Cambridge, Massachusetts, the nation's first garden cemetery. Mount Hope is filled with elaborate Victorian monuments, marble urns, granite obelisks, and ironwork. A cannon marks the site of the Grand Army Lot, a burial ground consecrated in 1864 for Civil War veterans.

The city's increasing number of rich entrepreneurs commissioned Bryant and other architects to design houses. Most of the clients preferred to build just south of Main Street in what is now called the **High Street Historic District** (a triangle defined by Union, Columbia, and Hammond streets). Rising above the district is the **Hammond Street Congregational Church,** built in 1853. Built in 1822, the **William Mason House** (62 High Street, private) is probably the oldest brick house in the district. Bryant's **George W. Brown House** (43 High Street, private) and **Pickering House** (39 High Street, private), both built in 1833–1835, are gable-roofed twins with Greek Revival porticoes.

Another of Bangor's historic residential neighborhoods is bounded by Essex, Center, Garland, and State streets. Developed in the 1830s, the **Broadway Historic District** includes several houses designed by architect Charles Bryant, including the Greek

Revival **Smith-Boutelle House** (private) on Broadway near Cumberland. The elaborate doorway, contained within a Doric portico, sports a top panel of anthemion leaves, a popular motif of the Greek Revival style. One resident of the house was Charles Boutelle, Civil War naval officer, publisher of the Bangor *Daily Whig and Courier,* and nine-term congressman. Among Boutelle's guests were three U.S. presidents—Garfield, Harrison, and McKinley. On Penobscot off Broadway is Bryant's **Ken-Cutting House** (private), a graceful Greek Revival double house with wrought-iron railings.

Perhaps the city's most beloved landmark is the 1898 **Bangor Standpipe and Observatory,** which dominates Thomas Hill, the highest elevation in the city, a hilly former Indian hunting ground. Probably the only Shingle-style standpipe in the nation, it handsomely shrouds a huge water tank (now used only in emergencies). The balustrade is lit at night. Also notable in the area is the massive, red brick **Bangor Children's Home.** Built 1868–1869 as an orphanage, it is now a day-care center and private school.

The **Bangor Public Library,** boasting nearly half a million volumes and renowned as a great repository of state and local history, was founded in 1845, but its present building on Hammond Street was built in 1912, after the fire that gutted the area. In fact, the neighborhood is known as the **Great Fire Historic District** for the reconstruction that occurred between 1911 and 1915. Among the library's neighbors are the **Bangor Savings Bank,** the **Bangor High School** (now an apartment building called the Schoolhouse), and the Romanesque **Graham Building.**

One of the earliest examples in the state of the Greek Revival temple style is the 1832 **Zebulon Smith House** (55 Summer Street, private), once one of a line of fashionable residences that announced the wealth of their owners. Smith was a jeweler and silversmith. Another Greek Revival structure is the **Nathaniel Hatch House** at 117 Court Street, with porticoes at both the front and back of the house. The history of the house's owners reflects the boom-time fluctuations of American mid-nineteenth-century society. Nathaniel Hatch, a prosperous banker, built the house in 1832–1833 and sold it soon afterward to Samuel Farrar, who worked with his father in lumber after ill health forced him to give up studying law. In 1857, when his successful business floundered, Farrar sold the house, packed up, and moved to Wisconsin. The house is currently run by the Bangor Housing Authority.

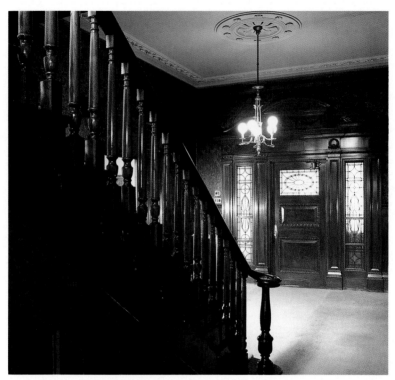

The mahagony-rich entrance hall of Isaac Farrar Mansion in Bangor.

Lumber baron and merchant Isaac Farrar ordered the finest materials for his house, which was the first known U.S. commission of English architect Richard Upjohn. The 1833 **Isaac Farrar Mansion** (166 Union Street, 207–941–2808) contains marble mantles, stained-glass windows, mahogany wainscotting, and much carved woodwork. It has been extensively remodeled. Across from it is the Greek Revival cottage that Upjohn designed in 1836 for lawyer Thomas A. Hill. Now headquarters of the Bangor Historical Society and Museum, the **Hill House** (159 Union Street, 207–942–5766) has a completely restored downstairs floor, the highlight of which is a grand double parlor, furnished to Victorian perfection. In the 1840s the house passed to Samuel Dale, mayor of Bangor, whose guests included Ulysses S. Grant. Among the rotating exhibits are nineteenth-century letters and diaries, photographs, and paintings, as well as household tools and utensils, many of them made in Bangor.

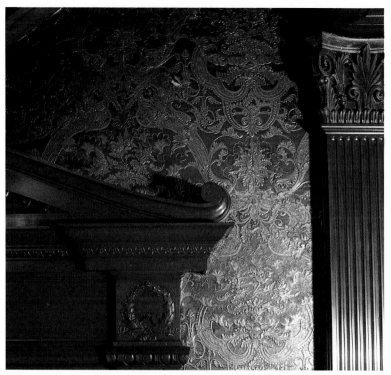

The ornate wallpaper in the Farrar entrance hall is original, dating from 1833.

In the front hallway of the Hill House is a desk that belonged to Hannibal Hamlin, a prominent Maine politician before he became Abraham Lincoln's vice president. Born in Paris Hill in 1809, he died in Bangor in 1891 and is buried in Mount Hope Cemetery. A farmer and lawyer based in Hampden, just south of Bangor, Hamlin entered politics as a Jacksonian Democrat. He served first in the state House of Representatives (1836–1841), was elected to the U.S. House of Representatives in 1843, and then to the Senate. His abolitionist views led him to resign from the Democratic Party, and in 1856 he was elected Maine's first Republican governor. The following year he was reelected to the U.S. Senate. Although chosen by Lincoln as his running mate in 1860, Hamlin was passed over in 1864 for Andrew Johnson, who became president upon Lincoln's assassination. The Maine electorate returned Hamlin to the U.S. Senate in 1869, where he served until 1881. Before retiring to Bangor, he served as U.S. minister to Spain.

In Bangor, Hamlin lived at 15 Fifth Street, in an 1848 mansard-roofed house that is now the official residence of presidents of the **Bangor Theological Seminary.** Moved to Bangor from Hampden in 1819, the seminary boasts significant buildings, including the 1827 **Old Commons Building,** the 1833 **Maine Hall,** and the 1858 **Chapel.** Bordering the seminary is the **Whitney Park Historic District.** Clustered around West Broadway between Union and Hammond streets, it was developed during the Civil War era by a generation of prosperous newcomers to Bangor. They built large houses in the popular Victorian styles such as Queen Anne and Shingle. One of the most exuberant is the Italianate **William Arnold House** (47 West Broadway, private) built by a local merchant in 1857. The **Penobscot Nation Museum** (207–827–6545) in Old Town exhibits a range of Indian artifacts including basketry, clothing, stone tools and sculpture, and birchbark artwork.

The heritage of Bangor's logging industry is the subject of exhibits at the **Maine Forest and Logging Museum** (Route 178 in Bradley, 207–942–4228), scheduled for completion in 1991. The centerpiece of the complex is a re-creation of Leonard's Mills, active in 1797. Exhibits explain the sawmill process—from northern wood harvesting, spring log drives, the establishment of logging camps, and forest management to the actual milling (the waterwheel driven by Blackman Stream). Froes, adzes, broad axes, pick poles, and other eighteenth-century tools are on display. The chronology ends with the modern lumber and paper industries.

At **Greenville,** summer residents got around Moosehead Lake on the *Katahdin,* one of Maine's last and largest steamboats. Built at the Bath Iron Works in 1914, the powerful vessel carried passengers and logs between various points on the forty-mile-long lake. Resort hotels such as the **Mount Kineo House** (207–695–2702) commandeered her services for popular excursions. She made her farewell passenger run in 1938 and her final run in 1976. Now a steamboat-era exhibit at the **Moosehead Marine Museum,** the *Katahdin* has been restored and outfitted with displays of her history.

KATAHDIN IRON WORKS

East of Greenville, on **Silver Lake,** are the Katahdin Iron Works, abandoned in 1890. The blast furnace and kiln remain, survivors of the once-fiery operation, the only one of its kind in the state. Katahdin was a factory town, built along with the ironworks in 1843—the workers' houses, town hall, train depot, school, stores, auxiliary farms, and boardinghouses are now gone. Taking raw materials from its mineral-rich location, Katahdin produced about twenty tons of pig iron a day in the early 1880s, sending it to markets by rail and river. For a while, the Katahdin furnace blasted nonstop, and the factory produced iron farm tools, parts for machinery, and wheels for railroad cars. After the 1880s, Katahdin could not compete with the newer and more centrally located technology in Pittsburgh, Pennsylvania. Of Katahdin's extensive operation, only one of fourteen kilns and the blast-furnace tower remain and have been renovated, massive and impressive monuments to the passage of boom-time prosperity and society.

LOCATION: Off Route 11, five miles north of Brownsville Junction.
HOURS: Memorial Day through Labor Day: 9–5 Daily. FEE: None.
TELEPHONE: 207–645–4217.

Chamberlain Lake is just above **Baxter State Park** (207–723–9616), established in 1931. Near the southeast corner of the park is **Mount Katahdin,** northern terminus of the **Appalachian Trail,** blazed by foresters in the 1920s. The 2,100-mile wilderness trail connects Maine's Baxter Peak to Georgia's Mount Springer.

South of Fort Kent, beginning at **Eagle Lake** and stretching southwest to Chamberlain Lake, lie the remains of a remarkable logging-transportation system in the **Tramway Historical District.** The steam-driven Tramway was engineered in 1902 to solve the problem of getting logs from lumbering areas to the waterways for transportation to markets.

In 1841 the waters of Chamberlain Lake had been diverted into the east branch of the Penobscot River. By the beginning of the twentieth century, lumber in the surrounding area had been depleted. The Tramway was developed to carry logs 3,000 feet over land from the timber-rich Eagle Lake area to Chamberlain Lake, which had links to the mills on the Penobscot and the overseas markets. A 6,000-foot steel cable formed a single loop between the two lakes, along which trucks were attached every 10 feet. The trucks ran along 22-inch-gauge rails, with the delivery line on a

OVERLEAF: *Mount Katahdin rises 5,268 feet above autumnal forests.*

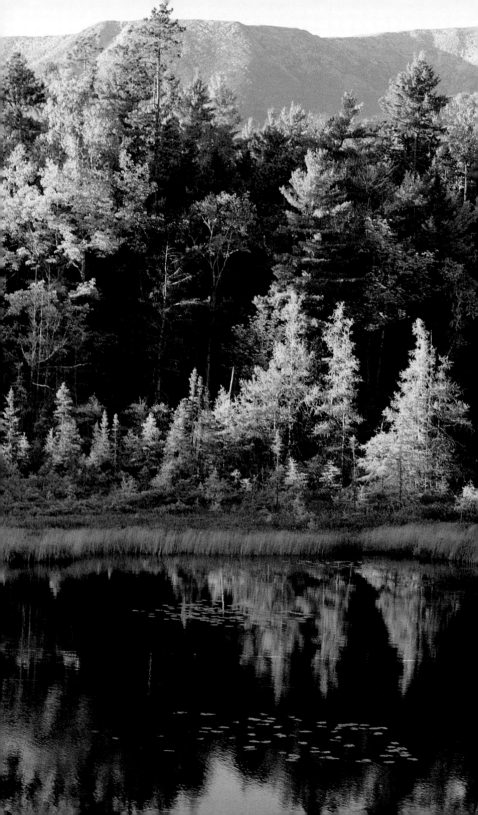

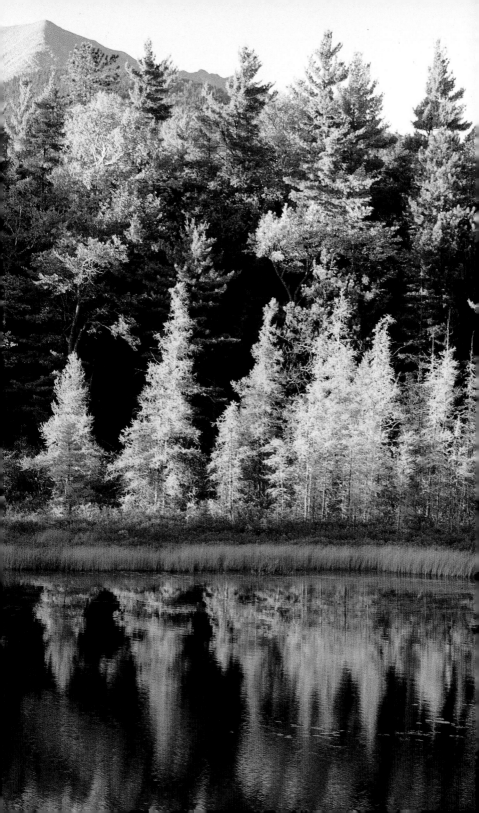

raised wooden structure directly above that of the return line. A 9-foot sprocket wheel was driven by steam at the Chamberlain end, drawing the cable and trucks along the route. A log spanned two trucks on its way to Chamberlain Lake, and the trucks returned empty and upside down to Eagle Lake. Although it was made obsolete by more powerful log haulers and locomotives, the Tramway was never destroyed, and its entire length remains virtually intact. Between 1927 and 1933 a railroad line ran each summer from the Tramway district to Umbazooksus Lake to continue feeding the lumber-mill market, this time to the west branch of the Penobscot River. The railroad engines were subsequently stored in Eagle Lake in a structure that later burned to the ground. The Tramway and the exposed engines of the railway are extraordinary relics of Maine's land, technology, and logging industry.

FORT KENT

Maine's northern border with Canada became a focal point of conflict between the United States and Britain beginning in 1755, when French-Acadians moved into the region known as the Madawaska Territory to escape increasing British domination in Canada. After the American Revolution, the United States and Britain competed for the region's wealth in game, lumber, and minerals. Each country trespassed against the other, creating disputes that continued over fifty years and culminated in the Aroostook War of 1838–1839. This purely diplomatic but potentially bloody confrontation resulted in the establishment of the St. John River as Maine's international border with New Brunswick, Canada.

In the winter of 1838–1839, military troops, sent by the governments of the United States, Great Britain, Maine, and New Brunswick, converged on the lumbering region of the Aroostook Valley. Each was determined to exercise control over the land rich in spruce, cedar, and white pine. Within six weeks officials had settled on an uneasy truce, and the troops withdrew. At the end of 1839, however, a Maine public-land agent hired a local force to establish and monitor the state's claim to the area. The militia, numbering thirty-six men, chose the meeting of the Fish and St. John rivers to locate the **Fort Kent Blockhouse** (Blockhouse Road and West Main Street, 207–834–3866), named for the then-governor of Maine, Edward Kent. New Brunswick and Great Britain

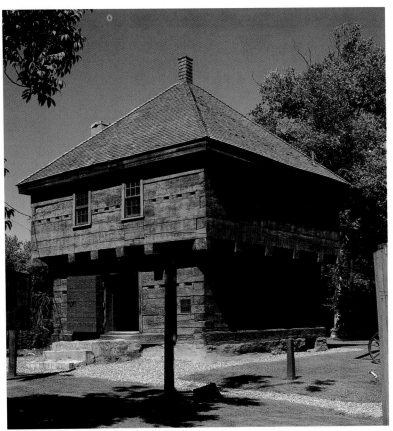

The stocky Fort Kent Blockhouse, a landmark of Maine's border disputes.

countered with an establishment twenty miles away, and the heated confrontation continued. In 1841 the U.S. government sought to end the persistent and potentially dangerous dispute by relieving the civil militia and installing federal troops at Fort Kent. The threat of serious conflict forced negotiations that ended in the Webster-Ashburton Treaty in 1842.

In 1843 the last of the federal troops left Fort Kent. It was sold into private hands in 1858 and was used as a family residence. The state purchased the blockhouse in 1891.

Built of thick, squared cedar logs, the blockhouse, with its prominent second-story overhang, most closely resembles fortifications erected a century before 1839, perhaps as a result of the lack of modern engineering expertise of the local civil militia when it began its task. Inside the rough-hewn structure are pictorial displays of the dispute era, as well as a selection of lumbering equipment.

In 1785 the Acadians landed upriver at St. David in the Madawaska area. They planted a cross on the southern shore of the St. John River to commemorate their safe passage from British persecution in Canada and their establishment in Maine. The **Madawaska Historic Museum** and **Acadian Cross Historic Shrine** (Route 1, 207–728–4518) now mark that point of entry; exhibits include a century-old Acadian schoolhouse and 150-year-old homestead.

VAN BUREN

Each year profitable timber harvests enliven towns up and down the St. John River—Hamlin, Grand Isle, Notre Dame, Lille, Cyr Plantation. One of the larger logging towns is Van Buren, named for President Martin Van Buren, who once visited here. Many of its loggers (as well as most of the river valley's farmers and business-men) are descendants of the original French Acadians. The local economy is based on lumbering, farming, and small businesses.

Van Buren's **Acadian Village** (Route 1, 207–868–2691) con-sists of reconstructed and relocated eighteenth- and nineteenth-century houses and cabins, barns, a railroad station, general store, church, and barber, shoe, and blacksmith shops. The houses are appointed with period furnishings and crafts; the barns, shops, and other buildings are set up with appropriate equipment from plows to blacksmith's anvils to barber chairs. The entire grouping gives visitors a look into early life on Maine's northern frontier.

At the junction of Route 1 and four state highways is **Caribou,** a shipping center for Aroostook potato farmers. Some of them are descendants of Scandinavians who came to northern Maine in the 1870s, settling in the communities they named **New Sweden** and **Stockholm.** Their history is preserved by the **New Sweden Histori-cal Society Museum** (off Route 161, 207–896–5639), whose exhib-its include two Swedish log cabins and a replica of an 1870 commu-nity hall. Immigrant artifacts, documents, and photographs also are housed in the **Stockholm Museum** (Main and Lake streets), which occupies the town's old general store and post office.

Just above Houlton, in **Littleton,** is the youngest and northernmost covered bridge in the state. The 150-foot **Watson Settlement Bridge,** spanning the Meduxnekeag Stream, was built in 1911.

HOULTON

Hub of three railroads—the Bangor and Aroostook, the New Brunswick, and the Aroostook Valley lines—the pioneer community of Houlton grew into a real market town in the 1890s, with impressive commercial buildings constructed along **Market Square.** Built in 1907, the **First National Bank** is of a particularly noble Grecian design. The **Aroostook Historical and Art Museum** (109 Main Street, 207–532–4216) occupies a 1903 Colonial Revival house, the finest residence of its time in Houlton. Surviving from the town's earlier days, and indeed the earliest surviving structure in Aroostook County, is the 1813 **Black Hawk Putnam Tavern** at 22 North Street. Now an office building, the structure served as the town's hotel during its frontier years. The original exterior has been preserved.

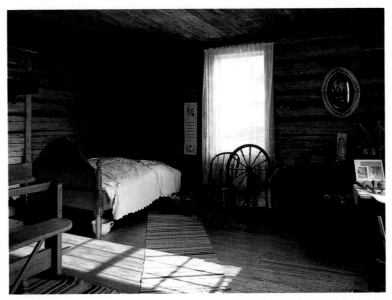

One of New Sweden's log cabins contains a spinning wheel and other belongings of the family who built it in 1894.

NOTES ON ARCHITECTURE

EARLY COLONIAL

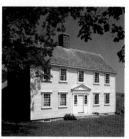

JOHN PERKINS HOUSE, ME

In the eastern colonies, Europeans first built houses using a medieval, vertical asymmetry, which in the eighteenth century evolved toward Classical symmetry. Roofs were gabled and hipped, often with prominent exterior chimneys. Small casement windows became larger and more evenly spaced and balanced on each facade.

GEORGIAN

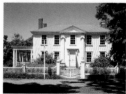

LADY PEPPERRELL HOUSE, ME

Beginning in Boston as early as 1686, and only much later elsewhere, the design of houses became balanced about a central axis, with only careful, stripped detail. A few large houses incorporated double-story pilasters. Sash windows with rectilinear panes replaced casements. Hipped roofs accentuated the balanced and strict proportions inherited from Italy and Holland via England and Scotland.

FEDERAL

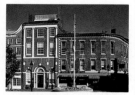

PORTSMOUTH ATHENAEUM, NH

The post-Revolutionary style sometimes called "Federal" was more flexible and delicate than the more formal Georgian. It evolved from archaeological discoveries at Pompeii and Herculaneum in Italy in the 1750s, as well as in contemporary French interior planning principles. A fanshaped window over the door is its most characteristic detail.

GREEK REVIVAL

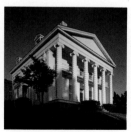

FOLLETT HOUSE, VT

The Greek Revival manifested itself in severe, stripped, rectilinear proportions, occasionally a set of columns or pilasters, and even, in a few instances, Greek-temple form. It combined Greek and Roman forms—low pitched pediments, simple moldings, rounded arches, and shallow domes—and was used in official buildings and many private houses.

COUNTRY VERNACULAR

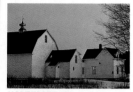

NORTHPORT, ME

The builders of many modest structures in northern New England were concerned only with function, not with stylistic considerations. Many farmhouses and barns do not fit easily into any stylistic designation, although they grew out of building traditions of the colonial period. One distinctive regional building type is the connected house and barn, which developed in the severe climate of Maine and New Hampshire. Simple wooden farmhouses are connected—by means of a rear ell, woodshed, carriage house, and outhouse—to the barn, an arrangement that ultimately proved to be a fire hazard.

GOTHIC REVIVAL

After about 1830, darker colors, asymmetry, broken skylines, verticality, and the pointed arch began to appear. New machinery produced carved and pierced trim along the eaves. Roofs became steep and gabled; "porches" or "piazzas" became more spacious. Oriel and bay windows were common and there was greater use of stained glass.

ITALIANATE

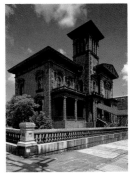

MORSE-LIBBY HOUSE, ME

The Italianate style began to appear in the 1840s, both in a formal, balanced "palazzo" style and in a picturesque "villa" style. Both had round-headed windows and arcaded porches. Commercial structures were often made of cast iron, with a ground floor of large arcaded windows with smaller windows on each successive rising story.

SECOND EMPIRE

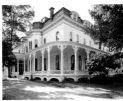

PARK-McCULLOUGH HOUSE, VT

After 1860, Parisian fashion inspired American builders to use mansard roofs, dark colors, and varied textures, including shingles, tiles, and ironwork, especially on balconies and skylines. With their ornamental quoins, balustrades, pavilions, pediments, columns, and pilasters, Second Empire buildings recalled many historical styles.

QUEEN ANNE

The Queen Anne style emphasized contrasts of form, texture, and color. Large encircling verandahs, tall chimneys, turrets, towers, and a multitude of textures are typical of the style. The ground floor might be of stone or brick, the upper floors of stucco, shingle, or clapboard. Specially shaped bricks and plaques were used for decoration. Panels of stained glass outlined or filled the windows. Gabled or hipped steep roofs, and pediments, Venetian windows, and front and corner bay windows were typical.

SHINGLE STYLE

The Shingle Style bore the stamp of a new generation of professional architects led by Henry Hobson Richardson (1838–1886). Sheathed in wooden shingles, its forms were smoothed and unified. Verandahs, turrets, and complex roofs were sometimes used, but they were thoroughly integrated into a whole that emphasized uniformity of surface rather than a jumble of forms. The style was a domestic and informal expression of what became known as Richardsonian Romanesque.

RICHARDSONIAN ROMANESQUE

Richardsonian Romanesque made use of the massive forms and ornamental details of the Romanesque: rounded arches, towers, stone and brick facing. The solidity and gravity of the masses were accentuated by deep recesses for windows and entrances and by rough stone masonry, stubby columns, strong horizontals, rounded towers with conical caps, and repetitive, botanical ornament.

RENAISSANCE REVIVAL OR BEAUX ARTS

Later, in the 1880s and 1890s, American architects who had studied at the Ecole des Beaux Arts in Paris brought a new Renaissance Revival to the United States. Sometimes used in urban mansions, but generally reserved for public and academic buildings, it borrowed from three centuries of Renaissance detail—much of it French—and put together picturesque combinations from widely differing periods.

ECLECTIC PERIOD REVIVALS

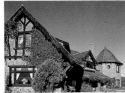

CASTLE IN THE CLOUDS, NH

During the first decades of the twentieth century, revivals of diverse architectural styles became popular in the United States, particularly for residential buildings. Architects designed Swiss chalets, half-timbered Tudor houses, and Norman chateaus with equal enthusiasm. Many of these houses were modeled on rural structures and constructed in suburban settings. Although widely divergent in appearance, they have similar plans, site orientations, and general scale, brought about by similarities in building sites and by clients' desires for spacious interiors.

I   N   D   E   X

PHOTO CREDITS

All photographs are by Paul Rocheleau except for the following:

Cover: George A. Robinson/ f/STOP
Half-title Page: Ken Burris/Shelburne Museum, Shelburne, VT
Title: Jeff Gnass Photography, Oroville, CA
Page 12: Clyde H. Smith/ f/STOP
19: Sheldon Museum
24: Brian Vanden Brink, Rockport, ME
25: Clyde H. Smith/The Stock Shop
24: Brian Vanden Brink, Rockport, ME
27: Douglas Armsden, Kittery Point, ME
45: Helga Photo Studio
46-47: T. S. Marr, Courtesy of Shelburne Farms, Shelburne, VT
48: Shelburne Museum, Shelburne, VT
53: Kindra Clineff/The Picture Cube
56: Clyde H. Smith/ f/STOP
59: Vermont Historical Society, Montpelier, VT
62: Helga Photo Studio
64: Helga Photo Studio
66-67: Helga Photo Studio
72-73: Fred M. Dole/ f/STOP Pictures
75: Helga Photo Studio
78: Mrs. Samuel B. Pettengill, Grafton Historical Society, Grafton, VT
83: Helga Photo Studio
87: From the Historic Photographic Collection of Strawbery Banke, Inc.

94: Bob Baillargeon/New England Stock Photo
95: Jonathan Blake/New England Stock Photo
97: Douglas Armsden, courtesy of the National Society of Colonial Dames in New Hampshire
101: Peter E. Randall, Portsmouth, NH
108-109: Craig Blouin/ New England Stock Photo
112-113: Eric Sanford Photography, Manchester, NH
115: Johnson's Photography, Bristol, NH
118-119: Library of Congress, LC-USZ62-1832
129: The Currier Gallery of Art, Manchester, NH
133: John Snowden/New England Stock Photo
143: George A. Robinson/ f/STOP Pictures
144: VISU—Photography/ Thomas W. Chase/New England Stock Photo
150: Clyde H. Smith/The Stock Shop
151: Collection of Paul Katz/ courtesy of the Hood Gallery, Dartmouth, NH
152-153: Peter E. Randall, Portsmouth, NH
158: Eric Sanford Photography, Manchester, NH
160: Gene Ahrens, Berkeley Heights, NJ
163: Library of Congress, LC-USZ62-39501
167: Voscar The Maine Photographer, Presque Isle, ME
168 (both): Douglas Arms-

den, Kittery Point, ME
170: Peter E. Randall, Portsmouth, NH
172: Douglas Armsden, Kittery Point, ME
174-175: Brian Vanden Brink, Rockport, ME
176: Brian Vanden Brink, Rockport, ME
181: Portland Museum of Art, Portland, ME
182: Jeff Gnass Photography, Oroville, CA
184: Brian Vanden Brink, Rockport, ME
187: Helga Photo Studio
189: Brian Vanden Brink, Rockport, ME
190: Brian Vanden Brink, Rockport, ME
194: Portland Museum of Art, Portland, ME/Gift of Elizabeth Foster Mann in memory of her father and mother, Maximilian and Elizabeth Dickson Foster, 1953
199: Michael Freeman
200-201: Michael Freeman
205: B. Cory Kilvert, Jr./ The Stock Shop
208: Library of Congress, LC-USZ62-1832
211: Clyde H. Smith/ f/STOP Pictures
215: Helga Photo Studio
222: Brian Vanden Brink, Rockport, ME
224: Brian Vanden Brink, Rockport, ME
226: Ira Block/The Image Bank
227: Portland Museum of Art, Portland, ME, Anonymous gift, 1980
229: Brian Vanden Brink, Rockport, ME

294

230: Brian Vanden Brink, Rockport, ME
231: Brian Vanden Brink, Rockport, ME
234-235: Fred M. Dole/ f/STOP Pictures
238-239: The Museum of Fine Arts, Boston, MA. Bequest of Martha C. Karolik for the Karolik Collection of American Paintings, 1815-1865
240: Helga Photo Studio
248 (lower right): Brian Vanden Brink, Rockport, ME
251: Clyde H. Smith/ f/STOP Pictures
252: Clyde H. Smith/The Stock Shop

255: Yale University Art Gallery, New Haven, CT, Stanley B. Resor, B.A. 1901, Fund
259: Helga Photo Studio
262: Lynn F. Gustin, courtesy of Fort Western, Augusta ME
276-277: Clyde H. Smith/ f/STOP Pictures
279: Voscar The Maine Photographer, Presque Isle, ME
282 (top left): Helga Photo Studio
282 (lower left): Douglas Armsden, Kittery Point, ME
282 (top center): Peter E. Randall, Portsmouth, NH

282 (right): Brian Vanden Brink, Rockport, ME
283 (top left): Brian Vanden Brink, Rockport, ME
283 (lower left): Douglas Armsden, Kittery Point, ME
Back Cover: Clyde H. Smith/f/STOP Pictures

The editors gratefully acknowledge the assistance of Honi Brett, Ann J. Campbell, Rita Campon, Ann ffolliott, Amy Hughes, Carol A. McKeown, Klaske Piebenga, Martha Schulman, and Patricia Woodruff.

Composed in Basilia Haas and ITC New Baskerville by Graphic Arts Composition, Inc., Philadelphia, Pennsylvania. Printed and bound by Toppan Printing Company, Ltd., Tokyo, Japan.